Medical Terminology
in Hospital Practice

Medical Terminology in Hospital Practice

A GUIDE FOR ALL THOSE ENGAGED IN PROFESSIONS
ALLIED TO MEDICINE

PAUL M. DAVIES

T.D., M.B., B.S., D.P.H., F.F.R., D.M.R.

*Consultant Radiologist, Guildford and Godalming Group Hospitals,
and Guildford Chest Clinic.*

Foreword by

PROFESSOR GEORGE J. CUNNINGHAM

M.B.E., M.D. F.C. Path.

*Professor of Pathology, Medical College of Virginia,
Richmond, Virginia*

*Late Sir William Collins Professor of Pathology,
Royal College of Surgeons of England*

WILLIAM HEINEMANN MEDICAL BOOKS LTD.
LONDON

First published 1969

S.BN 433, 07181, 8

PRINTED IN THE REPUBLIC OF IRELAND BY
HELY THOM LIMITED, DUBLIN

Foreword

THE success of his previous work for the benefit of radiographers has fortunately encouraged Dr. Paul Davies to write this present book, designed to be of help to a much wider group of those engaged in professions allied to medicine.

There is a wealth of literature on detailed aspects of special subjects. In the midst of this modern development, however, the general needs of members and students of these allied professions must be constantly borne in mind. Many people find the general approach difficult to explain in a comprehensible way. Although a specialist himself, the author has retained a broad general interest in medicine and, more important still, has managed to impart it most lucidly.

I am sure this work will fulfill the author's purpose and become increasingly used, by those whose skilled assistance is nowadays essential in so many different aspects of medical practice.

GEORGE J. CUNNINGHAM.

January, 1969.

Preface

THE acquisition of a sound basic knowledge of medical terminology, relevant to their work in the investigation and treatment of disease, is of considerable practical value to members of the nursing profession, and members of the professions supplementary to medicine and other paramedical professions.

This book has been written with the object of providing all those engaged in these professions, referred to in the sub-title of the work as "professions allied to medicine", with a guide to the current usage of meanings of a large variety of medical terms used in current general hospital practice.

Besides indicating the meanings of many terms employed in pathology, medicine, surgery, gynaecology and obstetrics, a number of short descriptions of common and important clinical disorders are given. It is, however, stressed that these descriptions are intended to present such facts as are considered likely to facilitate a good basic understanding of the nature of the conditions to which the terms under discussion refer. They do not thus purport to be comprehensive accounts of the diseases discussed, such as are given in the many excellent textbooks nowadays available to the reader.

P.M.D.

January 1969.

Acknowledgements

I HAVE been fortunate in receiving valuable assistance, in the writing of various parts of the text relating to their individual specialities, from Professor George Cunningham and from my colleagues in the Guildford and Godalming Hospitals: Mr. N. J. Barwell, Mr. D. W. Bawtree, Mr. P. S. Boulter, Mr. W. M. de C. Boxill, Dr. A. T. Broadbridge, Mr. M. Meredith Brown, Dr. L. G. Capra, Dr. S. G. de Clive-Lowe, Mr. W. G. Gill, Dr. J. M. Frew, Dr. F. E. Joules, Dr. R. B. McMillan, Mr. S. S. F. Pooley, Dr. J. L. Price, Dr. L. Rowley, and Dr. O. L. S. Scott.

I am also indebted to my wife for considerable help in the preparation of all phases of the book and to Mrs. Mary Clifton for her excellent typing of the manuscript.

My thanks are also due to Mr. Owen R. Evans, Managing Director of William Heinemann Medical Books Ltd., for his consideration and helpful advice and for permission to make extensive use of material from a previous work, *Medical Terminology for Radiographers* (Heinemann 1966).

The many sources of reference which I have consulted are listed in the Appendix at the end of the book.

Contents

Contents

PART I

Introductory

TERMS Referring to some General Aspects of Medicine, Medical Terminology and the Practice of Medicine and its Allied Professions.

1. MEDICINE, DISEASE AND MEDICAL TERMINOLOGY

AT the commencement of a study of medical terms it is most important to obtain a clear concept of the meanings of the words "medicine" and "disease".

Medicine is a term with three meanings, denoting:

(*a*) a drug—as in the expression "taking medicine".

(*b*) the clinical speciality of medicine, as practised by physicians and concerned with the treatment of patients with drugs and other non-surgical measures.

(*c*) *all aspects of the science of the prevention and treatment of disease*—this latter being the principal sense in which the term is used.

Disease *is a condition in which some abnormality of structure or function, or of both structure and function, is present in some part, or parts of the body.*

Thus a large part of medical science, being concerned with disease, comprises the study of abnormal conditions within the body.

However, the abnormal can only be appreciated in relation to a knowledge of normal conditions. Thus human **anatomy,** the study of normal body structures, and human **physiology**—the study of normal body functions, are integral branches of medicine and words relative to these subjects are classified as medical terms.

Medical Terminology is the study of words used to communicate facts and ideas particular to medicine, and is concerned with the origin, construction, past and present usage and meaning of such words.

The concern of the hospital worker is, however, for all practical purposes, with present usage and meaning of medical language and it is these aspects of medical terminology that are principally dealt with in this book.

It may, however, be of interest to note in passing that a special characteristic of the subject under discussion is the great number of words encountered which are of direct, or indirect, Greek or Latin origin. This has resulted from the physicians of ancient Greece, notable among whom was Hippocrates (born 360 B.C.), having been the first to introduce scientific methods into medicine; and later from the use of Latin as the international language for scholars throughout the Western world, following on after the decline of Greek civilization.

The Latin tongue obtained this dominant position through the rise of the power of Rome, but maintained it for many centuries after the fall of the Roman Empire (A.D. 476).

The term "disease" is of necessity of frequent occurrence in medical speech and writing, but an endeavour may be made to avoid undue repetition by employing other words, which, when used in the right context, are its synonyms (i.e. words with similar meanings), e.g. disorder, illness, sickness, morbidity, malady, pathological condition, morbid condition, ailment.

Some general descriptive terms which may be applied when discussing different forms of illness are:

Description of disease.	Meaning.
Congenital.	Present at birth.
Acquired.	Acquired after birth.
Acute.	Of rapid onset and progress.
Chronic.	Of slow onset and progress.
Functional.	Associated with abnormality of function but without demonstrable abnormality of structure.
Organic.	Associated with structural abnormality.
Silent.	Producing no symptoms or readily detectable signs.
Systemic.	Involving the body (i.e. the system) as a whole.
Local.	Involving only a part of the body (in contradistinction to systemic disease).

2. CAUSES AND CLASSIFICATION OF DISEASE

The causes of the abnormalities which constitute disease are many and varied. Some are known and others imperfectly understood or completely unknown. The study of the causation of diseases is called **aetiology.**

A useful classification which takes account of causal factors, in so far as these are known, is as follows:

Introductory

TYPES OF DISEASES

(a) **Congenital**—diseases which are present at birth as a result of:

(i) developmental errors occurring in various organs or tissues, e.g. cleft palate;

(ii) diseases acquired in intra-uterine life, e.g. congenital syphilis acquired as a result of maternal syphilitic infection; or

(iii) hereditary (familial) diseases due to abnormalities transmitted by genes (units of hereditary material) in reproductive cells, e.g. haemophilia, a familial disease associated with excessive haemorrhage.

(b) **Traumatic** (Injuries)—due to:

(i) Violence—e.g. fractures and dislocations.

(ii) Mechanical irritation, e.g. bed sores.

(iii) External physical agents, e.g. thermal burns, frost-bite, radiation injury.

(iv) External chemical agents, e.g. acid and alkali burns.

(c) **Infective**—due to infection with pathogenic micro-organisms (disease-producing germs), e.g. influenza, measles, tuberculosis, malaria; and **infestations**—due to worms, e.g. tape worm infestation.

(d) **Neoplastic**—due to the pathological process called neoplasia (new growth) which results in formation of benign and malignant tumours.

(e) **Metabolic** due to:

(i) Lack of essential food factors required for building and maintenance of body tissues, e.g. rickets, due to lack of Vitamin D.

(ii) Disorders of metabolism, i.e. the processes whereby absorbed foodstuffs are modified for tissue building and repair; and, whereby waste products are broken down into the forms in which they can be excreted from the body—e.g. gout, which is a disorder of the metabolism of uric acid.

(f) **Chemical poisonings**—due to entry of chemical poisons into the body, e.g. arsenic poisoning, lead poisoning.

(g) **Endocrine**—due to disorders in endocrine (ductless) glands, e.g. goitre, pituitary dwarfism.

(h) **Allergic**—due to various types of hypersensitivity, e.g. hay fever.

(i) **Psychiatric**—due to abnormal conditions of the mind, e.g anxiety states, depressive states, schizophrenia.

(j) **Iatrogenic**—due to treatments given for other diseases, the term meaning "produced by physicians", e.g. sensitivity reactions caused by administration of penicillin.

(*k*) **Idiopathic**—of unknown causation, e.g. idiopathic epilepsy, essential hypertension (high blood pressure).

3. MANIFESTATIONS OF DISEASE

The presence of disease may be revealed by:

(*a*) **Symptoms**—abnormalities which are appreciable by the patient himself, e.g. painful sensations, giddiness.

(*b*) **Signs**—abnormalities appreciable to an observer, e.g. pallor, elevation of body temperature.

Signs detectable by a medical practitioner during the course of an ordinary medical examination are often termed **clinical signs,** whereas those requiring specialized methods of detection may, according to the nature of these be designated as pathological signs, radiological signs, electro-cardiographic signs, etc.

It is desirable at this stage to consider the meaning of the term **clinical.** This word, although widely employed, is difficult of definition. It is derived from the Greek word for "a bed" and originally meant "at the bedside". It has now come to indicate those aspects of medical science most directly concerned with actual patients, e.g. a "clinical demonstration" is one in which patients are the main subject of the demonstration; a "clinic" is a building where patients attend for medical care, or alternatively, a session for medical diagnosis or treatment attended by patients, as in the expression "the Monday morning surgical clinic", etc.

During the course of a disease, signs and symptoms may not infrequently appear which are not due to the original condition, but are manifestations of some disorder whose occurrence is directly consequent upon the presence of the original disease. Such secondary disorder is referred to as a **complication,** e.g. pneumonia occurring as a complication of chronic bronchitis.

4. PRACTICE OF MEDICINE AND ALLIED PROFESSIONS AND TECHNICAL OCCUPATIONS

The practice of medicine is concerned with the prevention, investigation, diagnosis and treatment of disease; the alleviation of suffering; and with the furtherance of medical knowledge and medical education.

Those who are qualified to practise medicine are, by established usage, commonly known as **doctors,** although their official designation is that of **medical practitioners.**

Medical practitioners in the United Kingdom, in addition to holding certain qualifications, recognized by law, must also be **registered** by the General Medical Council, if they wish to practise. (*Note*: Newly-qualified doctors are first conditionally registered and must spend a year in approved **pre-registration posts** before full registration can be effected).

There are many careers within the medical profession but the majority of medical men or women are engaged primarily in:

(*a*) **General Medical Practice**—general medical practitioners; usually referred to as **general practitioners** (G.P's) or **family doctors.**

(*b*) **Specialist Practice** (e.g. surgery, pathology, radiology, etc.,— specialist medical practitioners, referred to as **specialists.** Senior specialists who hold established consultant posts in hospitals, government departments, etc., are designated as **consultants.**

[*Note* : The terms "registrar" and "house officer" often cause perplexity:

A **registrar** is a doctor who is acquiring specialist experience and holds a registrar post in a hospital speciality (e.g. medical registrar, surgical registrar).

A **house officer** is a junior doctor who is gaining experience within a hospital, before embarking on a career as a specialist, family doctor, etc. He, or she, is frequently resident in the "house", i.e. the hospital].

(*c*) **Preventive Medicine**—usually within Public Health services or in industry.

Doctors engaged in public health work have the professional assistance of public health inspectors and health visitors (qualified nurses with training in midwifery or obstetric nursing, and in preventive medicine).

From time immemorial those engaged in the profession of medicine have required nursing assistance with their more serious cases of illness and the help of midwives in maternity work. It is thus interesting to note, that it was not until the latter half of the nineteenth century that the need was generally appreciated for establishing nursing and midwifery as fully recognized professions, with organized systems of practical and theoretical training. Indeed, but for the work of Florence Nightingale, during and after the Crimean War (1854-56), the attainment of a proper professional status by the nursing profession, might have been even longer delayed.

During the earlier part of the twentieth century, the practice of these professions became regulated by law and their controlling bodies legally established. Thus the Central Midwives Board was set up in 1902, and the General Nursing Council in 1919, by Acts of Parliament.

From requiring direct help mainly in these two spheres, and that of pharmacy, progress has been such since the early years of this century, that trained and skilled assistance is now an essential feature in many branches of medicine. This is particularly so in relation to many of the more complex techniques employed in hospital practice, where teamwork is vital for efficient diagnosis and treatment, and medical staff head teams which are often composed of members of a variety of other professions and technical occupations allied to medicine.

In hospitals, hospital staff associated directly with the medical profession in the diagnosis and treatment of disease include:

(*a*) **Members of Professions allied to Medicine and other Professions connected with Medical Diagnosis and Treatment :**

Nurses and midwives, *chiropodists, clinical biochemists, clinical psychologists, *hospital dietitians, hospital pharmacists, hospital physicists, *medical laboratory technicians, medical photographers, medical social workers (formerly called almoners), *occupational therapists, opticians (ophthalmic and dispensing), orthoptists, psychiatric social workers, *physiotherapists, *radiographers (diagnostic and therapeutic), *remedial gymnasts, and speech therapists.

(*b*) **Staff in technical occupations connected with medical treatment and diagnosis**—these include:

Audiological technicians, cardiological technicians, dental technicians, electro-encephalography (E.E.G.) technicians, operating theatre technicians, pharmacy technicians, physics technicians, technicians in venereology, and X-ray dark-room technicians.

The roles of some of these hospital workers will be briefly indicated subsequently, whilst discussing various methods of diagnosis and treatment. No account of hospital practice can, however, be regarded as complete without emphasis on the importance therein of the work of medical secretaries.

The management of affairs relevant to the practice of medicine is termed **medical administration** and within an individual hospital the senior administrator may be either a medical man termed a **Medical Superintendent** or a lay official, usually designated as the **Hospital Secretary.**

It will be appreciated that efficient medical administration, with a proper management and co-ordination of supplies, catering, finance, engineering, building, maintenance and transport, is an essential

*Signifies a profession legally designated as a "Profession Supplementary to Medicine".

feature in the provision of hospital facilities for the diagnosis and treatment of disease.

5. DIAGNOSIS OF DISEASE

The term **diagnosis** denotes both the measures taken to identify a particular disease and also the statement of the nature of a particular disease, once its presence has been established.

The making of a diagnosis in a patient with manifestations of disease is a logical prelude to the commencement of a rational form of treatment. It may also render possible the giving of a **prognosis,** i.e. a forecast as to the duration and outcome of the malady.

The first diagnostic procedure is the taking of a **clinical history** from the patient whenever practicable, but otherwise from parents, relatives or others with knowledge of the facts pertaining to the patient's illness.

Following history-taking, the next step is the carrying out of a **clinical examination** to determine the presence or absence of clinical signs of disease. The extent of this will vary considerably according to the nature of the condition suspected.

A full clinical examination may comprise the employment of simple physical methods such as inspection, palpation, percussion and auscultation (listening with a stethoscope, e.g. to heart or bowel sounds); and may also include inspection of the interior of the eyes with an instrument called an **ophthalmoscope**; inspection of the outer parts of the ears and ear drums with an **auriscope,** estimation of the systemic blood pressure with a **sphygmomanometer,** and simple testing of the urine for abnormal constituents such as sugar and albumen, a protein substance.

At the end of his clinical examination the medical practitioner will decide whether he can make a firm diagnosis or a provisional diagnosis; whether he wishes to subject the patient to some form of specialized investigation before making or finalising a diagnosis, or whether he wishes for a "second opinion" on the patient's condition from a specialist or other medical colleague. He will also determine whether he wishes to institute treatment himself, refer the patient elsewhere for treatment, or delay treatment pending the results of further investigation.

In most cases of illness, other than emergencies which may be sent direct to hospital, the practitioner first examining the patient will be a family doctor.

It is the role of the hospital services to provide both in-patient and out-patient facilities for such patients who require investigations and treatments which are beyond the province of the family doctor, and also to provide facilities for dealing with all types of medical emergency (e.g. accidents, sudden illness, poisonings, etc.).

In referring a patient to hospital, the family doctor will decide, according to the nature or suspected nature of the patient's malady, as to which department he should be referred in the first instance.

Hospital specialities are conventionally grouped into **clinical departments** which are concerned with both investigation and treatment and are responsible for the overall care of patients referred to them, and **special** departments which deal with some specialized aspect of either investigation or treatment.

Nomenclature and organization of departments varies in different hospitals, but the following arrangement of principal departments may be regarded as fairly representative of a large general hospital dealing with all types of illness and with maternity work.

Clinical Departments.

| Medicine. | Surgery. (including Accident surgery). | Obstetrics and Gynaecology. |
| Ophthalmology (Eye diseases). | | Oto-rhino-laryngology (Ear, nose and throat diseases). |

Special Departments

| Pathology. | Diagnostic Radiology. |
| Physical Medicine | Radiotherapy. |

Occupational Therapy.

A variety of investigations may be performed by the clinical departments and many of these will be indicated subsequently (e.g. electrocardiography, electro-encephalography, sight testing, audiometry, etc.).

The two major special departments concerned with diagnostic measures are those of:

(*a*) **Pathology**—wherein a wide range of laboratory investigations are performed. These include examination of specimens from the patient by macroscopic (naked eye), microscopic, chemical, physical, bacteriological, and virological methods. Such specimens may consist of secretions of the body (e.g. sputum), excretions (e.g. urine), body fluids (e.g. blood), smears containing body cells (e.g. as in cervical cytology); or portions of body tissue removed during the course of a surgical operation or at biopsy.

(**Biopsy** is a diagnostic procedure in which a small fragment of tissue is removed from a living subject, specifically for microscopic examination. It is very frequently performed under local anaesthesia).

Pathology is the science of disease, and is that branch of medicine concerned with the investigation of disease processes in patients by methods such as those referred to above; and also with research into the basic nature of such processes and the study of their end-results at **autopsy** (post-mortem examination). Medical practitioners who specialize in this subject are termed **pathologists,** and their professional assistants are called **medical laboratory technicians.** Also working in departments of pathology are **clinical biochemists** who are mainly concerned with the branch of pathology known as **chemical pathology,** wherein investigations are made into abnormalities of chemical structure and of chemical processes in the body, caused by disease. (**Biochemistry** is the study of the chemical nature and functions of living tissues).

In addition to chemical pathology there are the following other branches of pathology: **morbid anatomy,** dealing with structural changes produced by disease and including **histopathology**—the study of minute structural changes by microscopy; **medical microbiology**— the study of pathogenic micro-organisms [thus including the studies of **bacteriology** (bacteria), **virology** (viruses) and **protozoology** (protozoa) (see p. 33)]; and **haematology**—the study of the blood and its diseases, allied to which is **blood transfusion serology** concerned with all aspects (e.g. grouping, cross-matching, taking of blood, etc.), of providing blood suitable and safe for transfusion.

(*b*) **Diagnostic Radiology**—radiology is the science of ionizing radiations (see p. 311), and medical radiology has two main branches —**diagnostic radiology** and **radiotherapy** (see p. 23).

Diagnostic radiological investigations consist chiefly of the taking of X-ray pictures called **radiographs** and visual examination of internal structures on a fluorescent screen, in the procedure termed **fluoroscopy** or **X-ray screening.**

The radiological demonstration of certain body structures necessitates the filling of their interior cavities with substances which are either considerably more opaque (e.g. barium) or more translucent (e.g. air) than surrounding body tissues. Such substances are called **contrast media,** and techniques involving their use comprise **contrast radiology.**

Another form of radiological investigation is the diagnostic use of **radioactive isotopes** (see p. 311), e.g. the estimation of the uptake of radioactive iodine by the thyroid gland.

A doctor who specializes in diagnostic radiology is known as a **diagnostic radiologist,** or more shortly as a **radiologist,** and the ancillary medical staff in his department consist of trained professional assistants called **diagnostic radiographers,** and **dark-room technicians,** who carry out the processing of X-ray films.

Neuroradiology, meaning radiology of the nervous system, is a branch of diagnostic radiology.

The investigation of disease by methods involving the use of **ultrasound** or by methods which record the emission of infra-red radiation from the body (**thermography**) may also fall within the scope of a diagnostic radiology department.

6. TREATMENT OF DISEASE

Treatment of disease may be by drugs (medicines)—medical treatment; by operation—surgical treatment; by physical methods—physiotherapy; by ionizing radiations—radiotherapy; by psychological methods—psychotherapy; by other therapeutic methods; and by various combinations of these different forms of treatment.

The aspect of medicine dealing specifically with treatment is called **therapeutics.**

The term **therapy** means treatment of disease.

Some general aspects of therapy and of obstetric care will now be discussed:

(*a*) **Medical treatment**—comprises mainly treatment by medicines, i.e. by drugs; but includes other non-surgical measures such as dietetic therapy, rest, re-assurance and often, of the highest importance, medical nursing care. The term "medical" is here used in its restricted sense as referring to the province of the physician, as opposed to that of the surgeon.

Drugs are used extensively in medical treatment and also as adjuvants in many other types of therapy. Some important types of drugs will be indicated later.

(*b*) **Surgical treatment** consists, in most instances, of treatment by **surgical operations** (i.e. procedures in which an instrument such as a scalpel is used to cut into body tissues for therapeutic purposes), and any pre-operative or post-operative measures necessary in conjunction with such operations. Certain non-operative techniques such as the closed reduction of fractures and dislocations may also be regarded as forms of surgical treatment.

The term **surgery** means "work by hand". Surgical operations, other than certain of those of a minor nature, fall within the province of the specialist **surgeons,** aided by other doctors who are specialist **anaesthetists.**

In the operating theatre, surgeons and anaesthetists are assisted by both theatre nursing staff and trained assistants called **operating theatre technicians.**

In the surgical wards, skilled and efficient surgical nursing is of prime importance in post-operative management of most patients who are subjected to operation, whilst in many it is also a leading factor in pre-operative treatment also.

(*c*) **Physiotherapy**—this means treatment by physical (i.e. natural) methods, comprising measures such as the therapeutic use of exercise, light, heat, and water. A hospital physiotherapy department is staffed by **physiotherapists** usually under the general direction of a medical practitioner who is a specialist in **physical medicine.** Physiotherapy has a wide application in both medical and surgical conditions, but finds its most extensive use in diseases and injuries of the loco-motor system (i.e. the bones, joints and muscles).

(*d*) **Radiotherapy**—comprising treatment by ionizing radiations (see p. 311) produced by apparatus such as superficial and deep X-ray apparatus, linear accelerators, betatrons, etc.; or ionizing radiations emitted spontaneously by radium, radio-cobalt, radiophosphorus, radio-iodine, and other radioactive isotopes.

This form of therapy is chiefly employed for malignant new growths but is also used for a number of non-malignant conditions (e.g. skin diseases, ankylosing spondylitis).

A doctor who specialises in radiotherapy is called a **radiotherapist** and his technical assistants are called therapeutic **radiographers.** An essential adjunct to a radiotherapy department, is a department of physics, under the direction of a **hospital physicist** and staffed also with **physics technicians.** This department is concerned with the planning of treatments prescribed by radiotherapists, the care and the calibration of apparatus; the construction of appliances for radium application, etc; the care of radio-active isotopes; and other tasks, among which are important duties relating to the protection of patients and staff against possible hazards arising from the diag-nostic and therapeutic uses of ionising radiations.

(*e*) **Psychiatric treatment**—includes the use, in patients with disorders of the mind, of (*a*) medical measures (e.g. sedative drugs, stimulant drugs, anti-depressant drugs, tranquillisers), (*b*) surgical measures (e.g. prefrontal leucotomy—nowadays performed only to a very small extent), (*c*) physical measures (e.g. electro-convulsive therapy), and (*d*) **psychotherapy,** and **group therapy**—forms of treatment for mental illness which do not involve medical, surgical, or physical methods.

The study of the mind is called **psychology** and the branch of medicine which deals with diseases of the mind is termed **psychiatry** and is practised by doctors who are specialist **psychiatrists.** In the investigation of some aspects of mental illness, and also in the giving of some forms of treatment and rehabilitation work, psychiatrists are assisted by **clinical psychologists,** whose training includes the obtaining of a University Honours degree in psychology. Also working within the field of mental illness and concerned with its social aspects are professional staff termed **psychiatric social workers.**

Whilst psychiatric out-patient clinics are a common feature of general hospitals, facilities for the in-patient treatment of mental disorders are provided, at the present time, mainly in special hospitals, termed **mental hospitals,** which aim at providing a therapeutic community where all staff of the hospital assist in treatment.

Terms relating to psychiatry will be further discussed in Part IV.

(*f*) **Other therapeutic methods**—these include:

(i) **Chiropody**—the specialized treatment of foot disorders given by **chiropodists;** professional staff who have been trained in **podology,** i.e. the branch of medicine concerned with the study of human foot in health and in medical and surgical disease conditions.

(ii) **Diet therapy**—the word "diet" means a customary or prescribed form of feeding and the control of patient's feeding for therapeutic purposes is termed diet therapy.

Therapeutic diets are planned and their provision is supervised by hospital dietetic departments, in charge of which are professionally trained **therapeutic dietitians.** The hospital dietitian is also concerned with advising out-patients regarding their diets at home.

Dietitians may also, in some instances, assume responsibility for general catering arrangements in a hospital, and hold appointments as a dietitian-catering officer.

(iii) **Occupational therapy**—treatment of disease by occupational activities in the form of work or recreation. This is given, on medical prescription, by **occupational therapists** and is of particular value to patients with physical disabilities and also to those with mental and nervous illnesses.

Occupational therapy is usually given in the form of **remedial therapy,** i.e. treatment designed to assist in the cure or relief of disease. It sometimes, however, comprises **diversional therapy** which is given to occupy the patient's mind and thus divert his thoughts from his symptoms.

(iv) **Orthoptic treatment**—is a process of mental training, involving the employment of special eye exercises, employed in the treatment of squint and other disorders of normal binocular vision.

Investigation and treatment of such conditions are carried out by **orthoptists,** working under the direction of ophthalmic surgeons or ophthalmic medical practioners.

(v) **Optical treatment**—is the correction of errors of refraction by spectacles or contact lenses. Sight testing and prescribing of spectacles and contact lenses may be performed by both medical practitioners and also by qualified **ophthalmic opticians,** who may also supply visual appliances. **Dispensing opticians** supply visual appliances but do not test sight.

(vi) **Speech Therapy**—is performed by **speech therapists** and, as described by Hatfield (1), comprises "the scientific treatment of persons suffering from disorders of speech and language. Suitable cases include stammerers; the cerebral palsied; persons with abnormalities of the peripheral organs of speech, e.g. cleft palate; children with anomalous speech development of functional origin; and patients suffering from neurological conditions affecting speech and language".

(vii) **Remedial Gymnastics**—involving exercise therapy and recreational therapy. This form of treatment, which is of particular value in connection with rehabilitation of the sick and injured is administered by professionally trained **remedial gymnasts,** and who, in a hospital, are members of a department of physical medicine.

Assessment of the results of treatment may be made by clinical methods, and from the results of various forms of special investigations similar to those used in diagnosis, e.g. by pathology and radiology. In selected types of disease (e.g. diseases of the skin, tumours, lesions in certain internal structures capable of being photographed by what are termed endoscopic cameras) valuable records regarding progress under treatment may be obtained from **medical photography.** Records produced by qualified medical photographers are also of great value in various forms of research and in visual methods of instruction employed in medical education.

In many instances, social factors relating to a patient's home condition, or his work, or provision for his dependants may be factors of considerable relevance to the treatment of his illness. It is the task of **medical social workers** (or in psychiatric departments, of **psychiatric social workers**), working in co-operation with the medical staff, to assist patients with such personal problems that create difficulties during illness.

(*g*) **Obstetric care**—the speciality of **obstetrics** deals with the management of pregnancy, childbirth, and the **puerperium** (the period immediately following childbirth, during which the uterus returns to its normal size and lactation commences).

In hospital, this speciality is usually linked in the same department with that of **gynaecology** which is concerned with diseases of the female reproductive system.

By obstetric care is meant the care of women during the different phases of the process of child-bearing, given either by **obstetricians,** i.e. doctors practising obstetrics; or by **midwives** who also practise this speciality; and within certain legally defined limits, may carry out such practice independent of medical supervision. The term "obstetrics" means literally "to stand before" and the name of the speciality presumably derives from the position taken up by the doctor or midwife while assisting during childbirth. Whilst medical or surgical treatment may be required for various types of obstetric disorder, the majority of so-called "patients" under the care of an obstetric department are normal healthy women and require supervision and assistance rather than therapy. In other branches of medicine, however, the word **patient** is generally understood as applying to a subject who requires investigation and treatment for some disease condition.

7. SOME DRUGS USED IN MEDICINE

A **drug,** as defined by Sears (2) is "any substance taken into the body, or applied to its surface, for the prevention or treatment of disease".

Thus, in medical terminology, the word has a much wider application than is usually appreciated by many of the general public, to whom it usually indicates a substance which is either a stimulant or a poison, or has dangerous habit-forming properties.

The prefix **pharm-** means "pertaining to drugs". The study of drugs is called **pharmacology,** and the study of drugs used in medicine is referred to as **materia medica.**

In a hospital, drugs are prepared, stored and dispensed in a department termed a **hospital pharmacy.** This is under the charge of a **hospital pharmacist,** under whom work **pharmacy technicians** (formerly known as dispensing assistants).

Important types of drugs used in medicine include:

(i) **Anaesthetics**—used to produce loss of local sensibility, especially to touch and pain, i.e. **local anaesthetics** (e.g. cocaine and its derivatives); or **general anaesthetics** which cause a general loss of sensibility accompanied by unconsciousness (e.g. nitrous oxide, ether).

The word **anaesthesia** means "without sensation".

(ii) **Analgesics**—pain relieving drugs (e.g. morphine, aspirin).

(iii) **Antibiotics**—substances produced by living organisms which can destroy or prevent growth and multiplication of various pathogenic microbes (e.g. penicillin produced by a mould).

(iv) **Antihistamines**—drugs with an action opposed to that of **histamine** (a substance whose action, when liberated in body tissues, is thought to be responsible for certain of the effects of hypersensitivity (allergic) reactions (e.g. phenergan, piriton).

(v) **Antiseptics** — chemical substances which render disease-producing microbes harmless by preventing their growth and multiplication (e.g. surgical spirit, hibitane).

(vi) **Aperients**—substances which, when taken by mouth, promote bowel evacuation. Mild aperients are known as **laxatives** (e.g. liquid paraffin) and stronger aperients as **purgatives** (e.g. senna, castor oil).

(vii) **Cytotoxic drugs**—the name of these means "cell poisoning" drugs. This class of drugs destroys cells and affects the cells of malignant tumours, and cells found in certain diseases of the blood, bone marrow, lymphatic and reticulo-endothelial systems, more readily than normal cells (e.g. nitrogen mustard, thiotepa).

(viii) **Disinfectants** (Germicides)—chemical substances which destroy pathogenic microbes (e.g. lysol, phenol).

(ix) **Hormones**—secretions of ductless glands and synthetic preparations identical with, or closely resembling these secretions (e.g. insulin, cortisone, oestrogens).

(x) **Hypnotics**—drugs which induce sleep, and many of which also have analgesic (pain-relieving) properties (e.g. morphine, barbiturates).

   (xi) **Steroids**—a class of chemical substance which includes certain hormones produced in the cortex of the suprarenal glands and called **corticosteroids** (e.g. cortisone, hydrocortisone) and certain synthetic drugs (e.g. prednisolone).

  (xii) **Sulphonamides**—a particular class of chemical substance which can prevent the growth and multiplication, within the human body, of a wide range of bacteria (e.g. sulphadiazine, sulphathiazol).

 (xiii) **Tranquillisers**—substances which diminish anxiety and excitability by a sedative action on the nervous system (e.g. chlorpromazine).

 (xiv) **Vaccines and sera**—used in the prevention and treatment of various types of bacterial and viral infection.

Many drugs, if taken into the body in amounts greater than those prescribed for medical treatment, will act as tissue poisons with resultant ill-effects which may, in many instances, be of a serious nature. The margin between the therapeutic dose and the amount which will cause drug poisoning is frequently small.

A large number of drugs with poisonous properties are in the United Kingdom subject to certain statutory provisions for the control of drugs and legally designated as **Schedule 1 (S1.) poisons,** or **Schedule 4 (S.4) poisons.**

Certain drugs classified as S.1 poisons possess habit-forming properties and are commonly referred to as **drugs of addiction.** Some drugs of addiction, designated by law as **dangerous drugs** (e.g. alkaloids of opium such as morphine and heroin; pethidine, cocaine, cannabis) are subjected to further control under the Dangerous Drugs Act and Dangerous Drugs Regulations. Other habit-forming drugs (e.g. amphetamines, L.S.D. 25), are controlled under the provisions of the Drugs (Prevention of Misuse) Act.

Treatment with chemical substances is called **chemotherapy.** The term was initially introduced in connection with the treatment of syphilis by arsenical compounds. In its modern usage it refers chiefly to the treatment of infections by sulphonamides; the use of hormones and cytotoxic drugs in malignant conditions and therapy with anti-tuberculosis drugs.

8. BRANCHES OF MEDICINE AND SURGERY

A type of basic departmental hospital organization was described on p. 20.

Introductory

Customarily there are a number of divisions within the major clinical specialities of medicine and surgery, the number and form of these varying according to the size of the hospital and the nature of its work.

Some of the principal divisions of Medicine and Surgery and the types of diseases or structures of the body with which they deal are:

Medicine		**Surgery**	
General Medicine.		*General Surgery.*	
Paediatrics	—children's diseases.	*Accident Surgery.*	
Chest Diseases	—lung diseases.	*Orthopaedic Surgery.*	—bone and joint surgery.
Dermatology.	—skin disease.	*Urology*	—surgery of the urinary system of both sexes and the male reproductive system.
Cardiology	—heart diseases.	*Cardiac Surgery.*	—heart surgery.
Neurology	—diseases of the nervous system.	*Facio-maxillary Surgery.*	—surgery of the face and jaws.
Geriatrics	—diseases of old age.	*Thoracic Surgery.*	—chest surgery.
Endocrinology	—diseases of the endocrine glands.	*Neurosurgery*	—surgery of the nervous system.
Physical Medicine—(see p. 23).		*Plastic Surgery.*	—surgical repair of damaged or absent tissues.
Psychiatry	—diseases of the mind	*Dental Surgery.*	—surgery of the teeth.
Venereal Diseases.		*Ophthalmic Surgery.*	—eye surgery.
		Ear, Nose and Throat Surgery.	

REFERENCES

(1) Hatfield, Frances M. (Personal Communication).
(2) Sears, W. G. *Materia Medica for Nurses.* Edward Arnold, 1966.

PART II

Medical Terms Referring to Certain General Pathological Processes

THE researches of pathologists have shown that certain series of changes, from the normal, may occur as common features in disorders which are otherwise of a different nature, and of widely different causation, e.g. changes due to inflammation are observed in disease conditions due to such differing aetiology as infection, mechanical irritation, burns, over-exposure to ionizing radiations, etc.

Thus changes of this type, common to many different forms of disease are known as **general pathological processes.** In contradistinction, abnormalities peculiar to individual diseases, or a group of related diseases, may be referred to as **specific pathological processes.** Where appropriate these latter will be referred to when discussing terms referring to various types of diseases in Parts III, IV and V.

A comprehension of the nature of a number of the more important general pathological processes, affords a valuable basis for the proper understanding of many medical terms.

This part of the book will accordingly give brief explanations of some of these processes—namely certain manifestations of damage to tissue cells; infection, antibody formation, inflammation and repair; some disorders of growth; cyst formation; some disorders of blood circulation, and the conditions of allergy and auto-immunity.

1. MANIFESTATIONS OF DAMAGE TO TISSUE CELLS.

NECROSIS

This term means death of tissue cells within a localized area.

If necrosis is accompanied or rapidly followed by putrefactive changes, the condition then becomes one of **gangrene.**

Putrefaction is a type of tissue decomposition which results from infection with putrefactive bacteria. According to the type of putrefaction present, gangrene may be either **moist** or **dry** in type.

DEGENERATION

This is a condition in which structural changes are produced in tissue cells as a result of damage initially insufficient to cause necrosis.

The changes may, however, progress to necrosis or, alternatively, if the causal factors cease to operate, they may sometimes regress with a return to normality of the affected cells.

Degeneration is of various types. One form is called **fatty degeneration** and is characterized by an alteration in affected cells, termed "fatty change". This change occurs in organs such as the liver, kidney and heart due to a variety of causes, among which are lack of adequate oxygen supply, dietetic deficiencies, certain chemical poisons such as chloroform, excess consumption of alcohol, and severe infections.

Other forms of degeneration include the conditions called **cloudy swelling** and **hyaline, fibrinoid, mucoid** and **amyloid degeneration.**

In the last named, an abnormal protein substance called **amyloid** appears in the walls of blood vessels and in the connective tissues of muscles and various internal organs. Its presence is associated with the clinical conditions known as **primary amyloidosis** and **secondary amyloidosis.** In the former, which is very rare, the disorder develops without apparent cause, whereas in the latter, it is secondary to some form of chronic infection (e.g. osteomyelitis, tuberculosis, syphilis, ulcerative colitis, renal (kidney) infection), or to Hodgekin's disease or rheumatoid arthritis.

PATHOLOGICAL CALCIFICATION

This term describes the abnormal deposition of calcium salts in the soft tissues of the body.

In the form of pathological calcification called **dystrophic calcification,** calcium salts are deposited in tissue cells which have been killed or injured by disease. This process is a common feature in sites of healed tuberculous infection and may also be seen as a result of certain other inflammatory conditions, in some types of neoplasm, in some forms of arterial disease (e.g. atheroma), and in old blood clots.

Calculi (stones) in the kidneys and also calcium deposits in a variety of other sites may occur as a result of another form of pathological calcification called **metastatic calcification.** This process occurs in certain disorders (e.g. hyperparathyroidism) in which there is an upset of calcium metabolism, resulting in high levels of calcium being present in the circulating blood.

When of sufficient size, areas of pathological calcification may be readily demonstrated on X-ray films.

2. THE PROCESSES OF INFECTION, ANTIBODY FORMATION, INFLAMMATION AND REPAIR

INFECTION

Infection is said to be present when pathogenic micro-organisms (disease-producing germs) have established themselves in the tissues of some part, or parts of the body, and are able to survive and reproduce themselves therein.

Micro-organisms (also known as microbes) are minute living organisms of such a size that they either can only be visualized under a microscope, or so small that they are ultra-microscopic, i.e. beyond the range of visibility of any known microscopic methods.

It will be appreciated that the presence of bacteria, known as **commensals,** living normally on the external and certain of the internal surfaces of the body (e.g. within the mouth, bowel, etc.) without causing harmful effects, does not constitute infection. Certain commensals can, however, develop pathogenic properties if they are carried to organs or tissues in sites different from those in which they normally exist, e.g. the *bacterium coli* is normally a commensal in the bowel, but if it gains access to the urinary tract it may cause severe bladder and kidney infections.

Infection results in tissue damage and, in the vast majority of instances, in the production of clinical signs and symptoms of infective disease.

In some types of infection, however, it is possible for an individual to acquire the infection without developing any signs or symptoms of its presence. This is known as **sub-clinical infection** and the affected subject is called a "**healthy carrier**" of the disease in question, as he carries its causative micro-organisms. These he may transmit to others, who may then develop clinical signs and symptoms. Cases with sub-clinical infection are not uncommon in epidemics of poliomyelitis (infantile paralysis), and a number of epidemics of typhoid fever have been traced to infection of water or food supplies by healthy carriers.

A person may also become a healthy carrier as a result of survival of pathogenic micro-organisms, within his body, after otherwise apparently complete recovery from an infective illness and disappearance of all clinical signs and symptoms.

Germs that are harmful are termed medically **pathogenic** (disease-producing) **micro-organisms** (microbes) or more shortly **pathogens.**

They are of four main varieties, namely, **bacteria, viruses, fungi** and **protozoa.** Minute organisms known as **rickettsiae** are of intermediate type between bacteria and viruses.

Bacteria are of different types, among which are **cocci, bacilli,** and **spirochaetes.** Bacteria liberate poisonous substances called **toxins.** These are two varieties, **exotoxins,** which diffuse out from living bacteria and **endotoxins,** which are only liberated when bacteria die.

Bacteria, fungi and protozoa are all visible by ordinary microscopic methods. Many viruses are visible by special methods of microscopy—but others are ultramicroscopic.

Examples of infective diseases caused by these various forms of micro-organisms are:

(*a*) **Bacteria**—pneumococcal pneumonia (*pneumococcus*), tuberculosis (*tubercle bacillus*); syphilis (*Treponema pallidum*).

(*b*) **Viruses**—common cold, measles, poliomyelitis.

(*c*) **Fungi**—ringworm, athletes foot.

(*d*) **Protozoa**—malaria.

Micro-organisms may gain access to the body by **inhalation** (being inspired into the respiratory tract), **ingestion** (being swallowed in food or drink), by **inoculation** through wounds in the skin and sometimes by penetration of undamaged skin. They may also enter the body through the external ear, anal canal, vagina and urethra.

Invading microbes, when they cause damage to tissue cells, provoke a localized reaction. An infection may produce local signs and symptoms due to the inflammatory reaction it evokes and also general signs and symptoms such as **pyrexia** (fever, i.e. elevation of body temperature above normal), **tachycardia** (elevation of the rate of heart beat above normal), **headache, anorexia** (loss of appetite) and **malaise** (a feeling of being generally out-of-sorts).

The body possesses **surface defence mechanisms** which seek to prevent entry of pathogens into its tissues. Thus the skin and, to a lesser extent, the mucous membranes lining its interior structures provide barriers to such entry. Among other such mechanisms are also the destruction of bacteria by the acidity of the gastric juices, removal of particulate matter by coughing, etc.

There are also **internal defence mechanisms** such as the tissue reaction called **inflammation** (see later), and those which result in the formation of protein substances which have an antagonistic action to many types of pathogens and are known as **antibodies.** The body also appears to possess a natural inherited resistance to certain types of infection.

33

2

ANTIBODY FORMATION

Antibodies are proteins, of the type called globulins, and may be produced in response to an attack of an infection (clinical or subclinical), or their formation may be artificially induced by the administration of vaccines by injection, by mouth, or, as in vaccination against smallpox, by superficial scarification of the skin or multiple pressure technique.

Vaccines may consist of: (i) living but attenuated (i.e. weakened) pathogens (e.g. B.C.G. vaccination against tuberculosis); (ii) dead pathogens (e.g. T.A.B.C. vaccination against typhoid and paratyphoid A. B. and C. fevers); (iii) modified bacterial toxins called **toxoids** (e.g. as in vaccination against tetanus); (iv) living organisms of low virulence related to the causal micro-organisms of the disease against which protection is required (e.g. vaccination against smallpox with calf lymph containing the virus of cowpox).

Substances, the administration of which cause antibody formation, are called **antigens.** The procedure of provoking antibody formation, by administration of antigens (in the form of bacterial or viral preparations), with the object of protecting the vaccinated subject against certain specific diseases, or groups of diseases is referred to as **active immunization.** The term **immunity** used in this context means "freedom from disease", but the protection obtained either naturally or artificially is only partial in many instances. The thymus gland is now thought to be concerned in some way with reactions productive of immunity.

Active immunization usually produces some degree of protection for a fairly long period of time. Immunity, of much shorter duration, but more rapidly obtained, may be conferred in respect of some diseases by administration of sera from immunized animals or human beings. This is termed **passive immunization,** e.g. as used in the prevention and treatment of measles by gamma-globulin from the serum of humans who are convalescing from measles, and thus have a high content of antibodies against the causal virus in their blood serum.

A number of antibodies also appear to occur naturally in the body without any apparent stimulus, such as infection or other antigenic cause, being responsible for their formation. These are termed **natural antibodies.**

It is thought probable that antibodies may be formed in certain cells of the lymphatic system.

Antibody formation is caused not only by bacterial and viral antigens but also as a result of entry into the body of other substances with antigenic properties, e.g. various types of foreign protein, incompatible transfused blood, tissue grafts from other individuals, etc. (see also under "allergy" and "auto-immunity").

INFLAMMATION

This process is the local reaction of the body to any form of damage to its cells.

Whilst the most common cause of inflammation is infection, it also occurs in response to cellular damage from many other types of injury, e.g. by mechanical trauma, external physical and chemical agents.

Several different types of inflammation are described. These are, however, all essentially variants of the same basic pathological process, which is defensive in nature and tends to localize the effects of the damage and where possible prevent their extension to other organs and tissues.

The inflammatory reaction results in the production of an **inflammatory exudate,** in the tissue spaces in the affected area. This consists of blood cells and plasma which leave blood through openings in the walls of capillaries. In acute inflammation, the exudate is rich in both cells and fluid, whereas in chronic inflammation it is predominantly cellular in type. Chronic inflammatory reactions are often accompanied by much formation of fibrous connective tissue, a change known as **fibrosis** (see later). White blood cells, of the types known as lymphocytes and plasma cells, predominate in the exudates due to chronic inflammation. Plasma cells may play some part in the formation of defensive substances called **antibodies** (see p. 34) and it is thought that lymphocytes may carry antibodies and release them at the site of disease.

White cells of the variety called polymorphonuclear leucocytes, or polymorphs, are found in great numbers in the exudate of acute inflammation and, as the reaction subsides, increasing numbers of mobile cells of the reticulo-endothelial system (see p. 195) called macrophages appear at the site of the reaction. Both polymorphs and macrophages possess the ability to take up foreign matter, such as the bodies of infecting micro-organisms, into their cytoplasm. This is called **phagocytosis** and the plasma in the inflammatory exudate possesses naturally occurring antibodies which render bacteria more readily susceptible to phagocytic action.

The property of phagocytosis is also possessed by static cells of the reticulo-endothelial system which are found in sites such as lymph glands, liver, bone marrow and spleen. These cells, which form an important secondary line of defence against infection, are designed to clear the lymphatic circulation and blood stream of invading microbes.

The course of an inflammatory reaction varies greatly, according to the nature of the tissue damage by which it is evoked. When the tissue damage is slight, it may subside at an early stage. This is spoken of as **resolution,** a term indicating a return to normal after a disease process. When tissue damage is marked, and results from bacterial infection, the reaction may proceed to **suppuration,** i.e. the formation of pus. **Pus** is a yellowish fluid composed of fluid from the blood, dead and living bacteria, white blood cells and dead tissue cells. It lies initially within a cavity in the tissue which is formed as a result of tissue destruction. A cavity which contains pus is known as an **abscess.** In many sites, abscess cavities, unless relieved by surgical incision, tend to enlarge and ultimately rupture, either on the surface of the body, or into some hollow cavity or hollow organ. An infective **sinus** is a track produced by pus when discharging itself from an abscess cavity. A sinus is open at one end only. An abscess may in some instances burst in two directions and then a track, with two open ends called a **fistula,** is formed. A fistula may lead from skin to mucous membrane or from one cavity of the body to another. An **ulcer** is an open sore caused by an inflammatory process breaking through the skin or a mucous membrane.

An area that is the subject of an acute inflammatory reaction appears red and hot, owing to its having a temporarily increased blood supply, an essential feature of the reaction. It is also swollen owing to the presence of an exudate in its tissue spaces and is painful and tender to the touch as a result of increased tension within these spaces and pressure on sensory nerve endings in the vicinity. Presumably the heat and redness caused by acute inflammation were responsible for the name of the process "inflammation" which means literally "a setting on fire".

When an inflammatory reaction, caused by bacterial infection, fails to destroy and to localize the invading micro-organisms, one or more of the following may ensue:

(*a*) Spread of infection into the draining lymphatics causing **lymphangitis** (inflammation of lymph vessels) and **lymphadenitis** (inflammation of lymph glands).

(*b*) Spread of the infecting micro-organisms by the blood to distant tissues where thay may cause **metastatic infections** (secondary infections).

When pyogenic micro-organisms are carried in large numbers in the blood and cause multiple secondary abscesses in various structures, the condition is described as **pyaemia. (Pyogenic** means "pus-producing").

The presence of multiplying pyogenic micro-organisms in the blood stream is termed **septicaemia** (blood poisoning).

REPAIR

Injuries (e.g. fractures, wounds, etc.) and also disease processes (e.g. inflammatory reactions) which cause death of body cells in localized areas produce a loss of continuity in tissues of affected regions.

When any such loss of continuity is produced, natural processes are quickly set in motion in an endeavour to restore tissue continuity. Such processes constitute what is termed **repair.**

(Note: cells and tissues killed by disease are subjected to the action of phagocytes. Phagocytic action is generally efficacious in removing small areas of necrotic material and in separating off larger areas from surrounding living tissue, e.g. as in the separation of a slough from a boil).

In some tissues the specialized cells retain their powers of multiplication through life (e.g. bone, surface epithelium of skin, fibrous tissue, liver) and repair thus achieved by multiplication of undamaged specialized cells. This is known as **regeneration.**

In other tissues (e.g. muscle, cartilage) the specialized cells lose their powers of multiplication in post-natal life. Regeneration is thus not possible and deficiencies are restored by ingrowth of surround fibrous connective tissue; a process termed **replacement fibrosis.**

A similar process is seen in the central nervous system where damage to specialized cells is repaired by **gliosis,** an overgrowth of the supporting special connective tissue framework called neuroglia.

In addition to replacement fibrosis, fibrosis may also occur in inflammatory exudates which fail to absorb normally and, being invaded by cells from surrounding connective tissue, are converted into fibrous connective tissue.

A third form of fibrosis is the overgrowth of fibrous tissue, which is seen as a concomitant of chronic inflammation.

Connective tissue when newly formed during repair is at first soft

37

and richly supplied with blood vessels. Later, however, it contracts and becomes changed into dense fibrous **scar tissue,** with a scanty blood supply. Contraction of large fibrous scars may cause marked deformities (e.g. contractures following severe burns).

Fibrosis in sites such as the pleural, pericardial and peritoneal cavities frequently results in bands of fibrous scar tissue joining opposing surfaces of these cavities. Such bands are called **adhesions** and may sometimes cause serious ill-effects (e.g. intestinal obstruction due to peritoneal adhesions).

The process of repair may be slowed, or, in some instances, prevented entirely by a number of factors amongst which are chronic infection, deficient blood supply, vitamin C. deficiency, presence of foreign bodies, and the necessity to attempt to bridge large defects by newly formed tissue.

Conversely, repair may be hastened by effecting close apposition of the sides of the gap in the tissues (e.g. as in the suture of an uninfected incised wound or surgical incision) and obtaining what is termed **healing by first intention** (primary union).

In contradistinction to healing by first intention, is **healing by second intention** (healing by granulation, secondary union), in which the tissue defect is gradually filled by ingrowth of granulation tissue which is converted into newly formed fibrous connective tissue.

(*Note :* **granulation tissue** consists of loops of capillary blood vessels, macrophages, occasional polymorphs and associated young connective tissue cells).

In some individuals overgrowth of fibrous tissue during healing may result in the production of tumour-like masses in scars, known as **keloids.**

3. DISORDERS OF GROWTH

Growth in excess of normal, due to increase in the size of individual cells, **hypertrophy,** or to increased cell-division, **hyperplasia,** may be seen as a manifestation of disease.

A complete failure of development called **agenesis** or **aplasia;** a failure of development of organs or tissues to normal size, **hypoplasia;** and a shrinkage in size of organs and tissues, termed **atrophy** may be also seen as a result of various morbid conditions.

Some forms of hypertrophy (e.g. muscular enlargement in athletes) and hyperplasia (e.g. increase in numbers of red blood cells in persons living at high altitudes) are, however, physiological and not pathological. A generalized tissue atrophy is, moreover, seen as a physiological process in old people, whose wizened appearance is well known.

Another form of growth disorder is called **neoplasia.**

NEOPLASIA

This term means "new growth" and refers to the formation of **neoplasms** or **tumours.** Neoplasms consist of masses of abnormal cells, which grow at the expense of surrounding normal body tissues and carry out no useful functions in the body. In pathology the term "tumour" is used as being synonymous with the term " neoplasm". In the widest sense, however, a tumour is any form of swelling.

Neoplasms fall into two major divisions, the **benign** (innocent) and the **malignant:**

(*a*) **Benign neoplasms**—are usually of slow growth. They tend to displace normal tissues and seldom cause serious effects unless they grow in, or press on, important organs. A capsule of fibrous tissue is often formed around them. They do not spread to distant organs and tissues.

(*b*) **Malignant neoplasms**—are often of rapid growth. They tend to infiltrate widely into surrounding tissues and often cause ulceration. They cause serious general effects in the body, and, unless successfully treated, will eventually cause death of the patient. They have a marked tendency to spread to distant organs and tissues, forming **metastases** (secondary growths) therein. In the type of malignant neoplasms called **carcinomas** such metastatic spread occurs both via the lymphatics and blood stream. In the type called **sarcomas,** distant spread is usually only via the blood stream. **Carcinomas** are malignant tumours of **epithelia,** whereas **sarcomas** are derived from various types of connective tissue (including bone and cartilage).

Diagnostic radiology is of vital importance in the diagnosis of many types of neoplasm, and radiotherapy, used either alone, or in combination with surgery, of vital importance in their treatment.

Drugs, of a type known collectively as **anti-cancer drugs** are also now playing an important part in the treatment of a number of different types of neoplasm. These substances are of two main types: **cytotoxic drugs,** e.g. nitrogen mustard, methotrexate, and **hormones,** e.g. oestrogens (female hormones) and androgens (male hormones).

The word **cancer** may be used as a synonym of "carcinoma" both words being derived from the Latin word for a "crab". In its wider sense the term cancer, however, includes both carcinoma and sarcoma, and other conditions such as leukaemia and various forms of diseases described as malignant reticuloses, which display certain features akin to those of the malignant neoplasms and are thus included with the category of disorders referred to as **malignancies,** or **malignant diseases.**

Carcinogenesis means "production of cancer" and cancer-producing agents are called **carcinogens.**

4. CYST FORMATION

Cysts are abnormal cavities, which may form in the body as a result of a number of widely differing pathological processes (e.g. developmental error, trauma, infection, obstruction of glandular ducts, neoplastic disease, etc.). They contain either fluid or semifluid material, or air, and possess a lining membrane.

5. DISORDERS IN BLOOD CIRCULATION

HAEMORRHAGE

Means bleeding, and may occur as a result of trauma or disease affecting the walls of blood vessels. A number of diseases of widely different causation may cause bleeding into the skin or internal organs. **Epistaxis** is bleeding from the nose; **haematemesis,** vomiting of blood; **haemoptysis**—coughing up of blood from the respiratory tract; **haematuria,** blood in the urine. **Melaena** is the passage of stools, which are coloured black, owing to the presence of altered blood from some portion of the alimentary tract. Haemorrhage from the pregnant uterus, during the later weeks of pregnancy but before delivery, is called **ante-partum haemorrhage.**

HYPERAEMIA

This term describes a condition in which there is an excessive amount of blood present in a part or parts of the body. **Congestion** is a synonymous term. **Local hyperaemia** may result from inflammation or obstruction of veins. **General venous congestion** is seen in right-sided heart failure, when the right ventricle of the heart can no longer adequately pump blood, returned from the veins, out into the pulmonary circulation.

ANAEMIA

Means the blood is lacking in either, or both, normal haemoglobin content or numbers of red cells; or that there is a deficiency in the total amount of blood in the body.

ISCHAEMIA (LOCAL ANAEMIA)

Means a localized deficiency of blood in a part of the body, e.g. **ischaemic heart disease**—due to disease of coronary arteries resulting in a diminution of the blood supply to the heart muscle.

THROMBOSIS

Means the formation of a **thrombus** (clot) in the interior of a blood vessel or the heart. The main cause of thrombosis is damage to the walls of blood vessels or the endocardial lining of the heart. Infection is a common cause of thrombosis, as is an arterial disease called **atheroma.** Thrombi which block the interior of large vessels may be demonstrated radiographically by arteriography or venography, as appropriate.

EMBOLISM

A portion or the whole of a thrombus may become detached and be carried in the blood stream to another part of the body. This process is called **embolism**, and the detached fragment of blood clot is called an **embolus.** An embolus, arising in the venous side of the circulation, is likely to become impacted within the pulmonary circulation. If large it may block the main pulmonary artery, or one of its main branches, causing sudden death or death in a few hours. If smaller it may deprive an area of lung tissue of its supply of arterial blood and thus cause necrosis of its cells. Such an area of dead tissue produced by an impacted embolus, is called an **infarct.**

Emboli may consist of material, other than detached thrombi, which have entered the circulation, e.g. masses of bacteria or tumour cells; air, and oil or fat globules.

Fat embolism sometimes occurs as a result of a fracture, and oil embolism as a result of an X-ray examination called hysterosalpingography, when this is performed with iodized oil as the contrast medium (see p. 174).

OEDEMA (DROPSY)

Is a condition of swelling of soft tissues, resulting from the presence of excessive fluid in their tissue spaces. The fluid consists of plasma from the blood stream and may accumulate in the tissues as a result of obstruction to veins, inflammatory conditions, and certain types of heart and kidney disease, protein deficiency, or allergic disorders. Oedema may also be caused by obstruction of lymphatic vessels. The swollen arm, that may follow radical amputation of the breast, is an example of lymphatic oedema. It is thought that this condition may well result from the extensive removal of lymphatic tissue, in this operation.

In patients with oedema, concomitant exudation of plasma in the peritoneal cavity or pleural cavities may occur; resulting in **ascites,** in the former instance, and **pleural effusion** in the latter.

6. ALLERGY (HYPERSENSITIVITY)

The term allergy means "altered reaction" and Dowling and Wells (1) state that "it is generally held to imply reactivity to an agent of any kind, which normally provokes no reaction".

It was noted on p. 34 that bacteria and viruses have what are called antigenic properties, i.e. they evoke by their presence in the body antibody-formation resulting in antigen-antibody reactions, with beneficial effects to an infected individual.

In contradistinction, allergic reactions are thought to be caused by the occurrence of abnormal antigen-antibody reactions which cause damage to tissue cells and resultant undesirable and sometimes dangerous clinical manifestations.

A variety of agents may act as antigens and provoke allergic reactions in susceptible individuals.

Among the clinical disorders in which allergy is a basic factor or thought to play some role are bronchial asthma, hay fever (due to hypersensitivity to grass pollens), eczema, food allergy (e.g. allergic disorder following ingestion of shell-fish), certain types of reaction following administration of various drugs (e.g. drug rashes caused by penicillin, or sulphonamides; serum sickness caused by injection of therapeutic sera; hypersensitivity reactions to iodine-containing contrast media).

It is also to be noted that many authorities regard acute rheumatism, and acute glomerulo-nephritis, as being primarily due to allergic reactions resulting from streptococcal infection.

One type of severe and sometimes fatal acute allergic reaction is seen in the condition called **anaphylactic shock,** in which the outstanding feature is a sudden general circulatory collapse.

Certain of the important effects seen in allergic disorders are due to the liberation of a substance called **histamine** within the tissues, causing dilatation of capillaries, arterioles and venules. In the treatment of allergic disorders such effects may be controlled by the administration of **antihistamine drugs.**

AUTO-IMMUNITY

Allied to allergy (see above) is the phenomena of **auto-immunity** wherein some factor, which is an integral part of the body, develops antigenic properties and provokes antigen-antibody reactions.

Such reactions are widely considered as being the basis of a number of diseases which are termed **auto-immune diseases,** although opinions differ as to what conditions may at present be so classified.

Some authorities consider that auto-immunity may play some part in the causation of rheumatoid arthritis and many more would regard the uncommon conditions called Hashimotos thyroiditis and disseminated lupus erythematosus as auto-immune diseases.

REFERENCE

(1) Dowling, G. B. & Wells, G. *Conybeare's Textbook of Medicine* (Ed. W. N. Mann), Livingstone, 1964.

PART III

Medical Terms Referring to Certain Infective Diseases

DISEASES caused by invasion of the tissues by pathogenic micro-organisms, i.e. bacteria, viruses, rickettsiae, fungi and protozoa, are called **infective diseases.** As they can be transmitted from one individual to another, by either direct contact or via some intermediate agent (e.g. infected water and food, insect carriers), they are sometimes referred to as **communicable diseases.**

The term **contagious** is of rather ill-defined usage, but is generally employed in respect of those infective disorders which are transmissible by direct contact.

Any system of classification of infective diseases is likely to lead to some overlapping of various groups. In this explanation of medical terms, the conditions referred to will be described under the following headings: infectious fevers, pyogenic infections, tuberculosis, venereal diseases; some other infective diseases.

Tropical infections will be referred to in Part V of the book, and some other types of infective diseases will be referred to in Part IV, when discussing terms referring to diseases of the various systems of the body.

It is important in the consideration of infective disease to make special note of the following:

- (*a*) the meanings of the terms infection, inflammation, and immunization (see Part II).
- (*b*) the use of the suffix **-itis** to indicate inflammatory conditions, e.g. parotitis, inflammation of the parotid salivary glands.
- (*c*) the terms **pyrexia, tachycardia, headache, anorexia** and **malaise** (see p. 33).
- (*d*) **septicaemia** (see p. 37).
- (*e*) **toxaemia**—the word **toxin** means a poison, and toxaemia is a condition wherein bacterial toxins, or other poisonous substances, are present in the general circulation causing effects such as malaise, weakness, furring of the tongue, pyrexia, etc.
- (*f*) **lesion,** a word meaning " injury" and conveniently employed to any form of structural damage, caused to body tissues by disease.

44

(*g*) **focus**—(plural: foci)—a term used in one of its senses to indicate an area of disease, e.g. as in "primary tuberculous focus".

Section A.—INFECTIOUS FEVERS

By common usage, those of the infective diseases which are termed " infectious " comprise a number of acute infective disorders which, being readily transmissible, show a tendency to appear periodically in **epidemics,** i.e. outbreaks which affect fairly large numbers of individuals and which sometimes have a wide geographical distribution.

A **fever** is a condition in which the body temperature is raised above the normal. The adjective "febrile" means "pertaining to a fever" and a fever may also be termed a **"pyrexia".**

Included among disorders which may be classified as infectious fevers are what are sometimes called "common childhood ailments", i.e. measles, German measles, whooping cough, mumps and chicken pox. Also included are a number of other conditions such as smallpox, diphtheria, scarlet fever, typhoid fever and cerebrospinal fever.

All these fevers possess what is called an **incubation period,** i.e. the time between acquiring the infection and the appearance of the first clinical signs and symptoms. These latter, which are often of a non-specific type, herald the approach of the main clinical features of the illness and are known as **prodromal symptoms** and **signs** (e.g. headache, dizziness, general malaise, pyrexia, tachycardia).

Another feature common to the majority of these diseases is the development, at some stage, of multiple inflammatory skin lesions, referred to in lay parlance as "spots", which form a **rash.** (Synonyms: **eruption, exanthem**).

A rash may consist of **macules**—spots or blotches which are not raised above the surrounding skin; **papules**—spots which are raised above the skin (sometimes referred to as "pimples"); **vesicles**—small blisters containing clear fluid and **pustules,** small blisters containing pus;—or mixed forms of these lesions. A rash may also be described as **petechial,** when it is comprised of small purplish spots called **petechiae,** which are due to blood effused beneath the epidermis; or as **purpuric** when haemorrhages beneath the skin produce large purple spots or patches.

The infectious fevers discussed in this section are all due to either bacterial or viral infection, and in many of them active and passive methods of immunization (see p. 34) are employed in their prophylaxis

45

(prevention). Immune sera may also be used in the treatment of some of these illnesses.

MEASLES (MORBILLI)

This is a virus infection with an incubation period of about 10 to 14 days. Its name probably originally meant "spots" and a prominent feature is the appearance of a widespread rash, usually on the fourth day of the illness.

Characteristic early features are conjunctivitis and the development of white spots in the mouth, the so-called **Koplik's spots.**

Bronchopneumonia and otitis media are the most frequent complications, and the former may be of very serious import in infants.

Active immunization may now be undertaken with measles vaccine. Those exposed to infection may be given temporary protection by **gamma-globulin** (an extract of blood serum containing antibodies against the causal virus) or **convalescent serum** (i.e. blood serum obtained from patients during convalescence from measles).

GERMAN MEASLES (RUBELLA)

The alternative name of "rubella" derives from the redness of the rash which develops in this virus disease. Another characteristic is glandular enlargement, which may be widespread. The incubation period is about 14 to 21 days.

The infection is generally mild but unfortunately, if contracted during the first three months of pregnancy, may lead to subsequent birth of a child with serious disabilities such as congenital heart disease, congenital cataract (opacity of the lens of the eye) and congenital deafness.

Temporary protection may be given during early pregnancy by administration of gamma-globulin.

WHOOPING COUGH (PERTUSSIS)

This is a bacterial infection due to an organism called *haemophilus pertussis*, and having an incubation period of about 8 to 14 days.

The infection causes a catarrhal inflammation of the upper respiratory tract and a dry cough which becomes paroxysmal in type. The fits of coughing often end with an inspiratory noise described as a "whoop".

Among the serious complications which may occur are bronchopneumonia, atelectasis (collapse) of segments of lung tissue, and

convulsions, i.e. fits in which abnormal movements occur owing to involuntary muscular contractions, and in which there may often be an accompanying loss of consciousness.

Antibiotics may be employed in treatment.

Prophylactic vaccinations may be carried out employing **"triple vaccine"**, which consists of a combined vaccine against whooping cough, diphtheria and tetanus.

MUMPS (EPIDEMIC PAROTITIS)

This is a virus infection which causes acute inflammatory changes in the parotid salivary glands (i.e. parotitis) and occasionally, in the usbmandibular salivary glands also.

The incubation period is about 14-21 days.

The disease is not itself serious but may, after puberty, produce serious complications among which are **orchitis** (inflammation of the testes), **oophoritis** (inflammation of the ovaries) and **pancreatitis** (inflammation of pancreas). Orchitis may result in sterility.

There is no specific treatment for mumps.

The name of the condition appears to derive from the abnormal appearance of the face, produced by the parotid swellings, the word "mumps" originally indicating an abnormal facial expression.

CHICKEN POX (VARICELLA)

This is a mild virus infection unconnected with chickens, but owing the second part of its name to the fact that, at one time, a disease with a rash exhibiting the formation of "pocks", i.e. spots of vesicular or pustular type, was referred to as a "pox".

Chicken pox has an incubation period of about 14-21 days and its causal virus is indistinguishable from that of herpes zoster (shingles).

The disease is characterized by a vesicular rash. It is sometimes, in the earlier stages of the disease, difficult to differentiate between the rashes of chicken pox and the much more serious condition of smallpox.

There is no specific treatment.

SMALLPOX (VARIOLA)

This virus disease may occur in the form of **classical smallpox (variola major)** which is serious and not infrequently fatal; and in a much milder form called **alastrim (variola minor)**.

The incubation period is 12 days. The rash is at first macular and

47

then goes through papular, vesicular and pustular stages (see p. 45), the latter being due to secondary bacterial infection of the vesicles. The difficulty which can occasionally occur in differentiating smallpox from chicken pox has been referred to when discussing the latter condition.

The infection is in its severer forms accompanied by marked pyrexia and considerable toxaemia. Myocarditis (inflammation of the heart muscle), bronchopneumonia and virus pneumonia are among the complications.

There is no specific therapy but penicillin, or other antibiotics, are of value in diminishing the effects of secondary infection and preventing complications.

A high degree of protection against smallpox can be obtained by active immunization with a vaccine of calf lymph, containing the live related virus which causes **cowpox (vaccinia).**

Vaccination against smallpox with vaccinia virus was first carried out, in England, in 1796 by Edward Jenner, a Gloucestershire physician.

DIPHTHERIA

The word "diphtheria" means "a membrane" and the name of this disease derives from the fact that the inflammatory exudate, formed at the site of infection, coagulates so as to form a characteristic false membrane.

The causal pathogen is a bacterium known variously as the *corynebacterium diphtheriae*, the *Klebs-Loeffler bacillus*, or the *diphtheria bacillus*.

Infection occurs most commonly in the throat, producing faucial diphtheria (i.e. so named from the pillars of the fauces, between which lies the tonsils), but can also develop in the nose or larynx, and rarely in the skin (cutaneous diphtheria).

In addition to local effects, damage in distant tissues may be caused by reason of the fact that the causal bacteria secrete a highly poisonous exotoxin, which is absorbed into the blood stream and is transported around the body.

Diphtheria exotoxin is particularly liable to affect the heart muscle, causing a toxic **myocarditis;** and the nervous system leading to disorders such as **palatal paralysis** (paralysis of the muscles of the soft palate); **ciliary paralysis** (paralysis of ciliary muscles, the muscles of the eye responsible for visual accommodation); **respiratory paralysis** and **peripheral neuritis** (a condition in which nerve damage causes various forms of sensory disturbance and weakness of motor muscles in the limbs). Peripheral neuritis is also referred to as **polyneuritis** or **peripheral neuropathy.**

The incubation period of diphtheria is 2 to 8 days. Treatment is with diphtheria antitoxin and penicillin.

Active immunization comprises vaccination with some form of diphtheria toxoid (i.e. toxin modified so as to render it harmless but retaining its antigenic properties), e.g. A.P.T., T.A.F. The toxoid may be incorporated in "triple vaccine", as noted when discussing whooping cough.

As a result of widespread active immunization, diphtheria is now very uncommon in the U.K. A skin test, called the **Schick test,** is employed to investigate the presence or absence of immunity to the disease.

SCARLET FEVER (SCARLATINA)

This is due to a variety of *streptococcus*, which differs from other types of streptococci, in that it secretes an exotoxin which produces the scarlet rash that gives this fever its name.

The incubation period is about 1 to 8 days. Treatment is with penicillin and complications during the course of the disease are uncommon. Acute nephritis or rheumatic fever may occur following an attack of scarlet fever and it is thought they may be due to a state of hypersensitivity, resulting from the streptococcal infection.

Scarlet fever may also be classified as a pyogenic infection (see later).

TYPHOID AND PARATYPHOID FEVERS (ENTERIC FEVERS).

"Typhoid" means "resembling typhus". "Typhus" means "a stupor" and both typhus fever (see p. 57) and typhoid fever are severe infections which may result in a stuporose or comatose condition of the patient.

The paratyphoid fevers A, B, and C, run a similar but generally milder course than typhoid fever. Together with typhoid, they constitute the **enteric fevers;** enteritis (i.e. inflammatory changes in the bowel) being a prominent feature in all these conditions, which are due to bacterial infection with intestinal pathogens known as *salmonellae*.

These fevers are spread by water, or food, which contains the causal bacteria as a result of contamination by the excreta of either patients suffering from the disease, or of "healthy carriers". The latter are individuals who have apparently recovered from an attack of the disease but continue thereafter, often for many years, to excrete typhoid or paratyphoid bacilli in their urine or faeces.

The main features of typhoid fever are initially a septicaemia (a condition in which the causal pathogens are present and multiplying in the blood stream); a fever producing a characteristic "step-ladder" temperature chart; a scanty rash consisting of "rose-spots"; diarrhoea with so-called "pea-soup" stools, commencing during the second week of the disease; and the development of a stuporose state.

Blood culture (i.e. the growing of any pathogens present in the blood on suitable bacteriological media) during the earliest stages of the infection, and, subsequently, performance of a test on the blood called the **Widal test** are important diagnostic investigations in enteric fevers.

The incubation period of this group of fevers is about 7 to 14 days.

Complications due to the enteritis are haemorrhage from ulcers in the small intestine and perforation of this part of the bowel. Other complications include cholecystitis (inflammation of the gall bladder).

An antibiotic called chloramphenicol is often of great value in treatment. Cases must be nursed with "barrier" precautions.

Active immunization with **T.A.B.C. vaccine** is employed with the object of reducing the incidence of the disease. These initials indicate the vaccine is constituted so as to produce antibodies against typhoid and paratyphoid fevers A, B, and C.

CEREBROSPINAL FEVER (MENINGOCOCCAL MENINGITIS)

This is a bacterial disease due to an organism called the *meningococcus*. The infection commences in the nasopharynx and from here the pathogens enter the blood stream causing a septicaemia. Later in most instances the infection becomes localized in the meninges, thus accounting for the alternative name of meningococcal meningitis. The disease used to be called **spotted fever,** as a purpuric rash not infrequently develops at an early stage of the disease.

Neck rigidity is an important sign of meningeal irritation due to inflammatory changes in the meninges.

The causative micro-organisms can be demonstrated by microscopy of stained films made from a sample of cerebrospinal fluid, obtained by lumbar puncture.

Complications include various paralyses of cranial nerves, broncho-pneumonia and hydrocephalus.

Treatment is by sulphonamide drugs, sometimes supplemented by penicillin.

Section B.—PYOGENIC INFECTIONS

Certain bacteria, such as the *staphylococcus, streptococcus, meningococcus, gonococcus, bacillus coli* and *bacillus proteus,* when they cause infection, provoke an inflammatory reaction which results in **suppuration,** i.e. the formation of pus. The word **pyogenic** means "producing pus" and thus infections characterized by purulent inflammatory exudates are frequently termed **pyogenic infections.** (**Purulent** means "consisting of pus").

The pathogens most commonly responsible for such infections are the staphylococcus and the streptococcus.

Two pyogenic infections, scarlet fever and meningococcal meningitis, have already been referred to as they may also be classified as infectious fevers. Gonococcal infection will be considered later when discussing terms relating to venereal diseases.

STAPHYLOCOCCAL INFECTIONS

These tend usually to take the form of localized abscesses. They may sometimes progress to **staphylococcal septicaemia** or **pyaemia,** but these latter conditions are not common.

Some important conditions caused by staphylococcal infection are:

(*a*) Skin and subcutaneous tissues: **furuncle** (a small abscess due to infection in a hair follicle or sweat gland known more widely as a **boil**); **carbuncle** (a condition akin to a boil but larger, consisting of a number of adjacent abscesses cavities within a localized area of inflammation); **paronychia** (infection of the tissues around a finger-nail, known also as a **whitlow**); **pulp infection of a finger; wound infections,** including also wounds involving other tissues besides the skin and subcutaneous tissues (a **wound** is a gap in an external or internal body surface caused by injury).

(*b*) Bone—**staphylococcal osteomyelitis** (inflammation of bone).

(*c*) Lung—**staphylococcal pneumonia** (inflammation of lung tissue).

Treatment of staphylococcal infections is by antibiotic drugs. Surgical treatment may also be required to drain abscesses.

STREPTOCOCCAL INFECTIONS

In contradistinction to staphylococci, streptococci tend to produce diffuse spreading inflammatory lesions.

Involvement of draining lymph vessels and glands, causing respectively **lymphangitis** and **lymphadenitis,** is not uncommon, and spread to the blood causing **streptococcal septicaemia** occasionally occurs.

Some important conditions caused by streptococci are:

(*a*) Skin and subcutaneous tissues—a spreading infection called **cellulitis,** the name meaning inflammation of cellular tissue.

A severe form of cellulitis is seen in the streptococcal infection called **erysipelas,** a term meaning " redness of the skin". (In olden days erysipelas was known as "St. Anthony's Fire").

(*b*) Pharynx—**streptococcal tonsillitis.** Infection of the throat with a certain type of streptococcus causes **scarlet fever** (see p. 49).

(*c*) Ear—**otitis media** (inflammation of the middle ear).

(*d*) Bone—streptococcal **osteomyelitis** (inflammation of bone).

(*e*) Heart—**subacute bacterial endocarditis** (see p. 70).

It is also considered by many authorities that the disease called **rheumatic fever,** and certain types of the kidney disorder called **nephritis** are manifestations of a state of hypersensitivity produced as a direct result of streptococcal infection in the tonsils or elsewhere in the pharynx.

(*f*) Female genital tract—**puerperal sepsis** (see p. 188).

Streptococcal infections are treated by antibiotics, and in some instances also by surgery.

Section C.—TUBERCULOSIS

The basic lesions in this disease are small nodules of chronic inflammatory tissue, which develop at sites where the invading pathogens establish themselves. These nodules are termed **tubercles** and the causative micro-organisms, which belong to a class of bacteria called acid-fast bacilli, are called *tubercle bacilli,* or alternatively *Koch's bacilli,* after Robert Koch, the famous German bacteriologist.

Tuberculosis means a condition in which tubercles are present.

A first infection with the disease constitutes **primary tuberculosis,** and the majority of individuals who live in civilized communities contract such an infection but, in most instances, in so mild a form that no recognizable ill-effects ensue. Common sites of primary tuberculosis are in the respiratory and alimentary tracts and their draining lymph glands. In subsequent years, sites of former lesions may be rendered apparent by small areas of pathological calcification in the lung and hilar lymph glands, or in lymph glands in the neck or mesentery.

Infection may be (i) with *"human type"* tubercle bacilli derived from inhalation of air, or ingestion of food, contaminated from the sputum of another human being with active tuberculosis, or (ii) with *"bovine type"* tubercle bacilli found in milk and milk products obtained from infected cattle.

The initial infective process, once it has subsided, gives the affected individual a varying degree of immunity against further tuberculous infection. Sometimes, however, primary tuberculosis may cause clinical signs and symptoms of some severity and also may produce **metastatic tuberculous infections.** These latter, result from tubercle bacilli entering the blood stream, or lymphatic channels, and thus being carried to distant organs and tissues where they produce secondary or (metastatic) infective lesions.

(*Note:* The word **metastasis** (plural: metastases) indicates a secondary lesion of a disease, occurring in a site at a distance from the first or primary centre of disease. Whilst it is used with reference to various infective disorders, this term finds its widest use in relation to malignant disorders).

Metastatic tuberculosis may supervene during the active stage of primary tuberculosis but occurs much more frequently as a result of reactivation of *tubercle bacilli,* which have been lying dormant in an apparently healed primary focus of infection. It is found in sites such as the lungs, bones and joints, kidneys, uterine tubes, peritoneum, meninges, etc., and, when tubercle bacilli are able to enter the blood stream in large numbers, it may occur in a generalized form called **miliary tuberculosis,** with disseminate lesions in many different organs.

In addition to reactivation of an old tuberculous focus, infection occurring subsequent to primary tuberculosis may result from re-infection, with *tubercle bacilli,* from a source outside the body. It is believed that re-infection may be a cause of the condition termed **post-primary pulmonary tuberculosis,** particularly in older subjects (see p. 95), but that this type of infection is more commonly due to reactivation of a former tuberculous lesion.

Metastatic tuberculosis infection and tuberculosis due to re-infection may both be described as forms of **secondary tuberculosis.**

Post-primary pulmonary tuberculosis can also produce metastatic tuberculous lesions through spread of bacilli by the blood and lymphatics. Extension of this type of disease, however, occurs more commonly through direct spread, in the sputum, of the *tubercle bacilli* to other sites, in the respiratory system and also the digestive system. This type of spread may cause complications such as tuberculous broncho-pneumonia, tracheo-bronchial tuberculosis, tuberculous laryngitis, intestinal tuberculosis, and tuberculous infection in the region of the anus. This latter is associated with fistula formation resulting in a condition known as **fistula-in-ano.**

(*Note:* tuberculosis is only one of a number of causes of fistula-in-ano).

Susceptibility to tuberculosis infection may be investigated by **tuberculin testing.** In this procedure a substance obtained from tubercle bacilli, and called tuberculin, is injected into the skin by intradermal injection as in the **Mantoux test,** or by a mechanical device making multiple minute punctures as in the **Heaf test.**

Negative reactors to tuberculin tests may be actively immunized by injection of an attenuated (weakened) strain of tubercle bacillus called the **Bacillus Calmette-Guérin.** This procedure is generally termed **B.C.G. vaccination.**

Measures to raise the general resistance to infection such as adequate rest, adequate diet and fresh air, are important in the treatment of tuberculosis. Chemotherapy with **antituberculosis drugs** such as streptomycin, isoniazid and P.A.S. (para-aminosalicylic acid) is extensively employed and surgery is required in some types of lesion.

Section D.—VENEREAL DISEASES

The word **venereal** derives from the Latin word meaning "love" and indicates that the commonest mode of transmission of these infective diseases is by sexual intercourse.

The two most important members of this group of disorders are called syphilis and gonorrhoea.

1. SYPHILIS

This infection may be congenital (due to infection of a foetus in-utero from the maternal blood-stream) or acquired and is due to a spirochaete (a type of bacterium) called *Treponema pallidum.*

ACQUIRED SYPHILIS

This disease is first manifested in the form of a primary stage. Subsequently other stages of infection may develop if it is untreated or inadequately treated. The various stages of acquired syphilis are described as:

(*a*) **Primary syphilis**—characterized by the development of a **primary sore,** or **chancre,** which is usually on the genital organs. It appears about a month after the infection is contracted.

(*b*) **Secondary syphilis**—appears about six weeks after the development of the primary sore. At this stage, dissemination of spirochaetes, by the blood stream, has resulted in generalized infection of the body tissues. Common manifestations are skin rashes, sore throat, pain in bones, etc. Sometimes localized nodular thickenings develop on bony surfaces. These are called **periosteal nodes** and can be demonstrated radiologically.

(*c*) **Latent syphilis**—a stage after healing of the secondary lesions, in which there are no clinical signs and symptoms of active disease. This stage may last many years.

(*d*) **Tertiary syphilis**—in this stage, lesions which are confined to a particular organ or tissue are often seen. The lesions are of many types: among them are swellings called **gummas,** syphilitic **osteitis** (inflammation of bone), syphilitic disease of the heart and aorta, manifestations of **neurosyphilis** (i.e. syphilitic infection of the nervous system) called **meningo-vascular syphilis.**

(*e*) **Quaternary syphilis**—two types of neurosyphilis may occur at this stage, namely, **tabes dorsalis** (locomotor ataxia) and **general paralysis of the insane** (dementia paralytica).

CONGENITAL SYPHILIS

A pregnant woman, who has syphilis in either active or latent form, can transmit the infection to her unborn child. This may result in either abortion, stillbirth, or the birth of a living child, whose tissues are widely infected with spirochaetes.

Thus, in congenital syphilis, there is no primary stage, and the manifestations of the disease are usually referred to as early and late.

Signs of **early congenital syphilis** usually begin to appear during the early weeks of life, e.g. loss of weight; inflammation of bone and cartilage around the nasal cavities causing a condition known by the descriptive name of **"snuffles",** inflammatory lesions in bone, fissures around the mouth, skin rashes.

In **late congenital syphilis** infection of bone is also common, as are inflammatory changes in the cornea of the eye, known as **interstitial keratitis,** and other eye lesions. Neurosyphilitic lesions may also occur. The permanent teeth may be deformed and the incisors may be of a type called **Hutchinson's teeth.**

THE WASSERMANN (W.R.) AND KAHN TESTS

These are tests which may be employed on samples of blood or cerebrospinal fluid to indicate the presence of syphilis.

Other tests used in the diagnosis of this condition are known as the **V.D.R.L.** (Venereal Disease Research Laboratory) and the **T.P.I.** (Treponema Pallidum Immobilisation) **tests.**

The treatment of syphilitic infection is principally by penicillin.

2. GONORRHOEA

In males, the initial result of this infection is an acute inflammation of the urethra with consequent production of a purulent urethral discharge. It is from this discharge that the name of the disease derives; 'gonorrhoea' meaning "a flowing of seminal fluid" although, in reality, the flow is of pus formed in the urethra.

Infection is due to a bacterium called the *gonococcus*, or alternatively the *neisseria gonorrhoeae*, and gonorrhoea is thus sometimes referred to as **neisserian infection.**

In females the disease usually begins as a urethritis (inflammation of the urethra) or cervicitis (inflammation of the cervix of the uterus).

Direct spread of pathogens along the genital tract to the prostate gland in the male, or the uterine tubes in the female, may cause respectively **prostatitis** (inflammation of the prostate gland) or **salpingitis** (inflammation of the uterine tubes).

Gonococci rarely spread by the blood stream but, if they do so, may cause metastatic inflammatory lesions in other structures such as **iritis** (inflammation of the iris diaphragm of the eye), **arthritis** (inflammation of joints), **bursitis** (inflammation of bursae), and **fasciitis** (inflammation of fasciae).

In males the urethritis may sometimes result in a localized area of narrowing in the urethra, called a **urethral stricture.**

Infants born to infected mothers may show evidence of an eye infection, called **ophthalmia neonatorum** about three days after birth. This condition, whose name means "eye inflammation of the newly born" can be due to organisms other than the gonococcus, e.g. staphylococcus. It can lead to blindness in the more severe types of case.

The treatment of gonorrhoea is primarily by penicillin, but other drugs may be required when the causative organisms belong to strains which do not exhibit a normal susceptibility to the action of this antibiotic, and are thus termed "penicillin-resistant".

3. OTHER VENEREAL DISEASES

The principal of these are:

(*a*) **Non-specific urethritis**—a disease of males which nowadays has a greater incidence in Britain than gonorrhoea. It occasionally occurs together with symptoms of conjunctivitis and arthritis in so-called **Reiter's syndrome.**

(*Note :* A **syndrome** is a combination of a number of symptoms which occur together).

(*b*) **Chancroid** (Soft sore)—due to *Ducrey's bacillus.*

(*c*) **Lymphogranuloma Venereum** (L.G.V.), also known as **lymphogranuloma inguinale**—a tropical infection due to a virus.

Section E.—SOME OTHER INFECTIVE DISEASES

Tetanus, typhus fever, actinomycosis, glandular fever and Weil's disease will be discussed briefly in this section. Coryza and influenza and certain other virus infections will be referred to when discussing infections of the respiratory tract. Infections which occur chiefly in tropical climates will be discussed in Part V.

TETANUS (LOCKJAW)

This disease is due to a bacterium, called the *clostridium tetani*, which lives normally in the intestines of horses and sheep. Infection is caused by soil, contaminated by the excreta of such animals, entering wounds. Such contamination is common in cultivated ground and in road dust. Active immunization with tetanus toxoid alone, or in the form of "triple vaccine" is a highly efficient method of prophylaxis.

Whilst tetanus produces a localized type of infection in a wound, the causal pathogens secrete a powerful exotoxin which spread both locally and to the central nervous system, producing muscle spasms and rigidity. The former usually commence in the muscles of mastication (eating). Spasm of these muscles is called **trismus** and results in inability to open the mouth; thus explaining the term '**lockjaw**' which is also used to describe the disease. The word "tetanus" is derived from a Greek word meaning "to stretch".

The onset of trismus is followed, after a varying interval, by the appearance of generalized muscle spasms which not infrequently result in death of the patient from exhaustion or cardiac failure, or complicating pneumonia.

Antitoxin and sedatives and muscle relaxants are employed in treatment and highly skilled nursing is of prime importance.

TYPHUS FEVER

The word typhus means a "stupor". There are various forms of typhus fever, such as **epidemic typhus** (transmitted by lice), **endemic typhus** (transmitted by rat fleas), and **scrub typhus** (transmitted by small parasitic insects of the variety called mites).

The most important of these is epidemic typhus, an acute and sometimes fatal fever, which tends to appear in epidemic form during wars and times of famine.

An **endemic disease** is one which characteristically occurs more or less constantly in a particular region or locality. Endemic typhus tends to remain confined to certain regions in the tropics, and subtropics, and does not show the widespread incidence which can develop in epidemic typhus, when conditions are suitable for the spread of this latter disease.

The above-mentioned forms of typhus are all caused by various types of rickettsiae (see p. 33). A number of other febrile rickettsial infections are often described as being members of the so-called typhus group of fevers, e.g. **Q fever, Rocky Mountain spotted fever, trench fever.**

In epidemic, endemic and scrub typhus, the diagnosis may be confirmed by a blood test for anti-rickettsial antibodies, called the **Weil-Felix reaction.**

ACTINOMYCOSIS

A **mycosis** is a disease caused by fungi. Actinomycosis is caused by a microbe called the **actinomyces bovis,** or **ray fungus.**

Infection with this organism leads to chronic inflammatory lesions in the tissues. The common sites for primary infection are the face and jaws, the intestine and the lung. Metastatic spread of the disease is not uncommon.

Pulmonary actinomycosis may be either primary or metastatic. Extension of disease to the chest wall and erosion of ribs are sometimes seen as complications of the lung lesions.

The ileo-caecal region is a common site for intestinal actinomycosis, and the early signs and symptoms of this condition may be confused with those of appendicitis.

The formation of small abscess cavities and multiple sinuses is a frequent feature of actinomycotic lesions. Actinomycotic pus contains characteristic small granules known as **sulphur granules** on account of their yellow colour.

WEIL'S DISEASE

A disease due to a spirochaete called the *leptospira icterohaemor-*

rhiae. As indicated by the name of this pathogen, jaundice (icterus) and haemorrhages into mucous membranes are prominent clinical features in the majority of cases. Kidney damage also frequently occurs and may lead to renal failure.

Infection is derived from food or water, contaminated with rat's urine, or less commonly from a rat bite. The causal spirochaete is a natural parasite of rats and is of world wide distribution.

Weil's disease is uncommon in Britain. It was named after Adolf Weil, a German physician.

PART IV

Medical Terms Referring to Diseases of the Various Systems of the Body and Obstetric Terms

THE various terms indicated on p. 44 as meriting special notice with reference to infective disease, are also highly relevant to a number of the descriptions in this part of the book. Also of considerable importance herein are the following:

(a) the prefixes:

dys- difficult, e.g. dysphagia—difficulty in swallowing.

haem- blood, e.g. haemorrhage—a flow of blood.

hydro- fluid, e.g. hydrothorax—fluid in the pleural cavity.

pneumo- air (or gas), e.g. pneumothorax—air in the pleural cavity.

py- pus; e.g. pyogenic—pus-producing.

(b) the suffixes:

-ectomy, removal, e.g. gastrectomy—removal of stomach.

-itis, inflammation, e.g. gastritis, inflammation of stomach.

-oma, tumour, e.g. epithelioma, epithelial tumour.

-scopy, visual examination, e.g. gastroscopy—visual examination of the interior of the stomach by a gastroscope.

-osis, a condition of, or indicating a degenerative condition, e.g. diverticulosis, a condition of diverticula and spondylosis, a degenerative disorder of the vertebrae.

-ostomy, making an opening into, e.g. gastrostomy, making an opening into the stomach.

-otomy, making an incision into or through a structure, e.g. laparotomy—making an incision into the abdominal cavity.

(c) the word **lesion,** meaning "an injury" and widely used to indicate any form of structural damage to the body tissues, caused by disease.

(*d*) the word **lumen** describing the space in the interior of any hollow structure e.g. the lumen of the intestine, indicating the space enclosed by the intestinal wall.

Section A.—THE CARDIOVASCULAR SYSTEM

1. SOME ANATOMICAL AND PHYSIOLOGICAL CONSIDERATIONS

The **cardiovascular system** is concerned with the circulation of blood throughout the body and consists of the heart and the blood vessels.

The circulation is maintained by the pumping action of the heart muscle which pumps blood into (*a*) the *pulmonary circulation*, wherein de-oxygenated blood is re-oxygenated whilst passing through the capillaries in the lungs; and (*b*) the *systemic circulation*, wherein oxygenated blood is carried to the various organs and tissues of the body. The main arterial trunk in this circulation is the *aorta* which arises from the left ventricle. All the blood passing through the systemic circulation returns to the right side of the heart, via the *superior vena cava* or *inferior cava*, and then passes through the pulmonary circulation and is re-oxygenated.

During its course some of the blood in the systemic circulation passes through (*c*) the *portal circulation* on its return journey to the heart. The main vessel of the portal circulation is the *portal vein*, which is formed by the union of the *superior mesenteric* and *splenic veins* and carries venous blood from the small and large intestine and the spleen, to the liver. Having passed through the liver capillaries, this blood is carried by the hepatic veins to the inferior vena cava.

The heart muscle is termed the *myocardium* and is lined by a membrane, the *endocardium*, which also covers the cusps of the heart valves. On its outer aspect the myocardium is covered by the inner and outer layers of a membrane called the *pericardium*.

In early foetal life the heart consists of a single tube which subsequently becomes folded and divided into the *right atrium* and *left atrium*, separated by the *interatrial septum*, and the *right ventricle* and *left ventricle*, separated by the *interventricular septum*.

The period during which the heart muscle contracts is called *systole*, and that during which it relaxes, *diastole*. The pressure maintained in the circulation by the pumping action of the heart is called the *blood pressure* and is normally about 40-60 millimetres of mercury higher in systole than in diastole.

The pumping action of the heart results in each period of systole causing an expansile impulse throughout the arteries. This impulse may be felt in superficial arteries (e.g. the radial, femoral and carotid arteries) and is known as the *pulse*.

The prefix **card-** and the adjective **cardiac,** mean "pertaining to the heart" but are sometimes also used with reference to the cardiac orifice of the stomach.

Blood vessels comprise *arteries*, *veins* and *capillaries*. Small arteries may be termed *arterioles* and small veins described as *venules*.

Arteries and arterioles possess three coats (*a*) the *adventitia*—an outer coat composed of fibrous and elastic tissue, (*b*) the *media*—composed of smooth muscle and elastic tissue, (*c*) the *intima*—composed of endothelium lining the *lumen* (interior) of the vessel.

The prefix **angio-** means "pertaining to a vessel", **arterio-** "pertaining to an artery"; **phlebo-** and **veno-** "pertaining to a vein".

2. SOME GENERAL ASPECTS OF CARDIOVASCULAR DISEASES

Diseases of the cardiovascular system may be congenital or acquired. Of the acquired disorders; whilst traumatic, infective and rarely neoplastic diseases can affect this system, of much greater incidence are a number of other disorders, many of which are of unknown or incompletely understood causation, e.g. hypertension (high blood pressure), coronary artery disease, and other forms of atheromatous disease, rheumatic heart disease, deep vein thrombosis. Heart disease occurring as secondary effect of chronic lung disease and known as **pulmonary heart disease,** is also common.

Among the clinical symptoms and signs which may be associated with heart disease are: **dyspnoea** (difficult breathing, shortness of breath) on exertion or at rest; pain in the chest on exertion; **oedema** (swelling) around the ankles and elsewhere in the soft tissues; **cyanosis** (blueness of the skin and mucous membranes); abnormalities in the rate and rhythm of the heart; cardiac enlargement and the presence of abnormal cardiac murmurs (heart sounds).

Various signs and symptoms due to disordered blood circulation may occur in regions affected by diseases of blood vessels, sometimes with accompanying pain.

The branch of medicine concerned with diseases of the heart is called **cardiology.** Qualified technicians who work in this speciality are called **cardiological technicians** and one of their duties is the carrying out of investigations by **electrocardiography** (see later).

3. SPECIAL METHODS OF INVESTIGATION

In ordinary clinical examination, **auscultation** (listening) with a stethoscope and **estimation of the systolic and diastolic blood pressure** with a **sphygmomanometer** are very important procedures in many types of cardiovascular disease, as may also be various forms of plain radiography and certain pathological investigations. In addition, certain specialized methods of examination may be employed and among these are the following:

(*a*) **Electrocardiography**—the suffix -**graphy** is derived from the Greek word for "writing" and in this context denotes the making of a record. This procedure involves the recording of minute electrical currents produced by contractions of various parts of the heart muscle. The recording may be effected so as to produce an image that can be recorded as a tracing on a screen or on photographic paper. This procedure is of great value in the investigation of many heart disorders, e.g. coronary thrombosis, disorders of cardiac rate and rhythm, heart block, etc.

(*b*) **Cardiac catheterization**—an investigation wherein a long, thin, flexible catheter (tube) is inserted into the lumen of a fairly large superficial artery or vein (e.g. femoral or brachial artery; an ante-cubital vein, femoral vein, etc.) and manipulated, under X-ray control, so as to enter either the left or right side of the heart.

Valuable information can be obtained by recording pressures within various heart chambers and great vessels, also by withdrawing samples of blood from such sites and analyzing their oxygen content.

Abnormal openings between various chambers of the heart (called **septal defects**) may also be demonstrated by cardiac catheterization and it is frequently convenient to combine this procedure with certain forms of contrast radiography (e.g. angiocardiography, coronary arteriography), the contrast medium being injected through the catheter at the conclusion of the other investigations.

(*c*) **Angiography**—this term describes various forms of X-ray investigation whereby blood vessels are filled with radiographic contrast media and demonstrated by fluoroscopy or by the taking of radiographs. Ciné-radiography is used in a number of instances.

Among such investigations are angiocardiography, coronary-arteriography, pulmonary arteriography, aortography, cerebral arteriography, peripheral arteriography and various forms of phlebography (contrast radiography of veins; also known as venography).

(*d*) Investigations on the circulation by injection of certain dyes and **radioactive isotopes** (see p. 311) which are used as **tracer materials.**

(*e*) Performance of various tests, which determine the response of the heart to exercise, and are called **exercise tolerance tests.**

4. CONGENITAL DISEASES OF THE HEART (CONGENITAL MORBUS CORDIS)

Congenital diseases of the heart comprise a group of conditions resulting from errors of development of the heart, and the great vessels arising from it. They vary greatly in severity, ranging from small isolated defects of little clinical significance to severe multiple abnormalities, resulting in early death of the patient. Their cause is unknown, although an association has been shown, in some cases, between infection with **rubella** (German measles) in early pregnancy and the subsequent birth of an infant with congenital cardiac disease. Maternal rubella in early pregnancy may also be followed by congenital deafness and congenital cataract. (A **cataract** is an opacity of the lens of the eye.)

Congenital cardiac lesions are frequently associated with congenital defects in structures elsewhere in the body.

In a number of types of congenital heart disease, a communication exists between the two sides of the heart permitting the passage of blood from one side of this organ to the other. This is known as a **shunt.** When a patient has a **right-to-left shunt,** de-oxygenated blood is passed into the left side of the heart and thus into the systemic circulation. This results in **cyanosis,** i.e. blueness of the skin and mucous membranes, and accounts for infants with a certain type of heart disease being described as "blue-babies".

Valuable information regarding the presence and nature of a shunt may be derived from cardiac catheterization and angiocardiography.

Some of the principal types of congenital heart disease will now be indicated. It should, however, be remembered that, in many instances, congenital defects may be multiple and a combination of different lesions may be found in the same patient.

(*a*) **Fallot's Tetralogy**—Fallot was a French physician and the term **"tetralogy"** indicates that a combination of four anomalies are found in this condition. These are: (i) stenosis (narrowing) of the pulmonary artery; (ii) a defect in the interventricular septum; (iii) an aorta which, instead of arising solely from the left ventricle, "overrides" the interventricular septum and thus receives blood from the right and left ventricle, i.e. there is a right-to-left shunt; (iv) an enlarged right ventricle.

The principal clinical features are cyanosis and shortness of breath. Radiographs may show the heart resembles a boot in shape, and that there is a deficiency of vascular markings in the lungs; this latter resulting from the narrowing of the pulmonary artery.

Suitable cases are treated by surgery.

(*b*) **Isolated Pulmonary Stenosis**—a condition in which a narrowing occurs at the pulmonary valve, or just below the root of the pulmonary artery in the portion of the right ventricle called the **pulmonary conus.** There is no shunt in this condition.

Cases with this defect vary considerably in severity. It may thus cause little disability or, alternatively, it may result in severe breathlessness and progress to cardiac failure. Selected cases are treated by an operation called **pulmonary valvotomy.**

(*c*) **Patent Ductus Arteriosus**—the **ductus arteriosus** is a vessel which during foetal life, when the lungs need very little blood, carries the majority of blood from the pulmonary artery into the aorta. When respiration commences, immediately after birth, the lungs need all the blood in the pulmonary artery, and the ductus thus normally closes shortly after birth.

Failure of closure constitutes the condition of patent ductus arteriosus. After birth the pressure of blood is higher in the aorta than the pulmonary artery; thus the direction of blood flow through the ductus is reversed and the anomaly results in an excess of blood in the lungs. It is to be noted that, although there is a shunt present, it is in this instance from left to right, so there is no cyanosis.

Breathlessness on exertion is the cardinal symptom but may be delayed until adult life is reached. Patients with a patent ductus show a special liability to develop an infective cardiac disease, called **subacute bacterial endocarditis.** On this account surgery is often advised for mild cases, as well as for those who suffer from disability due to the disease.

(*d*) **Co-arctation of the Aorta**—the term **co-arctation** means a narrowing, and in this condition there is congenital stenosis in the distal part of the arch of the aorta.

As a result of this stenosis, there is a high blood pressure in the head, neck and arms, and a low blood pressure in the lower part

3

of the trunk and legs. To remedy this deficient circulation in the lower part of the body, a **collateral circulation** is developed by enlargement of **anastomoses** (communicating channels) between arteries arising above and below the narrow segment of the aorta. As a result of this, one of the clinical signs of the condition is the presence of dilated arteries over the chest and back, and on X-ray films, a characteristic notching of the ribs may be seen, resulting from enlargement of the intercostal arteries.

The degree of aortic narrowing varies considerably and in some cases there may be no symptoms until late in life. In young subjects operation may be advised, the narrow area of the aorta being resected.

A number of patients with co-arctation of the aorta die as a result of haemorrhage from small **congenital aneurysms** at the base of the brain, which frequently occur in association with this disease. An **aneurysm** is a localized dilatation of a blood vessel.

(*e*) **Atrial Septal Defect** (Auricular Septal Defect)—in this disease there is a defect in the interatrial (interauricular) septum between the two atria of the heart. There is consequently a left-to-right shunt which increases the amount of blood in the right side of the heart and in the pulmonary artery. Breathlessness is the cardinal symptom of the disease. There is no cyanosis as the shunt is from left to right.

The onset of symptoms are often delayed until adult life is reached. Treatment is surgical in suitable cases.

Atrial septal defect may be found in combination with **congenital mitral stenosis** (narrowing of the orifice of the mitral valve, which lies between the left atrium and left ventricle). The combination of these two anomalies is known as **Lutembacher's syndrome,** after the French physician, R. Lutembacher. A **syndrome** is a combination of symptoms.

(*f*) **Ventricular Septal Defect**—there are two types of ventricular septal defects: (i) a small defect, which may cause an abnormal cardiac murmur, but which generally gives rise to no disability. This type is known as **"Maladie de Roger"**; (ii) a large defect in the interventricular septum, with a large left-to-right shunt. Like an interatrial septal defect this leads to an excess of blood entering the right side of the heart and pulmonary circulation. Certain types of interventricular septal defects may be closed surgically.

(*g*) **Dextrocardia**

A condition in which the apex of the heart is found on the right side (*Note:* **dextro-** means "right"). In uncomplicated cases the heart is a complete mirror image of the normal heart and the aortic knuckle is also found on the right side.

Dextrocardia is often found to be associated with a similar reverse position of the abdominal viscera, i.e. the liver lying in the left side of the abdomen, and the stomach in the right side. This is termed **transposition of the viscera.**

(*h*) **Some other types of Congenital Heart Disease.**

There are a great variety of different types of congenital disease. Some of the rarer forms are described by the following names:

Bicuspid aortic valve, congenital aortic stenosis (narrowing of aortic valve), **double aortic arch, Eisenmenger's complex, persistent truncus arteriosus** (the aorta and pulmonary artery possess a communication of varying size owing to failure in the development of the septum between them), **pulmonary atresia** (failure of development of the orifice of the pulmonary valve), **right-sided aortic arch, transposition of the great vessels** (the aorta arises from the right ventricle and the pulmonary artery from the left ventricle in this condition which is associated with septal defect), **tricuspid atresia** (failure of development of the tricuspid valve orifice between the right atrium and right ventricle).

5. INFLAMMATORY DISEASES OF THE HEART

The most important of these are **rheumatic heart disease,** an inflammatory condition whose exact cause has not been determined, and **bacterial endocarditis,** in which the inflammatory lesions develop as a result of infection.

Syphilitic aortic regurgitation is secondary to syphilitic inflammation of the aorta and will be referred to later when discussing diseases of arteries.

Inflammatory changes in the heart muscle may also develop as a complication of certain other infections (e.g. diphtheria, pyogenic infections, pneumonia, typhus, etc.) causing **myocarditis,** or in some instances a disorder referred to as **cardiomyopathy**; this latter term meaning "disease of the heart muscle". (*Note:* cardiomyopathy may be due to causes other than infection, e.g. chronic alcoholism, vitamin deficiency, etc.)

Inflammatory changes in the pericardium cause **pericarditis** and may result in the formation of a thick scanty inflammatory exudate —**dry pericarditis,** or the formation of an abundant fluid exudate—**pericardial effusion.** Among the causes of pericarditis are acute rheumatism, pyogenic infections, tuberculous infection and involvement of the pericardium by neoplastic (malignant) disease.

A sequel to pericarditis, especially to tuberculous pericarditis, may be fibrosis, contraction and pathological calcification within the pericardium; changes which impede the pumping action of the heart and constitute the disorder referred to as **chronic constrictive pericarditis.** This disorder is frequently amenable to surgical treatment.

RHEUMATIC HEART DISEASE

As stated by Duthie (1) the term **rheumatism** has been loosely applied to all conditions causing pain and stiffness in the muscles and joints.

Rheumatic heart disease, however, results from a specific type of rheumatic disorder termed **acute rheumatism** or a similar but less acute disorder called **subacute** rheumatism.

Lightwood and Brimblecombe (2) describe the term of acute rheumatism as referring to a group of conditions including **rheumatic fever** (polyarthritis), **rheumatic nodules, rheumatic carditis** (inflammation of the heart), **erythema marginatum** (a skin disease), and **chorea** (St. Vitus's dance, rheumatism of the nervous system).

The principal pathological features of acute and sub-acute rheumatism are the occurrence of foci of inflammation in the connective tissues of affected structures. These foci produce **arthritis** in the joints, **carditis** in the heart and **chorea** when they occur in the nervous system. In the majority of sites, the inflammatory changes resolve without causing permanent damage. This, however, does not occur in the heart, where serious damage often results from fibrosis. This develops during healing of the lesions and causes chronic heart disease. Moreover, as recurrent attacks of acute rheumatism are common, each new attack may cause further cardiac damage.

The cause of acute rheumatism has not been established, but many authorities regard it as a manifestation of allergy to streptococcal infection in the throat. Its chief incidence is seen in childhood.

Rest and the administration of salicylate drugs and penicillin are important treatment measures during the acute stages of the condition. Subsequently, small doses of penicillin may be given as a prophylactic against further streptococcal infection as this carries a high risk of causing recurrence of acute rheumatism.

Any type of cardiac involvement in acute and subacute rheumatism is referred to as **rheumatic carditis.** Different types of this condition may be described as **rheumatic endocarditis, myocarditis,** or **pericarditis,** according to the part of the heart principally involved. Sometimes in cases with marked involvement of the pericardium, an effusion may form between the two layers of pericardium. This is known as a **rheumatic pericardial effusion** and produces an appearance of gross cardiac enlargement on radiographs.

In the frequent instances when permanent cardiac damage follows rheumatic carditis, a number of different sequelae may develop, according to the extent and distribution of the lesions in the heart. The principal types of these are:

(*a*) **Chronic rheumatic valvular disease of the heart**—this is produced by fibrosis of the endocardial covering of the cusps of the cardiac valves. It may result in a valvular orifice becoming narrowed, i.e. in **valvular stenosis**; or, in thickened valve cusps becoming unable to close a valvular orifice properly, i.e. in **valvular incompetence.** Alternatively, there may be a combination of stenosis and incompetence. One or more valves may be affected.

The chief types of chronic valvular disease due to acute and subacute rheumatism are first, **mitral stenosis** (narrowing of the orifice of the mitral valve), and secondly, **aortic incompetence,** also known as **aortic regurgitation** (a condition in which the aortic valve cannot close properly). Much less common are **mitral incompetence, aortic stenosis** and **tricuspid valvular disease.**

Many cases of mitral stenosis are now amenable to surgical treatment; the stenosis being relieved by an operation called **mitral valvotomy.**

Radiologically, cases with chronic valvular disease frequently show alterations in the shape of the heart which differ according to the valve, or valves involved. There is often demonstrable cardiac enlargement, which, in advanced cases, may be very great. Pathological calcification in the mitral or aortic valves may sometimes be observed on fluoroscopy. In mitral stenosis the oesophagus becomes displaced by enlargement of the left auricle. This displacement is demonstrable on barium swallow.

(*b*) **Chronic myocarditis** (myocardial fibrosis) — a sequel of myocardial involvement leading to fibrosis of varying extent in the heart muscle. When the fibrosis is extensive the pumping action of the heart may be seriously impeded.

(*c*) **Adherent pericardium**—this condition is uncommon, but may be a sequel to marked involvement of the pericardium (whether resulting in an effusion, or not), in rheumatic carditis. The two layers of the pericardium become bound together, in places, by fibrous adhesions and this may seriously impede the heart's action and lead to cardiac enlargement. Pathological calcification may occur in the diseased pericardium.

(*d*) **Cardiac failure**—heart failure may occur during the active phase of rheumatic carditis or as a result of any one of its sequelae.

BACTERIAL ENDOCARDITIS

Bacterial endocarditis is a condition in which inflammatory changes occur in the endothelial coverings of the cardiac valves, as a result of direct invasion by pathogenic bacteria. It is of two types, acute and sub-acute:

(*a*) **Acute Bacterial Endocarditis.**—A rare condition in which acute endocarditis usually occurs in the course of a general septicaemia due to infection with organisms such as staphylococci, streptococci or pneumococci.

(*b*) **Subacute Bacterial Endocarditis.**—This disease is usually due to infection with a type of streptococcus called *streptococcus viridans*. This organism is found as a normal inhabitant of the upper respiratory tract. If, however, it gains access to the blood stream and invades the endocardium of the cardiac valves, it is capable of causing serious damage to these latter structures. Such damage is usually only seen in those whose heart is already abnormal as a result of, either previous rheumatic endocarditis, or congenital heart disease. The inflammatory changes result in deposits of fibrin and blood platelets on the surface of the valve cusps. Such deposits are called **vegetations.** Fragments of vegetations may become detached forming emboli in the blood stream, and these may lodge in sites such as the skin, kidneys, spleen and brain.

Among the clinical features are fever, wasting, anaemia, enlargement of the heart and spleen, abnormal cardiac murmurs and signs and symptoms due to embolism.

The diagnosis is initially made on clinical grounds but can often be confirmed bacteriologically by demonstrating the causal streptococci in a sample of blood. The test employed is called a **blood culture.**

Standard treatment is by prolonged therapy with antibiotic and anti-coagulant drugs.

6. CORONARY ARTERY DISEASE (CORONARY INSUFFICIENCY)

This disease, which appears to be of increasing prevalence, is a common cause of disability and death, especially in the male sex.

It is due to the development of atheroma (a degenerative arterial disease) in the coronary arteries, which arise from the ascending aorta and carry the blood supply of the heart muscle. The atheromatous changes produce areas of narrowing in the interiors of the arterial vessels in the coronary circulation, thus diminishing the supply of blood available to areas of the myocardium.

The term **ischaemia** has already been noted as indicating a localized deficiency of blood supply and coronary atheroma is the commonest cause of what is termed **ischaemic heart disease**; some authorities using this term and coronary artery disease as synonyms.

Clinically coronary heart disease is manifested by angina pectoris and by coronary thrombosis.

ANGINA PECTORIS (ANGINA OF EFFORT)

Angina is cardiac pain which occurs when the blood supply to the myocardium is inadequate to meet increased demands arising from some physical exertion. It usually commences in the chest but may radiate to other regions. It is characteristically relieved by rest, and an attack may be cut short by taking a tablet of drug called glyceryl trinitrate (trinitrin).

In selected cases of angina, surgical measures may be employed for relief of pain or to improve the myocardial blood supply.

True angina is sometimes mimicked by pain known as **pseudo-angina.** This latter may be caused by chronic inflammation of the oesophagus or by **Tietze's disease,** a condition in which there is a painful swelling of one or more rib cartilages.

CORONARY THROMBOSIS (CORONARY OCCLUSION, MYOCARDIAL INFARCTION, CARDIAC INFARCTION)

The pathology of this form of coronary artery disease is largely explained by its several alternative names, given above. Sudden occlusion (blockage) of a coronary artery by the formation of a thrombus (clot) in an area of narrowing, produced by atheromatous change in the arterial wall, deprives an area of myocardium of its blood supply. Arterial anastomoses (communicating channels) being poorly developed in the coronary circulation, the occlusion results in the death of an area of myocardium, the dead tissues being termed a **myocardial** or **cardiac infarct.**

The severity of the condition depends on the size of the vessel which is occluded. A small infarct may produce few signs and symptoms. A large infarct may be rapidly fatal. The dead muscular tissue of a cardiac infarct is, in the course of time, removed and converted into fibrous tissue, leaving an area of permanent weakness in the wall of the heart.

Coronary thrombosis usually presents a fairly characteristic clinical picture. Electrocardiography is a valuable procedure in this condition. Usually little information is obtained by plain radiology. This latter type of investigation will, however, demonstrate one rare sequel to coronary thrombosis, namely, the development of a localized bulging of the heart wall described as a **cardiac aneurysm.**

A treatment of coronary thrombosis comprises rest, and measures to relieve the pain which is associated with this condition. In many cases drugs, called **anticoagulants,** are given in order to try and prevent further clotting of the blood.

7. HYPERTENSIVE HEART DISEASE

The term **hypertension** used with reference to the cardiovascular system, and without qualification, indicates a blood pressure greater than the normal, in the systemic circulation (cf. pulmonary hypertension and portal hypertension).

Hypertensive heart disease is a disease of the heart, resulting from the increased load on the heart arising from the presence of a sustained high blood pressure.

Hypertension is, in the vast majority of cases, of unknown origin and usually of the type termed **essential hypertension,** the word "essential" indicating that it is a primary condition and not secondary to any known cause (cf. essential hypertrophic emphysema).

A proportion of cases of essential hypertension, in which the disease is especially severe and rapidly progressive, fall into a sub-group called **malignant hypertension.**

Hypertension, in some cases, is secondary to renal (kidney) disease and is then called **hypertension of renal origin.**

In most types of chronic hypertension there is widespread narrowing of small arterial vessels which causes increased resistance in the peripheral part of the circulation. The left ventricle, therefore, has to work harder to maintain its output against this resistance. As a result it hypertrophies and eventually areas of fibrosis may develop in the myocardium. Ultimately, the condition may progress to one of heart failure.

In the treatment of the more severe types of hypertension, drugs which lower the blood pressure and are thus known as **hypotensive**

drugs (e.g. mecamyline, guanethidine, rauwolfia, etc.) are widely employed.

It is to be noted that hypertension and coronary heart disease not infrequently co-exist in the same patient.

8. CHRONIC VALVULAR DISEASE OF THE HEART

This term is usually employed with reference to acquired disorders of the heart valve. Acute rheumatism has already been noted as a common cause of valvular disease, particularly of mitral stenosis and aortic regurgitation. Syphilitic aortitis has been indicated as causing syphilitic aortic regurgitation. The arterial disease, atheroma, which affects the coronary circulation in coronary heart disease can also affect the cusps of the aortic valve and is an important cause of aortic stenosis (narrowing of the orifice of the aortic valve).

9. DISTURBANCES OF CARDIAC RATE AND RHYTHM (CARDIAC ARRHYTHMIAS)

In health the average normal heart rate is, in a subject at rest, taken as 72 beats a minute. The beats are regularly spaced and of equal volume.

An abnormally rapid heart rate is called **tachycardia,** and an abnormally slow rate, **bradycardia.**

Terms used to describe abnormalities of rhythm include the following:

(*a*) **Extrasystoles**—premature contractions, which in the absence of organic heart disease are not of significance.

(*b*) **Paroxysmal Tachycardia**—intermittent attacks of tachycardia which may occur without apparent cause in some instances, but in others may be associated with coronary artery disease and other serious types of organic heart disease.

(*c*) **Atrial Fibrillation** (Auricular fibrillation)—an abnormality of cardiac rhythm resulting from irregular and intermittent very rapid contractions of muscle fibres in the atrial walls. The ventricles, as a result, also contract irregularly and often at an increased rate.

Atrial fibrillation is a common complication of rheumatic mitral stenosis and of heart disease associated with over-activity of the thyroid gland. It is frequently a precursor of heart failure.

The drug digitalis is extensively used in the treatment of fibrillation. Another drug called quinidine may be employed in selected cases.

(*d*) **Heart block**—contractile impulses in the heart commence in a structure called the *sino-atrial* node (the pacemaker of the heart), pass through the atrial walls to the *atrio-ventricular* node and are conducted to the walls of the ventricles via the *atrio-ventricular* bundle of His. Involvement of this latter structure, by various forms of disease processes (e.g. coronary artery disease, rheumatic heart disease) may cause partial or complete, temporary or permanent, interruption of the conduction of contractile impulses producing various degrees of the condition described as heart block. In **complete heart block** the contraction of the ventricles is quite independent of that of the atria.

Heart block is frequently complicated by periodic attacks of loss of consciousness called **Stokes-Adams attacks.** One method of treating patients with such attacks is by some form of battery-operated **cardiac pacemaker,** which has one of its electrodes either passed into the cavity of the right ventricle, or attached to the outer surface of the heart and thus paces the heart beat artificially.

10. CHRONIC PULMONARY HEART DISEASE

This type of heart disease is also referred as **cor pulmonale,** and is defined by Turner (3) as "right-sided heart disease secondary to disease of the lungs or pulmonary vessels".

It occurs when the right ventricle has to work against an increased resistance in the pulmonary circulation, such as may develop in a common lung disorder called emphysema, in various types of pulmonary fibrosis, and as a result of severe chronic bronchitis.

Patients with cor pulmonale ultimately develop right ventricular failure.

11. PULMONARY HYPERTENSION

This is a condition of raised blood pressure in the pulmonary circulation. It may be due to a variety of causes including certain types of heart disease and certain disorders in the lungs which obstruct the flow of blood through the pulmonary vessels (e.g. multiple pulmonary emboli, extensive pulmonary fibrosis). Typical changes in the pulmonary arteries may be demonstrable on radiographs.

12. THYROTOXIC HEART DISEASE

This term describes heart disease secondary to hyperthyroidism (thyrotoxicosis), i.e. overactivity of the thyroid gland. The disorder of cardiac rhythm called atrial fibrillation is common in this type of heart condition.

13. HEART FAILURE (CARDIAC FAILURE)

Heart failure is a condition that occurs when, as a result of disease, the heart can no longer pump out blood in amounts adequate to maintain the circulation. It may be of sudden or slow onset. According to its cause and severity it may prove rapidly or eventually fatal; or, alternatively, it may slowly recover. It should not be confused with **cardiac arrest,** a condition of complete cessation of the contractions of the heart muscle, which is fatal unless the heart beat can be restarted within a short period.

Heart failure usually develops in the first instance in one other ventricle and then, unless relieved, eventually involves the opposite ventricle also.

(*a*) **Left Ventricular Failure**

In this type, as a result of diseases which impose an undue strain on the left ventricle (e.g. hypertensive heart disease, a proportion of cases of coronary heart disease, aortic incompetence, co-arctation of the aorta, etc.), this structure dilates and blood accumulates in the pulmonary circulation. The lungs become congested and fluid may leak out of the pulmonary capillaries into the lungs causing **pulmonary oedema.** The patient is short of breath and often suffers from paroxysms of difficulty in breathing. These latter are called **cardiac asthma** on account of a superficial resemblance to attacks of bronchial asthma.

Fluid in the pleural cavity may also be found. This is termed a **hydrothorax,** and can be a feature of either left or right-sided ventricular failure.

In left ventricular failure the right ventricle has to work against an increased pressure of blood in the pulmonary circulation. If left ventricular failure is not relieved, it will therefore eventually result in super-added right ventricular failure.

(*b*) **Right Ventricular Failure**

This type of failure, as noted above, may be a sequel to left ventricular failure. It is also caused by diseases of the heart and lungs which impose an undue strain on the right ventricle [e.g. mitral stenosis; certain types of coronary and congenital heart disease; and diseases of the lungs, such as emphysema (see p. 97), which increase the resistance to the flow of blood through the pulmonary circulation]. When the right ventricle fails blood accumulates in the veins and capillaries of the systemic circulation. This results in cyanosis, oedema and enlargement of the liver. Effusion of fluid into the pleural and peritoneal cavities occurs in some cases. Pulmonary congestion is seen in certain types of right ventricular failure, e.g. when due to mitral stenosis. This causes shortness of breath and may be associated with haemoptysis.

The abnormality of the rhythm of the heart beat called **atrial fibrillation** is of frequent occurrence in right ventricular failure.

X-ray films are of value in cases of cardiac failure to demonstrate the size of the heart and state of the lung vessels. Pleural effusions may be demonstrated when present, and pulmonary oedema may produce X-ray signs.

Rest, the administration of a low salt diet, sedation and the administration of digitalis, are basic forms of treatment in heart failure. Drugs which increase the flow of urine and are thus called **diuretics** are employed to reduce oedema. Oxygen is given to patients with cyanosis and dyspnoea.

14. CARDIAC ARREST

This term describes the cessation of the pumping action of the heart and consequent halting of the circulation of blood through the blood vessels. It is accompanied by cessation of respiration and is thus frequently referred to as **cardio-respiratory arrest.**

The condition may be due to a variety of causes among which are diseases of the cardiovascular and respiratory systems (e.g. coronary thrombosis, pulmonary embolism, etc.), head injuries and chest injuries.

Clinically, cardiac arrest is evidenced by unconsciousness, absent pulses, absence of respiration and dilated pupils.

Persistence of the condition for more than about three minutes may lead to serious and permanent brain damage, the brain tissues being particularly sensitive to deprivation of a normal supply of oxygenated blood.

To be effective, resuscitation measures must therefore be instituted without any delay. Immediate measures comprise external cardiac compression (external cardiac massage) and artificial ventilation (artificial respiration) by the mouth-to-mouth or mouth-to-nose method. If these are not rapidly successful more complex procedures are required. These may involve internal cardiac compression (internal cardiac massage), intubation of the trachea, and intravenous or intracardiac injection of various drugs.

In patients who are shown by electrocardiography to exhibit abnormal contractions of the ventricles of the heart of a type called **ventricular fibrillation,** a procedure called **defibrillation** is required to restore normal cardiac rhythm. This involves the momentary passage through the heart of a high voltage electric current.

15. SOME TERMS USED WITH REFERENCE TO CARDIAC SURGERY

(*a*) **Hypothermia**—the use of this term in connection with cardiac surgery indicates a number of methods used in association with general anaesthesia, to obtain an appreciable lowering of body temperature. By such means the oxygen needs of the body are reduced, making it possible for the circulation to be arrested for a short period of time, during which cardiac surgery of short duration may be carried out. The word hypothermia means "low temperature".

(*b*) **Cardio-pulmonary By-pass** (Heart-lung machine).—A machine whereby the blood is drawn off the venous side of the systemic circulation, oxygenated and pumped back into the arterial side; the heart and lungs being by-passed. It is used for cardiac operations of long duration.

(*c*) **Blalock's operation**—one type of operation employed in the treatment of Fallot's tetralogy.

(*d*) **Valvotomy**—an operation designed to enlarge a narrowed cardiac valve orifice.

(*e*) **Open and closed cardiac surgery**—open cardiac surgery comprises surgical operations on the interior of the heart performed under direct vision. Other forms of heart operation, including those on the interior of the heart by indirect methods, comprise closed cardiac surgery.

(*f*) **Cardiac Pacing**—surgical measures concerned with the introduction into the body of cardiac pacemakers (see p. 74).

(*g*) **Cardiac Transplantation**—replacement of a diseased heart by a heart taken from a donor shortly after death. The first man-to-man cardiac transplant operation was performed in the Union of South Africa in 1967.

16. DISEASES OF ARTERIES

Arterial disease may be congenital, traumatic, inflammatory or due to other and unknown causes. That with the highest incidence is called **atheroma** or **atherosclerosis.** This latter name should not be confused with **arteriosclerosis** which means "hardening of the arteries" and is a term which is applied to any form of disorder in which arterial walls become thickened and hard in texture as a result of degenerative changes.

Some important arterial disorders are:

(*a*) **Atheroma** (Atherosclerosis)—the name of this disease derives from the Greek word for "gruel", a substance to which the atheromatous lesions in affected arteries were thought to bear some resemblance.

Atheroma is a degenerative condition of unknown origin, which is extremely common in middle-aged and elderly subjects. It may also occur in young people who suffer from diabetes mellitus.

The basic features of the disease are the patchy deposition of lipoids (fatty substances) and the occurrence of areas of thickening in the intima of affected arteries. These latter accordingly develop areas of narrowing within their interiors and this diminishes their blood carrying capacity. Moreover, the presence of atheroma predisposes to occlusion of arteries as a result of thrombosis, and may also lead to a complication called **aneurysm formation.** An **aneurysm** is a localized dilatation of a vessel wall, usually formed as a result of an area of disease stretching unduly under the pressure of the blood.

Clinical manifestations resulting from diminution or deprivation of blood supply may occur in tissues supplied by atheromatous arteries.

Among the clinical disorders due to atheroma are:

(i) **Angina** and **coronary thrombosis,** both resulting from atheroma of the coronary arteries (see p. 71).

(ii) Mental changes, **cerebral thrombosis** and **cerebral haemorrhage** due to atheroma of the arteries supplying the brain.

(iii) **Peripheral vascular disease** resulting from atheroma of the limb arteries (usually those of the lower limb) and often also from atheroma of the lower part of the abdominal aorta and external iliac arteries. The chief symptoms are coldness of the limb and a type of pain in the legs called **intermittent claudication.** This resembles angina, in that it appears with exertion and is relieved by rest.

Thrombosis is a not uncommon occurrence in peripheral vascular disease. In lower limb vessels it may sometimes lead to gangrene, especially in diabetic subjects.

(iv) **Aortic stenosis**—a form of chronic valvular disease of the heart in which the aortic orifice becomes narrowed as a result of atheroma involving the valve cusps.

(v) **Renal artery stenosis** (see p. 159).

Pathological calcification is common in atheromatous lesions, frequently to an extent which renders them visible on radiographs. Various forms of angiography are employed in the investigation of clinical disorders resulting from atheroma.

There is no specific treatment for atheroma. In certain sites the continuity of an artery occluded by thrombosis, may be restored by the surgical operations of **disobliterative endarectomy** or **arterial grafting. Amputation** (i.e. cutting off a limb) is the treatment for established gangrene.

(*b*) **Syphilitic Disease of Arteries**—Syphilitic infection in the walls of the thoracic aorta is a fairly common feature of tertiary syphilis. This condition is called syphilitic aortitis. It causes dilatation of the aorta and this may lead to stretching of the aortic valve ring, resulting in an inability of the valve cusps to close completely; a condition termed **aortic incompetence,** or, alternatively, **aortic regurgitation.**

Aneurysm formation is a not uncommon complication of syphilitic aortitis.

The arteries of the central nervous system may also be the site of syphilitic inflammation in the disorder called **meningo-vascular syphilis,** another manifestation of tertiary syphilis. Arteries supplying the meninges, brain and spinal cord may be affected and various different clinical conditions produced according to the site of the inflammatory lesions.

(*c*) **Aneurysm formation**—As noted when discussing atheroma, an aneurysm is a localized dilatation of a vessel usually resulting from undue stretching of a diseased area in its wall. The commonest cause of arterial aneurysm is nowadays atheroma; although aneurysms may also be due to syphilis or trauma, and in the cerebral circulation they may be of a congenital origin.

The stretching of a diseased area in the vessel wall produces a bulge which may enlarge into a rounded or fusiform swelling, producing in the first instance a **saccular aneurysm,** and the second a **fusiform aneurysm.** Saccular and fusiform aneurysms occur both in the aorta and peripheral arteries. Angiography plays an important part in their diagnosis. Aneurysms tend to rupture causing severe and often fatal haemorrhage. Surgery is thus the treatment of choice when practicable.

Of a different type to the above aneurysms is the **dissecting aneurysm,** which originates in the thoracic aorta, but which may extend so as to involve the abdominal aorta. It is formed when a tear occurs in intima (innermost coat) of the aorta, and permits blood to seep into the media and spread along this coat. This can only occur, however, when the media itself is the subject of degenerative arterial disease called **cystic medionecrosis.** The presence of a dissecting aneurysm is characterized by a tearing pain in the chest or abdomen. Plain X-ray films, followed by angiocardiography, are important procedures in diagnosis. Treatment is surgical, whenever possible.

(*d*) **Acute Arterial Block**—this is caused by blockage of an artery by an embolus from the heart, or by rapidly developing thrombosis in an atheromatous artery. The causal embolus or thrombus may be surgically removed. In the former instance the operation is called **embolectomy.**

(*e*) **Raynaud's Syndrome**—a condition of spasm in the arteries of the fingers due to a variety of different causes, among which may be mentioned cervical ribs, and atheroma. Maurice Raynaud was a French physician of the nineteenth century.

(*f*) **Some Other Arterial Disorders**—these include conditions with the following names:

   (i) **Arterio-venous fistula**—a communication between an artery and a vein due to trauma, or of congenital origin.
  (ii) **Frostbite**—due to exposure to severe cold.
 (iii) **Chilblains, erythrocyanosis, acrocyanosis, erythromelalgia**—all of which are various forms of abnormal response to cold.
 (iv) **Buerger's disease**—(thrombo-angiitis obliterans), **polyarteritis nodosa, temporal arteritis**—terms which denote uncommon inflammatory conditions of unknown causation.

17. DISEASES OF VEINS

(*a*) **Thrombophlebitis**—this is a disorder in which inflammatory changes in the walls of veins lead to thrombosis (clot formation). It may affect the superficial or deep veins. Occasionally pus formation may occur in the clot. The condition is then referred to as a **suppurative thrombophlebitis,** and may lead to pyaemia.

Of much greater incidence is the type of thrombophlebitis called **deep vein thrombosis** or **phlebothrombosis** which occurs in veins of the pelvis and lower limbs following surgical operations or childbirth, or sometimes in varicose veins, and not infrequently results in pulmonary embolism, through detachment of a fragment of clot (see p. 100).

(*b*) **Varicose Veins**—the word **varix** means "crooked". Varicose veins are dilated venous channels which pursue a tortuous course.

They occur most commonly in the lower limbs, and in the anal canal and around the anal margin. In these latter two situations they are known as **haemorrhoids** (piles), and are an important cause of bleeding from the lower intestinal tract.

Varicose veins in the lower limbs appear to be caused by a number of factors, amongst which are congenital weakness of the vein walls and prolonged standing. Pregnancy may also be a factor in their development. The condition commonly affects the superficial circulation but the deep veins may be affected. Before commencing treatment for varicose veins, it is often necessary to demonstrate the deep venous circulation by venography (phlebography).

In a region where varicosity of the veins is of a marked degree, the circulation may be interfered with to such an extent as to impair the nutrition of the surrounding tissues. This may lead to the development of a skin disorder called **varicose dermatitis.** Ulceration, known as **varicose ulceration,** may also result, and infection of the ulcerated area may produce localized periostitis in an underlying bone.

Non-suppurative thrombophlebitis is another complication of varicose veins.

REFERENCES

(1) Duthie, J. J. R. *The Practice and Principles of Medicine* (Ed. Sir Stanley Davidson). E. and S. Livingstone, 1966.
(2) Lightwood, R. and Brimblecombe, F. S. W. *Paterson's Sick Children.* Cassell, 1963.
(3) Turner, R. W. D. *The Practice and Principles of Medicine* (Ed. Sir Stanley Davidson). E. and S. Livingstone, 1966.

Section B.—THE RESPIRATORY SYSTEM

1. SOME ANATOMICAL AND PHYSIOLOGICAL CONSIDERATIONS

The respiratory system is concerned primarily with providing the blood with oxygen from inspired air, and with the removal of carbon dioxide from the blood and excretion of this waste product in expired air. This exchange of gases is effected in the lungs. Certain organs of the system have other functions also, e.g. voice production in the larynx, olfactory function of the nose (**olfactory** means referring to the sense of smell).

The respiratory system comprises:

(*a*) **The upper respiratory system,** consisting of the *nasal cavities, nasopharynx, oropharynx* and *laryngopharynx* (structures common to both the respiratory and digestive systems) and *larynx*. The *accessory nasal sinuses* open into the nasal cavities and infection of these structures is frequently associated with other respiratory disease.

(*b*) **The lower respiratory system,** consisting of the *trachea, bronchi, lungs* and *pleurae*.

The lungs and pleurae are contained within the thoracic cavity and between them is the space called the *mediastinum*. This latter contains numerous important structures, amongst which are the following: The heart and origins of the great vessels; the greater part of the oesophagus; portions of the vagus, phrenic and left recurrent laryngeal nerves; the lower part of the trachea and the origins of the two main bronchi; the thoracic duct and numerous lymph glands and lymphatic vessels; and the thymus gland.

In a number of diseases of the lower respiratory system, associated pathological changes are found affecting structures in the mediastinum.

The right lung contains three major subdivisions known as *lobes,* and the left lung has two lobes. Each lobe is divided further into *broncho-pulmonary segments,* composed of large numbers of small structures called *lobules*. Each lobule communicates with a small bronchus and consists of a number of minute air sacs called *alveoli*.

The alveoli are surrounded by a network of connective tissue referred to as the *interstitial tissue* of the lungs.

The regions on each side where the main bronchi, and main branches of the pulmonary artery enter the lungs are known as the *hila* (singular: hilum). Situated in the hila are the *hilar lymph glands,* into which drain lymph from the lungs. Efferent vessels from these glands pass to the *mediastinal lymph glands*. Enlargement of hilar and mediastinal lymph nodes is a frequent concomitant of a number of lung diseases.

Some prefixes used with reference to the respiratory system are: **rhino-** pertaining to the nose; **laryngo-** pertaining to the larynx; **tracheo-** pertaining to the trachea; **broncho-** pertaining to a bronchus or bronchi; **pleuro-** pertaining to the pleura; and **pneumono-** pertaining to lung.

2. SOME GENERAL ASPECTS OF RESPIRATORY DISEASES

Diseases affecting the respiratory system may be congenital traumatic, infective, neoplastic, or due to a variety of other causes, or idiopathic (of unknown causation).

Among these with the highest incidence are different forms of upper respiratory tract infection, bronchitis, asthma, pleurisy, traumatic lesions of the lung, pneumonias, neoplasms of the bronchi and pleura, dust diseases of the lung, and a degenerative disorder called emphysema.

Among the clinical symptoms and signs which may be associated with respiratory disease are **rhinorrhoea** (running from the nose), **epistaxis** (bleeding from the nose) soreness of the throat, hoarseness of the voice, pain on swallowing and breathing, cough, dyspnoea, cyanosis, **haemoptysis** (coughing of blood), **stridor** (a harsh sound produced on inspiration or expiration).

Certain diseases of the respiratory system fall within the province of the oto-rhino-laryngologist (Ear, nose and throat specialist), others within that of the general physician or of the chest physician. Diseases of the lower respiratory tract that require surgical treatment are generally referred to a specialist in chest surgery termed a thoracic surgeon.

It is to be noted that a serious degree of lack of adequate oxygenation of the blood, developing either in acute or chronic form, may occur in certain lung disorders causing **respiratory failure** or **ventilatory failure.** Complete cessation of respiratory function is termed **respiratory arrest.**

The occurrence of heart disease secondary to disease of the lungs or pulmonary vessels has already been noted (see under "chronic pulmonary heart disease").

3. SPECIAL METHODS OF INVESTIGATION

(*a*) **Radiological investigation** — this is extensively used in the investigation of chest diseases. Plain films and fluoroscopy may be supplemented by methods such as (i) **tomography** (layer radiography), a method which produces radiographs of selected thin layers within the interior of the body, and blurs out the images of structures in layers other than the one selected, (ii) **bronchography**—contrast radiography of the bronchial tree, (iii) **pulmonary angiography**— contrast radiography of the blood vessels of the lungs.

(*b*) **Visual inspection with special instruments**—inspection of the interior parts of the respiratory passages by the procedures called **rhinoscopy** (nose); **pharyngoscopy** (pharynx); **laryngoscopy** (larynx); **bronchoscopy** (trachea and main bronchi).

The termination **-scopy** denotes a visual examination; and the termination **-scope,** the instrument with which such examination is performed, e.g. bronchoscopy, with a bronchoscope.

(*c*) **Examination of sputum**—by the naked eye, and by microscopic and bacteriological methods.

(*d*) **Respiratory Function Tests** — these comprise various tests designed to estimate the efficiency of the respiratory organs. They involve use of methods such as **spirometry** (i.e. estimations of volumes of inspired and expired air); **blood gas analysis** (i.e. measurements indicating amounts of oxygen and carbon dioxide in the blood); and other tests.

4. DISEASES OF THE UPPER RESPIRATORY TRACT

(*a*) Congenital Disorders

(i) **Deviation of the Nasal Septum**—in this disorder the nasal septum is bent and may cause obstruction of one or both nasal passages. It is treated surgically if it causes symptoms. Besides being due to congenital causes, this abnormality can also result from trauma.

(ii) **Choanal Atresia**—a rare disorder in which developmental failure results in blockage of one or both *choanae,* i.e. the posterior openings of the nasal cavities into the nasopharynx.

(*b*) **Traumatic Disorders**—among these may be mentioned the introduction of extraneous objects into the body, which become lodged in the nasal cavities, pharynx or larynx. Such objects are termed **foreign bodies,** and when they become immovably fixed in a certain site they are said to be **impacted.** Children not infrequently push small objects into their nasal cavities. The commonest pharyngeal foreign bodies found in adults are meat and fish bones.

(*c*) **Infective Diseases**—these provoke inflammatory reactions which, according to their sites, are termed **rhinitis, sinusitis, pharyngitis** and **laryngitis.** Among these diseases are:

(i) **Coryza** (common cold)—a virus infection causing inflammation of the mucous membranes lining the nose and nasopharynx. During the course of the infection the mucous membranes may become further infected by pathogenic bacteria, which are then referred to as **secondary invaders.** Such secondary invasion can result in spread of infection to other parts of the upper and lower respiratory tracts, and also along the Eustachian tube to the middle ear on one or both sides. Grant (1) describing such spread, gives the following complications that can occur: sinusitis, Eustacchian catarrh, otitis media (inflammation of the middle ear), laryngitis, tracheitis, bronchitis, lobular pneumonia.

The name "coryza" derives from the "running nose" which is the most prominent clinical feature of this condition.

(ii) **Influenza**—a virus infection causing fever, inflammation of the upper respiratory tract, and severe aching in the back and limbs. Secondary infection with pathogenic bacteria during the course of this disease, may cause **pneumonia** (inflammation of the lungs).

(iii) **Sinusitis**—inflammation of the accessory nasal sinuses. This occurs most frequently in the maxillary sinuses (maxillary antra) but may develop in any of the other nasal sinuses in acute or chronic form.

Infective material from diseased sinuses frequently descends into the lower respiratory tract, where it may lead to infection within the bronchi or lungs.

Sinusitis is not always due to pathogenic micro-organisms. It quite frequently occurs as an allergic manifestation and may complicate hay fever.

(iv) **Adenovirus Infections**—due to members of a group of viruses called the *adenovirus group,* which cause inflammatory conditions in the upper respiratory tract.

(v) **Enlarged Adenoids**—swellings of collections of lymphatic tissue in the nasopharynx. Such swellings develop as a result of chronic infection and are usually associated with chronic tonsillitis. If surgical treatment (adenoidectomy) is required, tonsillectomy is usually performed at the same time.

Enlarged adenoids are a common cause of mouth-breathing and may cause deafness by blocking the pharyngeal openings of the Eustachian tubes.

(vi) **Tonsillitis**—the tonsils are masses of lymphoid tissue covered by mucous membrane and lying between the pillars of the fauces in the lateral walls of the oropharynx. They are frequently the site of acute or chronic infection and in the latter instance may require surgical removal.

Streptococcal infection is a common cause of acute tonsillitis and may lead to serious complications in the form of the subsequent development of acute nephritis or acute rheumatism. Streptococcal tonsillitis is sometimes difficult to differentiate from faucial diphtheria.

Scarlet fever is a manifestation of a special type of streptococcal tonsillitis.

Acute infection of the tonsils may sometimes lead to the formation of a **peritonsillar abscess** commonly known as a **quinsy,** characterized by a large swelling of the soft palate on the affected side, difficulty in swallowing and severe pain in the throat.

(vii) **Laryngitis**—the word denotes inflammation of the larynx.

Acute laryngitis is frequently of infective origin but may result from other causes, e.g. inhalation of irritant fumes. **Chronic laryngitis** is sometimes due to a tuberculous or syphilitic infection but develops much more often as a result of causes such as excessive use of the voice, heavy tobacco smoking, etc.

Hoarseness and loss of voice are prominent features in both acute and chronic laryngitis.

(viii) **Retropharyngeal Abscess**—the prefix **retro-** means "behind" and the term describes an abscess in the soft tissues behind the pharynx. It usually occurs in infancy as a result of infection of retropharyngeal lymph glands consequent upon a throat infection.

(*d*) **Neoplasms**—these may occur in any part of the upper respiratory tract. They include the following:

(i) **Benign**—the most common of these is a tumour called a **papilloma of the vocal cords,** which arises from mucous membrane covering the cords. It causes hoarseness of the voice, and if it attains a large size, may also cause dyspnoea.

(*Note:* The localised soft tissue swellings found in the nose, and called **nasal polypi** are regarded as tissue overgrowths and are not considered to be truly neoplastic in nature.)

(ii) **Malignant**—**carcinomas** of the **maxillary antrum, ethmoid cells, pharynx** and **larynx.** Carcinomatous growths arising from the vocal cords, or elsewhere within the larynx, are often described as **intrinsic laryngeal carcinomas.** In contradistinction, carcinomas which arise around the upper margins of the larynx, e.g. in sites such as the epiglottis, are sometimes referred to as **extrinsic laryngeal carcinomas,** although many authorities classify them as pharyngeal carcinomas.

A high degree of malignancy is a usual feature in malignant tumours of the nasopharynx, some of which are carcinomas, whilst others belong to the other great class of malignant tumours termed sarcomas, e.g. **nasopharyngeal lymphosarcoma.**

(*e*) **Other Diseases**

Hay Fever—an allergic disorder of the upper respiratory tract, so called because it is produced as a result of hypersensitivity to various types of pollen, the majority of which are grass pollens.

The principal clinical features are rhinorrhoea (running from the nose) and conjunctivitis.

Allied to hay fever, but resulting from sensitivity to other substances, is another allergic disorder called **perennial rhinorrhoea,** or **perennial rhinitis.**

5. DISEASES OF THE TRACHEA

The only common disease of the trachea is an acute inflammatory disorder called **acute tracheitis.** This may accompany various inflammations of the upper respiratory tract. It also not infrequently occurs in association with acute bronchitis when the condition is described as **acute tracheo-bronchitis.**

6. DISEASES OF THE BRONCHI

(*a*) **Bronchitis**—this term denotes the presence of inflammatory changes in the mucous membrane lining the bronchi. The description **bronchiolitis** is applied to inflammation of the smallest branches of the bronchial tree which are known as **bronchioles.**

(i) **Acute Bronchitis**—this is usually due to infection but can develop as a result of exposure to irritating dust and gases. Common clinical features are cough, fever and a tight feeling in the chest. The disease frequently follows an infection of the upper respiratory tract and may progress to broncho-pneumonia. Measles and whooping cough are common causes of acute bronchitis in childhood.

(ii) **Chronic Bronchitis**—is an extremely common disease in middle and old age. It may be a sequel to acute bronchitis or may be chronic in type from the start. In many instances there is no apparent cause, but in others factors such as exposure to fumes and dust, tobacco smoking and chronic sinusitis appear to play some part.

The chief symptoms are cough and **expectoration** (spitting) and, in advanced cases, shortness of breath. In early cases symptoms often disappear in the summer, but recur each winter. Many sufferers from chronic bronchitis develop a lung disorder called **emphysema** (see later).

Attacks of acute bronchitis and bronchopneumonia are frequent complications of chronic bronchitis and the disease may eventually lead to respiratory failure and to pulmonary heart disease.

(*b*) **Bronchiectasis**—the name of this disorder signifies the presence of abnormally dilated bronchi, or bronchioles, in the lungs; the ending-**ectasis** indicating a state of widening or expansion.

Such dilatation of bronchi is very liable to develop in areas of lung which, as a result of bronchial obstruction, becomes the site of persistent collapse. This latter condition is described in more detail on p. 91.

Among the many causes of bronchial obstruction, those associated with the subsequent development of bronchiectasis include inflammatory exudates and plugs of mucus in acute pulmonary infections; pressure from enlarged tuberculous glands, pulmonary fibrosis, and bronchial carcinomas.

Abnormal strain on bronchial walls in collapsed areas of lung; distension of the bronchi beyond an obstruction by infective secretions; and weakening of bronchial walls as a result of infective processes, have all been postulated as factors in the development of different varieties of bronchiectasis.

Bronchial dilatation may be reversible, in its early stages, if the bronchial obstruction responsible for its development can be effectively relieved.

The main clinical feature of bronchiectasis is the coughing up of purulent sputum. Haemoptysis is fairly common and the fingers often show an abnormality called **clubbing**, i.e. they show expansion of their ends and abnormal curvature of the nails. Clubbed fingers also occur in a number of other lung diseases and in certain heart disorders.

The presence of bronchiectasis is proved by demonstration of dilated bronchi by bronchography (contrast radiography of the bronchial tree).

Surgical removal of portions of lung affected by bronchiectasis is carried out in younger subjects, when the disease is localized.

(*c*) **Bronchial Asthma**—this disease is usually referred to as **asthma;** its name indicating the gasping for breath, which is the most prominent clinical feature and results from spasm of plain muscle in the walls of the smaller bronchi. (See also "cardiac asthma", p. 75).

The disorder is frequently familial (i.e. occurring in members of the same family) and often first appears in childhood. It is often associated with chronic bronchitis and the development of emphysema.

The cause is often obscure and factors which may operate in different cases include hypersensitivity (allergy) to various substances (e.g. dusts, pollens, face powders, eggs, milk, certain drugs, etc.); psychological disturbances and bronchial infection.

Sufferers from asthma are not infrequently subject to other allergic disorders such as hay fever and eczema. Asthmatic attacks are usually of fairly short duration. Rarely, however, a single attack may persist for longer than twenty-four hours, producing a condition termed **status asthmaticus.**

The combination of asthma and chronic bronchitis is sometimes referred to as **chronic asthmatic bronchitis.**

Attacks may be relieved by adrenalin, given by injection or inhalation, and when severe by aminophylline or steroids. When hypersensitivity to a known agent appears to be a factor, an attempt may be made to counteract this by a process called **desensitisation.**

Breathing exercises are of considerable value to asthmatic subjects.

(*d*) **Bronchial Neoplasms**—bronchial adenoma and bronchial carcinoma are discussed later (see p. 101).

7. DISEASES OF THE PLEURA

The majority of diseases of the pleura are secondary to disease in the lungs, or elsewhere in the body. Primary disorders of the pleura are uncommon.

(*a*) **Pleural effusion**—the term **effusion,** indicates an exudate of fluid from blood capillaries. In this condition the fluid collects in the space between the parietal and visceral layers of the pleura, i.e. in the pleural cavity.

Effusion into the pleural cavity may result from inflammation or malignant deposits in the pleura; or from transudation of fluid in conditions which cause oedema, such as heart failure and nephritis (inflammation of the kidneys). Bleeding into the pleura may occur as a result of injury to the thorax.

The presence of fluid in the pleural cavity is also indicated by the term **hydrothorax.** When the fluid is blood the condition is called a **haemothorax;** and when it is pus, a **pyothorax,** or, more commonly an **empyema.** A **hydropneumothorax** is a mixture of fluid and air within the pleural space; air or other gas within this space constituting a **pneumothorax.**

(*b*) **Pleurisy** (Pleuritis)—a condition of inflammation of the pleura, resulting from either infection or trauma, and producing an inflammatory exudate in the pleural cavity.

The exudate may be scanty and of thick consistency, when the condition is described as being one of **dry pleurisy;** or of fluid consistency when **pleurisy with effusion,** or **pleural effusion,** is said to be present. A dry pleurisy may develop into a pleural effusion. If a pleurisy is due to infection with pus-producing micro-organisms, a pleural effusion may become purulent, thus developing into an **empyema.**

Pleurisy may be unilateral or bilateral, and of greatly varying extent and location. Among its causes are: pneumonia, pulmonary tuberculosis and other lung infections which involve the pleura. Osteomyelitis of the ribs, and tuberculosis which commences primarily in the pleura are other causes. Pleurisy is also seen in association with certain infective lesions below the diaphragm (e.g. sub-phrenic abscess), and with fractured ribs.

During the course of pleurisy-with-effusion, the fluid may become walled off, in a localized part of the pleural cavity, as a result of the development of fibrous adhesions. A pleural effusion which is thus confined is known as an **encysted effusion.**

Both dry pleurisy and pleural effusion produce well-marked clinical features. Pain, due to pleurisy, must among other conditions be distinguished from that due to pain in the thoracic muscles from a virus disease called **Bornholm disease** (**epidemic myalgia**).

X-ray examination may yield no evidence of a dry pleurisy, but is important in showing the site and extent of a pleural effusion, and the presence of, or absence of, associated lesions within the chest. The nature of the fluid present in the pleural cavity is not, however, revealed by radiology. Thus pathological examination of a sample of fluid obtained by aspiration through a needle, is an essential investigation in many cases of pleurisy with effusion. With large effusions **chest aspiration** may also be necessary as a therapeutic measure. Aspiration of the chest is also called **paracentesis thoracis.**

(c) **Pneumothorax**—this has been already defined as a condition in which air, or other gas, is present in the pleural cavity. It may result from rupture of the lung through disease—when it is called a **spontaneous pneumothorax;** from injury to the lung or chest wall; from accidental puncture of the lung during aspiration of a pleural effusion; or from the operation of **thoracotomy,** in which an opening is made into the thorax.

An **artificial pneumothorax** used to be widely used as a form of treatment of pulmonary tuberculosis.

A pneumothorax of any appreciable size is readily shown by radiography. Pleural effusion frequently occurs in cases of pneumothorax, the condition then becoming one of hydropneumothorax.

The commonest causes of spontaneous pneumothorax is rupture of an emphysematous bulla (see p. 98).

(d) **Pleural Neoplasms**—(see p. 101).

8. DISEASES OF THE LUNGS

These may be congenital; traumatic, infective; neoplastic; due to cyst formation; due to the inhalation of harmful gases or dusts; allergic; or idiopathic. Pathological changes in the lungs not infrequently develop as a secondary result of heart disease.

Before proceeding to discuss terms relating to individual lung diseases and groups of such diseases, it will be useful to indicate the nature of three specific pathological processes which occur in a variety of different types of pulmonary (lung) disorder, viz.:

(i) **Pulmonary collapse**—a condition in which a portion of lung, or sometimes a whole lung becomes airless and thus collapses down, as a result of obstruction of the bronchus which supplies it with air. According to the site of the bronchial obstruction, the collapse may be lobar, segmental or lobular in type.

The term **atelectasis** which means a condition of incomplete expansion is frequently used as a synonym for pulmonary collapse, but in the stricter sense indicates lung tissue which has failed to expand normally, e.g. as in congenital atelectasis. (*Note:* the derivation of "atelectasis" is from **"a-"** meaning "without" and **"-ectasis"** meaning "expansion").

(ii) **Pulmonary consolidation**—a condition in which an area of lung acquires a solid or semi-solid consistency owing to the air in its alveoli being replaced by substances such as an inflammatory exudate (e.g. in pneumonia) or a mass of tumour cells.

(iii) **Pulmonary fibrosis**—a condition in which areas of normal lung tissue becomes replaced by overgrowth of fibrous connective tissue. It may be localized or diffuse and may occur in areas where the pulmonary alveoli have been damaged by disease, e.g. severe pneumonias, pulmonary tuberculosis, etc. It may also develop as a manifestation of radiation damage (**radiation fibrosis**) and as a reaction to the presence of various harmful dusts in the lungs in certain of the diseases called pneumoconioses.

CONGENITAL DISORDERS

Congenital abnormalities of clinical significance are not very common in the lungs. They include conditions such as (*a*) **pulmonary hamartoma**—this is described by Kerley(2) as a tumour-like malformation. Its name is derived from a Greek word meaning "to err" (see also p. 101); (*b*) **congenital cystic disease of the lungs;** (*c*) **Agenesis of the lung**—a condition in which there is a failure of development of the whole of a lung or part of a lung.

TRAUMATIC DISORDERS

The lungs may be damaged in both what are termed **penetrating** (open) and **non-penetrating** (closed) **chest injuries;** this distinction being made according to whether, or not, the injury causes an open wound which penetrates into the interior of the thoracic cavity and may thus permit the entry of external air into the thorax.

With penetrating wounds there is damage to the pleura which may cause an associated haemothorax or pneumothorax.

Non-penetrating chest injuries may result in **lung contusion** (bruising of the lung) and sometimes in a localized collection of effused blood, called a **haematoma of the lung.** Sometimes they may also cause laceration of the pleura and lung tissue, with the development of a haemothorax or pneumothorax, particularly if one or more ribs are fractured by the trauma.

Development of a pneumothorax may be associated with leakage of air into the neighbouring soft tissues causing a condition called **surgical emphysema.**

Penetrating and non-penetrating chest injuries may be associated with tears of the diaphragm. Severe chest injuries may require surgical treatment (e.g. tracheostomy, thoracotomy) and oxygen administration. In some cases what is termed **intermittent positive pressure ventilation** (I.P.P.V.) may be administered by a mechanical respirator.

INFECTIVE DISEASES

(*a*) **Pneumonias**—the term pneumonia indicates an inflammation of lung tissue. The word **pneumonitis** has a similar meaning but is used much less frequently.

Pneumonias comprise a group of infective lung diseases, the vast majority of which are of infective origin and are of two main types:

(i) **Specific Pneumonias**—due to specific pathogenic bacteria, e.g. **pneumococcal pneumonia, staphylococcal pneumonia, streptococcal pneumonia, tuberculous pneumonia, pneumonia** due to *Friedlander's bacillus*; due to viruses, e.g. **influenzal pneumonia, measles pneumonia, chickenpox pneumonia, pneumonia** in **ornithosis,** or due to rickettsiae, e.g. **pneumonia** due to **Q fever.**

Ornithosis is primarily an infection of birds and the disease **psittacosis** which is a type of this condition may be derived from contact with infected parrots or budgerigars.

(ii) **Non-specific pneumonias**—these are due to a mixture of pathogenic organisms. The most important are the **aspiration pneumonias** which, as their name denotes, are due to aspiration of infective material from the upper respiratory tract (e.g. accessory nasal sinuses) or bronchi. Oswald & Fry (3) also list the following other types of non-specific pneumonias: **pneumonia distal to a bronchial obstruction, recurrent pneumonia, secondary pneumonia.**

The basic pathological feature of pneumonia is the occurrence of pulmonary consolidation (see p. 91). This may involve the whole of one or more lobes, or segments; or may involve numerous lobules, in one or both lungs, in a patchy manner. Clinically, pneumonia is often described according to the type of consolidation encountered, as **lobar, segmental** or **lobular pneumonia.** Lobular pneumonia is also called **broncho-pneumonia.**

The consolidation in pneumococcal pneumonia is generally of lobar type, and that of aspiration pneumonia generally lobular in distribution.

Pneumonia can occur at any age, but is seen most commonly in children and elderly subjects. Common clinical features are cough and shortness of breath, together with elevation of the temperature and pulse rate. Dry pleurisy is a frequent accompaniment and causes pain in the chest.

Among the main complications of pneumonia are:

(i) Heart failure.

(ii) Pleural effusion.

(iii) Empyema.

(iv) Suppuration in the lung causing the condition of **lung abscess.**

(v) Pulmonary collapse which may persist and lead eventually to bronchiectasis.

(vi) Failure of resolution of the consolidation and the development of pulmonary fibrosis in the affected area of lung.

(vii) Spread of infection by the blood stream, causing infective lesions in other structures, e.g. pneumococcal arthritis and meningitis in pneumococcal pneumonia.

The diagnosis of pneumonia is usually made on clinical evidence. Sputum examination may be employed to demonstrate the nature of the infecting organism and the sensitivity of the latter to various antibiotic drugs may be investigated when desirable. X-ray examination is of value both in demonstrating the extent and distribution of the pulmonary consolidation, and also in the assessment of progress under treatment and the investigation of complications.

Treatment is by rest, sedation and the administration of drugs such as penicillin and other antibiotics. The administration of oxygen may be necessary in severe cases.

Note: In addition to pneumonia of infective causation there is another type of lung inflammation called **chemical pneumonia,** which can be caused by inhalation of irritant gases or mineral oils (e.g. paraffin).

93

(*b*) **Lung Abscess**—an abscess is a cavity containing pus, and results from infection of tissues by pyogenic bacteria.

Abscess cavities in lung tissue may be single or multiple. They may develop as a result of pneumonia, particularly staphylococcal pneumonia, or arise from a number of other causes. Among these are inhaled foreign body and the lodgement in the lungs of septic emboli from septic infective lesions in other parts of the body.

At an early stage of its development, a lung abscess usually develops a communication with a bronchus and the patient then starts to cough up purulent sputum. This communication also enables air to enter the cavity, and rising above the pus within the cavity, causes the formation of a "fluid level" which may be readily demonstrated by X-ray films, taken with appropriate positioning.

Treatment of a lung abscess is generally by postural drainage and the administration of antibiotics. Surgery is sometimes necessary when conservative measures fail.

(*c*) Pulmonary Tuberculosis

(i) **Primary pulmonary tuberculosis**—as noted in Part III, the lung is a common site for primary tuberculous infection. The initial lesion in lung tissue is termed a **primary focus** or **Ghon focus,** after a pathologist called Anton Ghon.

The presence of the primary focus characteristically results in associated, and often marked, inflammatory changes in draining lymph glands at the hilum of the affected lung. This combination of primary focus and hilar adenitis (lymph gland inflammation) is called a **primary tuberculous complex,** and in later years its site may be rendered evident as a result of pathological calcification in both the lung and gland lesions.

In some instances primary pulmonary tuberculosis does not produce any recognizable clinical effects. However, it can present as a severe infection and it can also, sometimes, produce serious complications. These include: pulmonary collapse (due to pressure of enlarged hilar glands on a bronchus and sometimes leading to bronchiectasis); pleural effusion; tuberculous broncho pneumonia; metastatic lesions in other structures (e.g. bone and joint tuberculosis, tuberculous meningitis, etc.); miliary tuberculosis.

A skin condition called **erythema nodosum** may occur in association with primary lung tuberculosis, as may an uncommon eye disorder called **phlyctenular conjunctivitis.**

The treatment of primary pulmonary tuberculosis, and its complications, is primarily by chemotherapy with anti-tuberculous drugs.

(ii) **Post primary Pulmonary Tuberculosis** ("adult type" pulmonary tuberculosis, adult phthisis)—this condition is thought to occur as a result of reactivation of a dormant tuberculous infection or less commonly a re-infection, with tubercle bacilli, in an individual who has previously had primary tuberculosis in the lung, or in some other site.

This disease can commence in childhood or in old age. Most cases, however, first develop in adolescence or early adult life.

The inflammatory reaction, produced by the infection, is chronic in nature. In some cases it produces much exudation. In others it is associated with considerable fibrosis. Tissue destruction is marked in many of the severer types of disease producing air-containing cavities within the lungs.

Some degree of fibrosis occurs during the healing of all types of tuberculous lung lesions and pathological calcification is common in areas of healed disease.

Occasionally the disease is seen in acute form, giving rise to a pneumonic type of inflammation termed **tuberculous pneumonia.**

Common symptoms and signs of post-primary tuberculosis are cough, haemoptysis, loss of weight, loss of energy, night sweats, evening pyrexia and amenorrhoea (absence of menstrual periods).

Radiological examination is essential in both the investigation of suspected cases and in the assessment of the progress under treatment of diagnosed cases. Examination of the sputum for *tubercle bacilli,* and frequently sputum culture are also highly important investigations.

The **Mantoux** and **Heaf skin tests** are positive in nearly all patients with active or healed tuberculous lesions.

In the more developed countries, improved hygiene and nutrition, together with the extensive use of anti-tuberculous drugs, have led to a considerable decrease in the incidence of pulmonary tuberculosis and also diminished the incidence of complications in sufferers from the disease.

Some of the complications of post-primary pulmonary tuberculosis, which may result from direct spread of tubercle bacilli, were referred to in Part III where it was noted this type of infection may also produce metastatic tuberculous lesions, as a result of spread of tubercle bacilli via blood vessels and lymphatic channels.

The treatment of pulmonary tuberculosis comprises rest and measures to improve the general health and, in all patients with active disease, chemotherapy with **anti-tuberculosis drugs** (strepto-mycin, P.A.S., and isoniazid).

(*d*) **Other Pulmonary Infections**—these are all rare. They include:

(i) **Pulmonary mycoses** (i.e. fungus infections of the lungs) among which are **pulmonary actinomycosis** (see p. 58), **aspergillosis** (due usually to infection from pigeons), **histoplasmosis, pulmonary blastomycosis, torulosis,** etc.

(ii) **Pulmonary hydatid disease**—see p. 133.

(iii) **Pulmonary amoebiasis**—see p. 301.

(iv) **Pulmonary syphilis.**

NEOPLASMS

Neoplasms of the lung will be discussed later, together with bronchial and other intrathoracic new growths.

CYSTS

Cysts are cavities, with a lining membrane and containing fluid, semi-fluid material or air. They may form in the body as a result of either developmental error or acquired disease.

Congenital cysts may occur in the lung in an uncommon disorder called **congenital cystic disease of the lungs** which, in some of its forms, has to be distinguished from a type of bronchiectasis known as **cystic bronchiectasis.**

Cyst formation may result from a number of pulmonary infections and may sometimes complicate pneumonia, especially when due to staphylococci. Infective cysts due to hydated disease may sometimes occur in lung tissue.

Very large cysts known as **pneumatoceles** (pneumoceles) or **giant air cysts** may be found in the lungs.

Multiple small cysts, with widespread distribution occur in a rare condition called **honeycomb lung** (cystic lung). This appears to be an acquired disorder of unknown basic causation. It may be seen in association with a number of uncommon disorders such as sarcoidosis, xanthomatosis, scleroderma, and a rare familial disorder called tuberose sclerosis. It may also develop in a type of fibrosis of the lungs called chronic diffuse interstitial pulmonary fibrosis (fibrosing alveolitis).

PNEUMOCONIOSES

The Greek word "konios" means "dusty" and the pneumoconioses comprise a group of lung diseases caused by the inhalation of harmful dusts. In the great majority of instances, exposure to the harmful dust occurs during the course of the patient's daily work. These diseases are consequently also referred to as **occupational diseases of the lungs.**

Some types of pneumoconioses are as follows:

Asbestosis (from asbestos fibres); **bagassosis** (from dust from sugar cane fibre); **berylliosis** (from beryllium-containing dust); **coal workers' pneumoconiosis** (from coal dust); **byssinosis** (from cotton dust); **farmers' lung** (dust from mouldy hay); **siderosis** (from iron-containing dust), **silicosis** (from silica-containing dust).

The names of other pneumoconioses include: **aluminium fibrosis, graphite pneumoconiosis, kaolin workers' pneumoconiosis, stannosis** (from dust containing tin), **suberosis** (from cork dust).

The two most important types of pneumoconioses are:

(a) **Coal Workers' Pneumoconiosis**—a condition due to the inhalation of a coal dust in high concentration and especially prevalent in the South Wales coalfields. Aggregations of coal dust form nodules within the lung and the condition may lead to the development of pulmonary fibrosis of varying degree. In severe cases this latter may take the form of **"progressive massive fibrosis"** (P.M.F.) wherein large areas in the upper parts of the lungs become replaced by masses of fibrous tissue, which may later break down with the formation of cavities.

It is thought by some authorities that the massive fibrosis may be the result of atypical tuberculous infection complicating the disease.

Chronic bronchitis, emphysema, and eventually pulmonary heart disease, leading to right-sided heart failure, are common complications of coal-workers' pneumoconiosis.

This disease produces characteristic appearances on X-ray films.

(b) **Silicosis**—an occupational disorder due to the inhalation of dust containing a high proportion of fine silica particles. It may develop in those engaged in occupations such as rock drilling, sandblasting, stonemasonry, pottery, metal grinding, quarry working, etc.

Continued inhalation of fine silica particles into the lungs results eventually in widespread pulmonary fibrosis. The chief clinical feature is breathlessness. Radiographs show first mottling due to nodules of silica and later, also demonstrate abnormal appearances resulting from the fibrosis.

IDIOPATHIC DISEASES

(a) **Pulmonary emphysema**—used without qualification, the term **emphysema** is used to describe a lung disease, of unknown origin, in which there develops a diffuse enlargement of the smaller air spaces

4

of the lungs. This enlargement may result from dilatation of the alveoli and smaller air passages, or from destruction of their walls. In either event it results in the lungs losing their normal elasticity. This leads to a condition of chronic over-inflation of the lungs which thus increase in size, pushing the chest wall outwards and diaphragm downwards, and causing the development of a so-called "barrel-chest".

In severe cases, rupture of the walls of distended alveoli results in the formation of cyst-like spaces of varying size known as emphysematous bullae; the word **bulla** meaning "a bubble". The word "emphysema" is derived from a Greek word meaning "to inflate".

Emphysema is a common cause of pulmonary heart disease and is frequently associated with chronic bronchitis.

The principal clinical feature of emphysema is shortness of breath; at first only on exertion but later, as the disease progresses, also at rest.

The disease produces characteristic X-ray appearances. There is no specific treatment and the condition runs a slowly progressive course, usually terminating in right-sided heart failure. In the less advanced cases, considerable benefit may be obtained from breathing exercises.

The type of emphysema referred to above may be described more fully as **hypertrophic pulmonary emphysema** or **chronic essential emphysema.**

Other types of pulmonary emphysema are distinguished by names such as **compensatory emphysema, obstructive emphysema,** etc.

It is also to be noted that the term **surgical emphysema** is used to denote conditions in which, as a result of injury or surgical operations, air finds its way into superficial or deep soft tissues, e.g. surgical emphysema of chest wall due to traumatic pneumothorax; mediastinal emphysema due to perforated oesophagus.

(*b*) **Sarcoidosis**—is the name of a chronic inflammatory disease of unknown cause. The characteristic lesions, when examined under the microscope, bear some resemblance to the chronic inflammatory foci found in tuberculosis. They occur in sites such as the skin, uveal tract (i.e. the iris diaphragm, ciliary body and choroid coat of the eye), lungs, lymph glands, bones, and in other organs and tissues. In bone they cause a condition called **osteitis multiplex cystoides.**

In the individual patient, sarcoid lesions may be localized to one particular organ or widespread throughout the body. The disease usually commences in adults under forty years of age.

The term **"sarcoid"** means "flesh-like" and has the same derivation as the name of the malignant neoplasm of connective tissues called a sarcoma. These two conditions are, however, otherwise quite unrelated.

Sarcoidosis of the lungs usually follows upon sarcoidosis of the hilar lymph glands and the involvement of these structures is frequently associated with a skin disorder called **erythema nodosum.** In the majority of cases the intrathoracic lesions clear up completely, but sometimes the lung changes lead to widespread pulmonary fibrosis and eventually to pulmonary heart disease.

Both the hilar gland and lung lesions produce abnormal appearances in chest radiographs.

A skin test called the **Kveim test** is positive in a majority of subjects with sarcoidosis. In patients who have lesions in the skin or in superficial lymph glands the presence of the disease may be confirmed by biopsy.

A large proportion of patients with the disease show a negative Mantoux test, although some authorities regard the disorder as being a manifestation of an atypical type of tuberculous infection.

There is no specific treatment for sarcoidosis but many patients are greatly benefited by the administration of steroids.

(*c*) **Hyaline Membrane Disease**—a condition in which difficulty in breathing is caused in newly born babies owing to the presence of abnormal material, referred to as **"hyaline membrane"**, lining the alveoli of the lungs and the terminal air passages. It is thought that this membrane is formed from fluid that has exuded from the blood owing to abnormal permeability of the walls of the lung capillaries.

Treatment is directed to relief of symptoms, there being no specific therapy.

Hyaline membrane disease together with a number of other disorders which cause difficulty in breathing, developing within a few hours of birth, produce what is referred to as the **respiratory distress syndrome.**

(*d*) **Other Idiopathic Lung Diseases**—among these are:

(i) **Idiopathic pulmonary haemosiderosis**—a condition in which haemosiderin (an iron-containing pigment derived from the haemoglobin of the blood) is deposited in the lungs.

(ii) **Loeffler's syndrome**—a condition in which transient areas of consolidation in the lungs are accompanied by **eosinophilia,** i.e. a rise in the circulating blood of white cells of the variety called eosinophil leucocytes (eosinophils).

(iii) **Pulmonary lesions in Collagen Diseases**—see p. 300.

PULMONARY EMBOLISM

As referred to when discussing general pathological processes in Part II, the process of embolism comprises the detachment of a fragment of a thrombus (i.e. the embolus), from its original position within the lumen of a vein or artery, and its carriage in the blood stream until it becomes arrested. Venous emboli are very much commoner than arterial emboli. A fragment of blood clot detached from a thrombus within a vein will be carried through venous channels to the right side of the heart. From its origin from some site of deep vein thrombosis, such as a leg or pelvic vein, during the course of its carriage to the right ventricle, the embolus will progress through successively larger blood vessels. Once, however, it is pumped out of the right ventricle into the pulmonary circulation it will traverse arterial blood vessels of progressively diminishing calibre. Thus, unless it is extremely minute it will eventually enter an artery or arteriole, which is too small for it to pass through and become impacted therein.

The seriousness of pulmonary embolism varies in accordance with the size of the detached fragment of thrombus (blood clot) which becomes arrested within the pulmonary circulation. Thus a large thrombus may occlude the pulmonary artery itself, or one of its two main branches (massive pulmonary embolism) causing sudden death or death within a few hours. If smaller, it may deprive an area of lung of its arterial blood supply, causing death of the tissue cells therein; the dead tissue being referred to as a **pulmonary infarct** and the causal process being termed **pulmonary infarction.** A very small embolism may cause only slight clinical signs and symptoms and produce negligible lung damage.

The occurrence of pulmonary embolism is often evidenced by sudden pain in the chest. Such pain frequently persists owing to the development of pleurisy over the area of the infarct. Haemoptysis is also a frequent feature of the condition and, if a large infarct is produced, there is often shortness of breath.

Infected emboli may cause abscess formation within the lungs.

Radiographs of the chest often give useful information in cases with suspected pulmonary embolism.

Lung emboli may be single or multiple.

In cases of so-called massive pulmonary embolism, **embolectomy,** i.e. surgical removal of the impacted thrombus may be considered. Less severe cases are treated with antibiotics, anticoagulants and rest.

Measures employed to prevent the occurrence of **deep vein thrombosis** (e.g. physiotherapy, getting of patients out of bed at an early stage after surgical operations) are of value in diminishing the incidence of pulmonary embolism and infarction.

9. INTRATHORACIC NEOPLASMS

Intrathoracic neoplasms may arise from the pleural membranes, bronchi, lungs or structures within the mediastinum.

PLEURAL NEOPLASMS

Primary pleural neoplasms are rare, but a malignant tumour called an **endothelioma of the pleura** is occasionally encountered. Metastic neoplasms from carcinomas elsewhere in the body, especially from the lung and breast, are frequent and are a common cause of pleural effusion.

BRONCHIAL AND PULMONARY NEOPLASMS

Benign tumours of the lung and bronchi are uncommon, but do occasionally occur; that with the highest incidence being a tumour of the lining epithelium of a bronchus, called a **bronchial adenoma.**

As has been pointed out by Kerley (4), most cases considered to be benign lung tumours are probably varieties of hamartoma and not true neoplasms.

A **pulmonary hamartoma** is, as described by the same author, a tumour-like congenital malformation and of common occurrence in Great Britain.

Primary and secondary malignant neoplasms are common. The majority of the former are bronchial carcinomas, often incorrectly referred to as lung carcinomas.

(*a*) **Bronchial carcinoma**—this is a tumour which has been much in the news for a number of years because of its frequent incidence, and the strong probability that heavy cigarette smoking is a factor in its causation.

It occurs much more often in men than in women and shows its maximum incidence in middle age.

Bronchial carcinoma usually arises in one of the larger bronchi near the hilum of the lung. It may, however, develop in a small peripheral bronchus. The growth commences in the bronchial mucosa and may grow so as to block the bronchial lumen, thus causing collapse of a segment, or lobe, or of the whole lung, according to the size of the blockage. Outward spread may also occur through the bronchial wall into the lung.

Spread of the disease by the lymphatics, to first the hilar and then the mediastinal lymph glands, is often a fairly early feature in the disease. Glandular metastases may involve the phrenic nerve and cause paralysis and elevation of the diaphragm on the affected side. Pleural effusion is a common complication as is broncho-pneumonia. Blood-borne spread is usually a late feature, but when it occurs, the bones, the brain and other parts of the lungs are common sites for metastases.

Cough and haemoptysis are the most frequent early symptoms. Radiological appearances are diverse in nature according to the site, size of the growth, its mode of spread and the presence, or absence, of intrathoracic complications such as spread to the hilar glands, pneumonic changes and pleural effusion. Tomography is often of great value in demonstrating early lesions.

Bronchoscopy is an important investigation in suspected early cases of bronchial carcinoma. When the tumour is accessible, a biopsy is carried out. It is also sometimes possible to confirm the diagnosis by microscopic demonstration of cancer cells in the sputum, or in the fluid obtained by aspiration of a pleural effusion.

Thoracotomy (surgical opening of the chest) is sometimes necessary as a diagnostic measure.

Treatment is by surgical removal of the tumour and surrounding area of lung, either lobectomy or pneumonectomy being performed, when the diagnosis is made before the growth has spread outside the lung. More advanced growths are treated by radiotherapy or the administration of drugs such as nitrogen mustard or other cytotoxic drugs.

(*b*) **Pulmonary metastases**—the lungs are the commonest site in the body for the occurrence of blood-borne metastases from malignant neoplasms, other than from those neoplasms arising in the area of drainage of the portal vein. Primary tumours arising in this latter area, as might be expected, produce their first blood-borne metastases most commonly in the liver.

Pulmonary metastases are usually multiple. Their presence is evidenced clinically by symptoms such as cough, haemoptysis and shortness of breath. Sometimes, however, they may be demonstrated on routine radiographs before they produce any clinical signs or symptoms. Metastases in the lungs frequently grow so as to involve the overlying pleura. Such involvement frequently results in pain in the chest and the formation of a pleural effusion.

On radiographs, metastases produce opacities which are generally rounded in shape. These opacities may be very large and produce the picture of "cannon-ball metastases" or very small and very numerous causing a widespread mottling in both lungs known as **miliary carcinomatosis.**

Carcinomatous metastases can also permeate lymphatic vessels in the lungs, causing a condition called **lymphangitis carcinomatosa.**

MEDIASTINAL NEOPLASMS

A variety of types of neoplasm may occur within the mediastinum, but with the exception of carcinomatous metastases, none of them are very common and some are very rare.

Some of the principal neoplasms and related disorders which affect mediastinal structures are:

BENIGN

(i) Arising from the nervous system: **neurofibroma**—a tumour of the sheath of a spinal nerve; **ganglioneuroma**—a tumour of the sympathetic nervous system.

(ii) Arising from abnormally persisting embryonic tissue—**dermoid; benign teratoma.**

MALIGNANT

(i) Occurring in lymph glands: **carcinomatous metastases; lymphadenoma** (Hodgkin's disease); **lymphosarcoma,** a malignant neoplasm of the lymphatic system; **reticulosarcoma,** a malignant neoplasm of the reticulo-endothelial system; **leukaemic deposits** in lymph glands.

(ii) Arising in abnormally persisting embryonic tissue—**malignant teratoma.**

(iii) Arising in the thymus gland—**malignant thymoma.**

Mediastinal tumours are frequently demonstrable on X-ray films of the chest. Enlargement of the mediastinal shadow due to a benign or malignant neoplasm must, however, be differentiated from enlargement due to certain non-neoplastic disorders, such as: tuberculous mediastinal lymph glands; aneurysm of the thoracic aorta; retrosternal goitre (enlargement of the thyroid gland downward behind the sternum); mediastinal cysts; and simple enlargements of the thymus gland.

10. SOME SURGICAL OPERATIONS ON THE RESPIRATORY SYSTEM AND CHEST

(*a*) **Adenoidectomy and Tonsillectomy**—Surgical removal of the adenoids and the tonsils, respectively. These two operations are frequently combined.

(*b*) **Antral Puncture**—Puncture of the maxillary antrum through the nasal cavity by means of a trochar and cannula. A **trochar** is a pointed metal rod, used as a perforator. It is enclosed, except for its point, in a hollow metal tube called a **cannula.** When the antral wall has been perforated, the trochar is removed and fluid or pus in the antrum can then be aspirated through the cannula and the antrum can be washed out.

(*c*) **Caldwell-Luc Operation**—An operation for making an opening into the maxillary antrum through the vestibule of the mouth. The incision is made through the alveolar process of the maxilla in the molar region.

(*d*) **Decortication of the Lung**—An operation in which diseased and thickened pleura is stripped off underlying lung. It is one form of treatment for chronic empyema.

(*f*) **Drainage Operations for Empyema**—These comprise **drainage by rib resection,** wherein access to the abscess cavity, in order to institute drainage of pus, is obtained by removal of an overlying portion of rib; and **intercostal drainage** wherein drainage is accomplished by inserting a large catheter, into the abscess, through an intercostal space (i.e. a space between two ribs). A trochar and cannula are employed to insert the catheter.

(*g*) **Laryngectomy**—Removal of the larynx.

(*h*) **Laryngofissure**—An operation to give access to the interior of the larynx, by splitting the thyroid cartilage vertically in the midline.

(*i*) **Lung Resection**—Removal of a part of a lung, or the whole of one lung. The latter procedure is termed **pneumonectomy.** Removal of a lobe is called **lobectomy,** and removal of a broncho-pulmonary segment is termed **segmental resection.**

(*j*) **Phrenic Crush**—Crushing of the phrenic nerve in the neck to effect a temporary paralysis of one side of the diaphragm.

(*k*) **Rib Resection**—Removal of a rib. Partial rib resection is frequently undertaken in order to drain empyema cavities.

(*l*) **Thoracoplasty**—An operation in which portions of a varying number of ribs are removed, thus permitting the chest wall to fall in. It used to be much employed in cases of chronic pulmonary tuberculosis, with the object of effecting partial collapse of lung tissue, thereby limiting the functional activity of diseased areas.

(*m*) **Thoracotomy**—Making an opening into the thoracic cavity.

(*n*) **Tracheostomy**—Making an opening into the trachea to relieve respiratory obstruction arising in the upper respiratory system and inserting a tube to maintain the airway.

REFERENCES

(1) Grant, J. W. B. *The Principles and Practice of Medicine* (Ed. Sir Stanley Davidson). E. and S. Livingstone, 1966.
(2) and (4) Kerley, P. A. *A Textbook of X-ray Diagnosis* (British Authors). H. K. Lewis, 1962.
(3) Oswald, N. C. and Fry, J. *Diseases of the Respiratory System.* Blackwell Scientific Publications, 1962.

Section C.—THE DIGESTIVE SYSTEM

1. SOME ANATOMICAL AND PHYSIOLOGICAL CONSIDERATIONS

The digestive system comprises (*a*) the *alimentary canal* which consists of the *mouth, oropharynx, laryngopharynx, stomach, small intestine (duodenum, jejunum* and *ileum)* and *large intestine (caecum, vermiform appendix, colon, rectum,* and *anal canal),* and (*b*) the *accessory digestive organs,* namely the *teeth, salivary glands, liver, pancreas, gall bladder* and *bile ducts.*

The term **digestion,** from which the system is named, indicates the processes whereby foodstuffs are broken down into substances which can be absorbed from the intestines and used for tissue building and repair. The digestive system is concerned with the digestion of foodstuffs, the absorption into the body of digested food and of water, and the excretion of undigested food in the faeces.

Ingested food is propelled through the alimentary canal chiefly by a type of muscular action referred to as **peristalsis.**

Digestion is effected by the active substances called *enzymes* (digestive ferments) which act on specific classes of foodstuffs and are secreted by the salivary glands, glands in the walls of the stomach and small intestine, and then by the pancreas, e.g. *pepsin* which is secreted in the stomach and acts on proteins; *amylase,* a pancreatic secretion which acts on fats.

The digestion of fatty foodstuffs is aided by the action of *bile,* which is secreted by the liver and is concentrated in the gall-bladder. Besides secreting bile, the liver also has a number of highly important functions concerned with the metabolism of the body.

The following are among the word components referring to organs of the digestive system: **gloss-** tongue; **gastr-** stomach; **enter-** intestine, particularly the small intestine; **sigmoid-** sigmoid colon; **proct-** rectum; **hepat-** liver; **chole-** bile; **cholecyst-** gall bladder; **cholangi-** bile ducts.

2. SOME GENERAL ASPECTS OF DISEASES OF THE DIGESTIVE SYSTEM

Diseases affecting this system may be congenital, traumatic, infective, neoplastic, due to cyst formation, metabolic, due to chemical poisons, allergic or idiopathic—all of which are associated with structural changes, i.e. **organic diseases.**

So-called **functional diseases,** i.e. diseases in which the symptoms and signs appear to arise as a result of functional disorder without demonstrable structural changes, are especially frequent in the digestive system and may produce symptoms which closely resemble those of organic diseases such as peptic ulceration, chronic appendicitis, and the milder types of colonic inflammation.

Disorders of the digestive system may give rise to a variety of signs and symptoms according to the part of the system affected. Some of these are as follows: pain arising from various parts of the system and including cramp-like pains in the abdomen due to spasm of plain muscle and described as **colic** (e.g. intestinal colic, biliary colic, appendicular colic): soreness of the mouth and throat, **dysphagia** (difficulty in swallowing), heartburn, nausea, flatulence: **anorexia** (loss of appetite), vomiting, abdominal discomfort, abdominal distention, **haematemesis** (vomiting of blood), **melaena** (passage of stools which are black owing to presence of altered blood): diarrhoea, constipation, rectal bleeding, **jaundice** (yellow colouration of the skin and mucous membranes), **steatorrhoea** (passage of stools containing excessive amounts of fat).

Symptoms such as flatulence, anorexia, vomiting, intestinal colic, and abdominal discomfort, are frequently referred to as being due to **indigestion,** a term of rather ill-defined usage indicating disordered digestion. The term **dyspepsia** is a synonym of "indigestion".

Disorders affecting the stomach and intestine are often referred to as **gastro-intestinal disorders.**

3. SPECIAL METHODS OF INVESTIGATION

(*a*) **Radiological investigation**—this may take the form of plain X-rays or contrast radiography.

The commoner types of contrast radiography of the digestive system and the parts of this system they are designed to demonstrate are:

Barium swallow—oesophagus; **barium meal**—stomach and duo-denum; **barium meal "follow-through"**—jejunum, ileum and, some-times, also, large intestine; **barium enema**—large intestine; **cholecystog-raphy**—gall bladder; **cholangiography**—bile ducts; **intravenous cholangio-cholecystography** (I.V.C.)—bile ducts and gall-bladder.

(*b*) **Pathological Investigations**—these are very diverse. Included among them are (i) **gastric analysis,** i.e. analysis of gastric secretions obtained by aspiration of the stomach contents through a Ryle's gastric tube, and often performed after giving a test-meal of gruel or after injection of histamine; (ii) **examination of the faeces for occult blood** by chemical tests or tests involving the use of radioactive isotopes. The word "occult" means concealed, and **occult blood** is blood which is not evident to the naked eye; (iii) **bacteriological examination of the faeces** in suspected gastro-intestinal infections; (iv) **Estimation of the fat content of the faeces** in suspected malabsorp-tion syndromes (see p. 129); (v) **biopsy**—this may be performed under direct vision in the mouth and through special instruments (see para. (*c*) below) in the oesophagus, stomach, sigmoid colon and rectum. **Small intestine biopsy** may be performed by specially designed biopsy tubes or by means of a small hollow capsule, containing a spring loaded knife-blade and called a **Crosby capsule. Liver biopsy** may be performed by inserting a biopsy needle through the lower chest wall directly into the liver; (vi) investigation of pressures within the bowel and the pH of the intestinal contents given by swallowed **telemetry capsules** which contain small transmitters designed to provide information at a distance from the body; (vii) **liver function tests**—used to investigate various of the many functions of the liver. There are a multiplicity of these tests. The names of just a few of them are: **estimation of the serum bilirubin; Van den Bergh test; estimation of serum proteins** by **flocculation tests** or a method called electrophoresis, estimation of the serum transaminase; (viii) **pancreatic function tests,** e.g. **estimation of the blood amylase** (a pancreatic enzyme).

(*c*) **Visual inspection by special instruments**—the interiors, or parts thereof, of the following organs may be examined visually by procedures involving the use of special instruments: the pharynx—by **pharyngoscopy;** the oesophagus—by **oesophagoscopy;** the stomach—by **gastroscopy;** the sigmoid colon—by **sigmoidoscopy;** and the rectum by **proctoscopy.** The instruments employed have similar names to the procedure, their names ending with the suffix **-scope,** e.g. proctoscopy is performed with a proctoscope.

(*d*) **Gastric photography**—this may be accomplished by passing a specially designed gastric camera into the interior of the stomach, which may then be photographed using a special colour film. The position of the gastric camera during the taking of the various exposures, may be controlled by fluoroscopy (X-ray screening).

4. DISEASES OF THE MOUTH AND TONGUE

CONGENITAL DISORDERS

The most important of these are gaps along normal lines of developmental fusion in the upper lip and palate, giving rise to the conditions called **cleft lip** (hare lip) and **cleft palate.** The reasons for the occurrence of developmental defects of this type are unknown.

Cleft lip and cleft palate may occur independently or both be present in the same patient. Both interfere with feeding and cleft palate causes defective speech. The treatment of both conditions is surgical.

INFLAMMATORY CONDITIONS

Inflammation of the mouth is called **stomatitis,** and of the tongue, **glossitis. Gingivitis** means inflammation of the gums.

A type of stomatitis due to fungus infection, and known as **thrush** or **moniliasis,** is not uncommon in infants. Another type of stomatitis is called **Vincent's angina.** This usually occurs only in debilitated individuals. Both spirochaetes and micro-organisms called fusiform bacilli are found in the ulcerative lesions which characterize this condition, but it is not certain if these organisms are the actual cause of the ulcers.

Glossitis is of various types and chronic inflammatory changes in the mucosa of the tongue may result in the development of a precancerous condition called **leucoplakia.** The prefix **leuco-** means "white" and this name is descriptive of the white patches which constitute the earlier lesions of the disorder.

NEOPLASMS

Benign tumours are not common in the mouth and tongue but carcinomas are of fairly frequent occurrence and may arise in the mucous membrane covering the lip, cheek, tongue, floor of mouth and the gums.

Collectively, such neoplasms are known as **buccal carcinomas;** the word **buccal** meaning pertaining to the mouth or cheek. The great majority of these are of the type of growths known as **epitheliomas;** or alternatively **squamous-celled carcinomas** as they arise from epithelium of the squamous type. (*Note:* The external surface of the body is covered by, and all its internal cavities are lined by, cellular tissue called **epithelium**).

Early spread by the lymphatics is often seen in buccal carcinomas, but blood-borne metastases are not common. Pneumonia is a frequent complication in advanced cases.

Surgery and radiotherapy, singly or in combination, are employed in the treatment of buccal carcinomas and their metastases in the cervical lymph glands. In suitable cases, however, these latter may be removed by a surgical operation called a **block dissection of the neck.**

CYSTS

Among these are the condition called **ranula,** a cyst in the floor of the mouth below the tongue, and **thyroglossal cyst,** a cyst of congenital origin found in the midline of the tongue or neck arising from remnants of an embryonic structure called the thyroglossal duct.

5. DISEASES OF THE SALIVARY GLANDS

These include the formation of calculi (stones) called **salivary calculi,** inflammatory conditions referred to as **sialitis,** and neoplasms. The virus disease called mumps is one form of acute sialitis. Chronic sialitis may lead to dilatation of the terminations of small ducts within, in a salivary gland. This disorder is termed **sialectasis,** and in the parotid and submandibular (submaxillary) salivary glands it may be demonstrated by a form of contrast radiography called sialography.

Lesions in the salivary glands are also prominent features in two rare disorders called **Mikulicz's syndrome** and **Sjogren's syndrome.**

The most important neoplasm in the salivary glands is the so-called "mixed parotid tumour".

"Mixed" Parotid Tumour (Parotid adenoma)—this is a benign neoplasm of epithelial origin. Formerly it was thought to belong to the class of mixed tumours which contain several different types of tissue (cf. dermoids and terratomas), and it has retained its old name. It may rarely develop malignant changes.

The tumour is slow growing. Treatment is by complete surgical removal of the growth. Post-operative radiotherapy is advantageous.

6. DISEASES OF THE PHARYNX

The nasopharynx is part of the upper respiratory tract. The oropharynx and part of the laryngopharynx are common to the respiratory and digestive systems. Some reference has thus already been made to a number of diseases of the pharynx (i.e. pharyngitis, adenoids, tonsillitis, quinsy, and certain carcinomas have already been referred to when discussing diseases of the upper respiratory system).

The hypopharynx, i.e. the lower part of the laryngopharynx, is part of the digestive tract and among the disorders found in this region are impaction of swallowed foreign bodies (especially meat and fish bones), pharyngeal pouch, and post-cricoid carcinoma.

PHARYNGEAL POUCH (PHARYNGEAL DIVERTICULUM)

This condition is thought to arise as a result of the presence of a small area of congenital weakness between muscles in the lower part of the pharynx. With advancing years a bulge of mucous membrane through this weak area develops. This at first forms a small pouch, which tends to gradually increase in size, until ultimately it may become very large. Large pouches cause **dysphagia,** i.e. difficulty in swallowing, as a result of their pressing on nearby portions of the lower pharynx and upper oesophagus. The presence of a pharyngeal pouch is readily demonstrable by barium swallow.

An alternative name for the condition is **pharyngeal diverticulum.** It is to be noted that pouches, or diverticula, may arise in other parts of the alimentary canal and are of fairly frequent occurrence in the colon.

NEOPLASMS OF THE HYPOPHARYNX

Benign neoplasms are rare in the hypopharynx. Carcinoma arising in the region behind the cricoid cartilage of the larynx is not uncommon.

Post-cricoid carcinoma is chiefly a disease of females showing its maximum incidence in middle age. Early lymphatic spread is often a feature of this tumour. The growth frequently develops as a sequel to Plummer-Vinson syndrome (see p. 202).

Dysphagia is the cardinal symptom.

Pharyngoscopy with biopsy, and barium swallow, are important diagnostic investigations.

Treatment is mainly by radiotherapy, few patients being suitable for surgery.

7. DISEASES OF THE OESOPHAGUS

These include congenital abnormalities, foreign body in the oesophagus, rupture of the oesophagus as a result of trauma or disease, burns from hot or corrosive liquids, an inflammatory condition called reflux oesophagitis, diverticula, carcinoma, and a disorder called achalasia of the cardia.

CONGENITAL ABNORMALITIES

The oesophagus is a hollow muscular tube. In rare instances, as a result of developmental error during early intra-uterine life, the upper and lower portions of the oesophagus may be separated by an area, of varying length, where the interior lumen is absent or narrowed.

In the former instance the upper segment of the oesophagus has a blind ending and the condition is called **atresia of the oesophagus.** In the majority of patients with this abnormality, the lumen of the lower segment of this structure is connected by a fistula (i.e. a track with two open ends) with the trachea and the disorder is then described as a **tracheo-oesophageal fistula.** Affected infants vomit their first feed and all subsequent feeds. The diagnosis may be confirmed by failure to pass a soft rubber catheter down the oesophagus and further established by a form of contrast radiology called a dionosil swallow. Treatment is by urgent surgery.

In patients where the defect results in narrowing, instead of complete atresia, the disorder is called a **congenital oesophageal stricture** or **stenosis.**

Congenital oesophageal strictures are much less common than acquired oesophageal strictures. The latter can result from burns from corrosive liquids, but more often develop as a result of reflux oesophagitis (see later).

Another type of developmental error may result in the oesophagus being abnormally short. In patients with **congenital short oesophagus,** the junction between the oesophagus and stomach lies within the thorax and there is thus a **congenital partial intrathoracic stomach,** also referred to as a **congenital hiatus hernia.**

A **hernia** is a protrusion of a structure through the wall of the cavity in which it is normally contained. A protrusion of the stomach through the oesophageal hiatus of the diaphragm is called a **hiatus hernia.**

Hiatus hernia is a fairly common condition. In the majority of cases, however, whether presenting in childhood or in adult life, the disorder is thought to be acquired (see below). Both the congenital and acquired varieties are demonstrable by barium swallow but are indistinguishable radiologically.

REFLUX OESOPHAGITIS AND HIATUS HERNIA

Reflux oesophagitis is a disease in which inflammation of the mucosa of the oesophagus results from reflux of acid gastric juice from the stomach. Its basis is inefficiency of the sphincter mechanism at the cardia (i.e. the opening at the joint of junction of the oesophagus and stomach); this latter condition being known as **incompetence of the cardia** or as **lax cardia.** Reflux oesophagitis occurs most frequently in childhood during middle and old age, and during pregnancy.

Heartburn is the commonest symptom. There may also be pain behind the sternum, which may mimic anginal pain, when it is called **pseudo-angina** (see p. 71). Vomiting, dysphagia and haematemesis may also be features of the disease.

The oesophageal inflammation may cause a localized spasm of the circular muscle coat of the oesophagus, resulting in a spastic narrowing in the lower part of the lumen of this organ. When inflammation is severe, fibrosis may occur in the oesophageal wall and initially spastic narrowing may develop into a permanent fibrous **stricture of the oesophagus.**

Reflux oesophagitis is often associated with the presence of a **sliding hiatus hernia,** an acquired condition in which a portion of stomach of varying size protrudes intermittently or permanently through the oesophageal hiatus in the diaphragm and, as a result, the cardiac orifice of the stomach lies intermittently or permanently within the thorax. The anatomical abnormality in this disorder is thus similar to that of a congenital short oesophagus with associated partial intrathoracic stomach (congenital hiatus hernia).

Laxity of the oesophageal hiatus and raised intra-abdominal pressure are thought to be factors in the causation of sliding hiatus hernia.

(*Note:* In addition to the congenital and sliding varieties of hiatus hernia, a third type of hiatus hernia, known as a **paraoesophageal hernia** sometimes occurs. This is an acquired condition in which the oesophagus is of normal length and the cardia lies below the diaphragm).

Barium swallow is essential in all cases of suspected reflux oesophagitis and suspected hiatus hernia. Oesophagoscopy is also frequently indicated.

Treatment is medical in the majority of patients with both conditions; surgery is, however, indicated when medical treatment does not relieve the severe symptoms of oesophagitis or when there is a large hiatus hernia or an oesophageal stricture. This latter complication may also be treated by dilatation of the stenosed area by cylindrical rods called **bougies.**

CARCINOMA OF THE OESOPHAGUS

Carcinoma may originate anywhere in the oesophagus, but occurs most frequently at the extreme upper and lower ends, and in the middle third of this viscus. It is predominantly a disease of old age, and much commoner in males than in females.

Dysphagia is the chief symptom and results from narrowing of the oesophagus. Barium swallow, oesophagoscopy and biopsy are all important diagnostic procedures in suspected cases.

Surgical excision may be practicable with early growths, particularly with carcinomas of the lower end of the oesophagus. The majority of cases are unsuitable for surgery and are treated by radiotherapy. In some cases a tube of silver wire, called a **Souttar's tube,** may be inserted into the stenosed area to maintain a patent channel, through which the patient may be fed. Alternatively, it may be necessary to open the abdomen and introduce a rubber tube into the stomach for feeding purposes. This operation is called a **gastrostomy.**

ACHALASIA OF THE CARDIA (CARDIOSPASM)

This is a condition of narrowing of the lower end of the oesophagus, due to spasm of circular muscle fibres in this region. The spasm is thought to result from degeneration of certain nerves in the oesophageal wall, and causes a failure of normal relaxation of the cardiac sphincter during swallowing. This gives the disease its name of **achalasia;** this term meaning "a failure to relax".

Solids and fluids are held up above the spastic area and, as a result, the oesophagus above this area becomes dilated and lengthened.

Dysphagia is the chief symptom. Illingworth (1) states that achalasia is believed to originate most often in early adult life, but the onset of symptoms may be delayed for several years.

Oesophagitis and bronchopneumonia are common complications. The condition produces characteristic appearances at barium swallow.

Treatment may be by instrumental dilatation of the spastic area or by surgery. (See "Hellers operation").

8. DISEASES OF THE STOMACH AND DUODENUM

CONGENITAL ABNORMALITIES

(*a*) **Congenital Pyloric Stenosis**—in this condition, as indicated by its name, there is a stenosis (narrowing) of the pylorus (the opening between the stomach and duodenum) due to hypertrophy of the circular muscle fibres in the region of the pyloric sphincter. The stenosis produces a varying degree of obstruction to the passage of gastric contents from the stomach into the duodenum.

The disease is much commoner in male than in female children. The cardinal symptom is vomiting which, however, does not usually occur until about three weeks after birth and is projectile in type. There is often a palpable swelling in the abdomen caused by the thickened muscle at the pylorus, and peristaltic waves passing from left to right, may often be observed in the upper abdomen, after administration of a feed.

Barium meal is a valuable investigation when the clinical diagnosis is in doubt.

A proportion of cases are treated with antispasmodic drugs but in the majority, treatment is surgical division of the thickened pyloric muscle **(Ramstedt's operation).**

(*b*) **Congenital duodenal atresia**—a condition in which development error results in the presence of an area where the lumen of the duodenum is absent. As a result of this there is vomiting from birth. The vomitus (vomited material) is bile-stained as the atresia occurs below the level where the common bile duct enters the duodenum.

INFLAMMATORY DISEASES

(*a*) **Gastritis**—this term means inflammation of the stomach and is used to describe a group of acute and chronic inflammatory disorders with rather ill-defined signs and symptoms, but in some instances producing clinical pictures which bear a similarity to those of either peptic ulceration or carcinoma of the stomach.

Names used to describe different varieties of gastritis include **acute simple gastritis, acute erosive gastritis, antral gastritis, chronic gastritis, chronic atrophic gastritis, phlegmonous gastritis, chronic hypertrophic gastritis.**

The simple type of acute gastritis is extremely common and can be caused by over-indulgence in alcohol, dietary indiscretion, food poisoning, or acute infective conditions such as influenza. It is evidenced by clinical features such as nausea, anorexia, vomiting and abdominal pain and discomfort.

(*b*) **Peptic Ulceration**—An ulcer has already been defined as an open sore caused by an inflammatory process breaking through the skin or a mucous membrane. In sites where pepsin, an enzyme found in gastric juice, comes in contact with mucous membranes, a type of ulcer, called a peptic ulcer, may develop.

Thus peptic ulcers are found mainly in the stomach and duodenum and are referred to respectively as **gastric** and **duodenal ulcers.** The commonest site for their occurrence is the first part of the duodenum. They can also occur in the jejunum usually as a sequel to certain types of operation which establish a direct communication between the stomach and jejunum (i.e. certain forms of partial gastrectomy and gastrojejunostomy). Rarely, also, peptic ulceration may be found in the lower oesophagus.

Peptic ulcers are common and may be acute or chronic in type. They are sometimes seen in children but their greatest incidence is in middle-age. Their cause is unknown. Occasional cases of acute peptic ulceration are associated with steroid therapy (e.g. for rheumatoid arthritis); hypersensitivity to aspirin, or severe burns.

Acute gastric and acute duodenal ulcers may cause symptoms of indigestion but, not infrequently, first reveal their presence as the result of the ulcerative process producing either severe bleeding; or causing perforation of the overlying wall of the stomach, or duodenum, with resultant leakage of gas and fluid into the peritoneal cavity, i.e. a condition of **perforated peptic ulcer.**

An appreciable degree of bleeding from a peptic ulcer will result in **melaena** (the passage of stools, coloured black owing to the presence of altered blood). Haemorrhage from a gastric ulcer frequently also causes **haematemesis** (vomiting of blood). Haematemesis can occur also from a duodenal ulcer but considerably less frequently.

Chronic gastric and duodenal ulcers may also cause bleeding or perforation but these complications are rarely the first evidence of their presence. Dyspepsia and pain after meals are usually the chief symptoms and vomiting is a feature in some cases.

Chronic peptic ulceration may result in the development of fibrosis in, and around, the ulcerated area. With ulcers in the region of the pylorus, contraction of fibrous tissue may lead in time to narrowing of the pylorus. This complication is called **pyloric stenosis** and is of serious import as it impedes gastric emptying, thus leading to vomiting of the stomach contents with consequent dehydration and loss of weight.

An ulcer in the body of the stomach may in the same way lead to fibrosis which ultimately produces a deformity with the descriptive name of **"hour-glass" stomach.**

Occasionally a carcinomatous growth may develop in a chronic gastric ulcer but this happens infrequently. (*Note:* carcinoma does not develop in connection with chronic duodenal ulceration).

Acute gastric and duodenal ulcers are generally difficult to demonstrate radiologically as they tend to be small and shallow. A high proportion of chronic peptic ulcers may, however, be shown by a barium meal examination. This investigation can also reveal complications such as pyloric stenosis and neoplastic change.

Clinically, perforation of an ulcer is characterized by severe abdominal pain of sudden onset, and by shock. Plain radiographs, taken with appropriate positioning, will generally reveal gas that has escaped through the perforation into the peritoneal cavity and thus confirm the diagnosis.

Gastroscopy is a useful investigation in suspected cases of chronic gastric ulceration. In some centres a gastric camera may also be employed as a diagnostic aid.

In many instances information of value may also be obtained by performing a test meal with gastric analysis.

Treatment of an uncomplicated peptic ulcer may be medical or surgical. Usually medical treatment is given an adequate trial in the first instance. Most cases of haematemesis are treated medically in the first instance, but surgical intervention may be required if the bleeding does not stop within a reasonable period of time. Perforated ulcers may be treated by either immediate operation or by gastric suction and administration of fluids through an intravenous drip. Surgical treatment is necessary in cases of "hour-glass" stomach and pyloric stenosis.

(c) **Duodenitis**—means "inflammation of the duodenum". Some authorities regard duodenitis as a distinct clinical disorder with characteristic radiological appearances. Other authorities disagree with this view.

(d) **Gastro-enteritis**—food poisoning has been referred to as a cause of gastritis. Very frequently when inflammation of the stomach is due to this cause, concomitant inflammatory changes are produced in the bowel. These latter are referred to as "enteritis" and the disorder is thus called **gastro-enteritis.**

Food poisoning may result from ingestion of food or drink contaminated by pathogenic bacteria, or from the ingestion of certain chemical poisons (e.g. arsenic). It may also occur as a manifestation of hypersensitivity to certain foods (e.g. shellfish) in individuals with food allergy.

Important causes of bacterial food poisoning are bacilli of the *Salmonella* group, certain strains of staphylococci, and a bacillus called *Clostridium Welchii.* An uncommon causal organism, but one which causes a very serious and often fatal illness, is the *Clostridium botulinus* which is responsible for the infection known as **botulinum.**

(e) **Pyloric stenosis**—narrowing of the pylorus, with resultant obstructive signs and symptoms, may be due to fibrosis caused by the inflammatory changes of gastric or duodenal ulceration.

By no means all cases of this condition are, however, of inflammatory origin. As already noted it may be due to developmental error as in congenital pyloric stenosis, and as will be indicated later, it may be produced by a carcinoma arising in the distal part of the pyloric antrum of the stomach.

Pyloric stenosis is also seen in an idiopathic disorder of adults called **chronic hypertrophic pyloric stenosis.**

NEOPLASMS

Benign neoplasms of the stomach are rare and any type of duodenal new growth is exceedingly uncommon. On the other hand, gastric carcinoma has a high incidence in males and is of fairly frequent occurrence in females.

Carcinoma of the Stomach—the maximum incidence of this disease is in middle age and the commonest site for its origin is in the mucosa of the pyloric antrum. It can, however, develop in the mucosal lining in any other part of the stomach. It can arise as a sequel to a chronic gastric ulcer but this does not happen very frequently.

The growth, as it progresses, may either infiltrate the stomach wall around its site of origin, produce a large tumour which projects into the lumen or the stomach, or cause malignant ulceration of the gastric mucosa.

According to the site of the growth, complications such as obstruction of the cardia, "hour-glass" deformity of the body of the stomach, and pyloric stenosis may develop as local spread of the malignant processes takes place. Perforation sometimes occurs but is not common.

Lymphatic metastases are often an early feature in the disease and when they occur in the cleft in the under surface of the liver, known as the porta hepatis, they may cause jaundice by pressing on and obstructing the bile ducts. (*Note:* **Jaundice** is a yellow colouration of the skin and mucous membranes due to excess of bilirubin, a bile pigment, in the circulation).

A gastric carcinoma causes symptoms and signs such as anorexia, loss of weight, pain in the epigastrium, vomiting, anaemia, and sometimes haematemesis and melaena. In advanced cases there may be a palpable mass in the epigastrium.

The most important single diagnostic measure is barium meal examination, although, unfortunately, the radiological detection of the disease in its earlier stages is extremely difficult. Gastroscopy is also often a valuable investigation and gastric photography may be helpful. However, sometimes, **diagnostic laparatomy** (the opening of the abdomen by surgical incision, as a diagnostic procedure) may be advisable when, in spite of negative radiological and gastroscopic findings, there is a strong suspicion on clinical evidence that a carcinoma of the stomach is present.

The treatment of a gastric carcinoma, diagnosed in an operable stage, is by radical surgery, and in advanced cases some form of palliative surgery is often advocated to relieve vomiting.

SOME OTHER GASTRIC AND DUODENAL DISEASES

These include: (*a*) **foreign bodies** in the stomach and duodenum; (*b*) gastric and duodenal **diverticula** (pouches); (*c*) **volvulus of the stomach**—a condition in which the stomach becomes twisted around one of its axes; the word "volvulus" indicating a twisting, but being originally derived from a Latin word meaning "to roll"; (*d*) **acute dilatation of the stomach**—a rare post-operative condition; (*e*) **chronic duodenal ileus**—a condition of chronic partial duodenal obstruction resulting from pressure of the superior mesenteric artery (and its containing fold of mesentery) on the third part of the duodenum; (*f*) duodenal obstruction associated with malrotation of the gut (see p. 120).

9. DISEASES OF THE SMALL AND LARGE INTESTINE

The intestine is referred to also as the "bowel" or the "gut". The small intestine comprises the duodenum, jejunum and ileum; but, for purposes of description, it is convenient to consider disorders of the duodenum together with those of the stomach, as has been done herein. The ensuing description will thus refer more particularly to diseases of the jejunum, ileum and large intestine.

CONGENITAL ABNORMALITIES

A variety of developmental abnormalities may affect the intestines. Some of the more important are:

(*a*) **Meckel's Diverticulum**—is a narrow tube, which communicates with the lower ileum and arises from a failure of closure of a duct (the vitelline duct), which is present at a certain stage of foetal life. Whilst not very uncommon, the presence of this abnormality rarely causes trouble. Sometimes, however, the diverticulum may become inflamed producing an illness similar to an attack of acute appendicitis. Also, there may be bands, attached to the diverticulum, which can cause intestinal obstruction through pressure on an adjacent loop of small bowel.

(*b*) **Hirschsprung's Disease** (Congenital megacolon)—a condition wherein a narrowed segment of bowel is found in the pelvic colon. This forms a partial obstruction to normal downward passage of faeces into the rectum. As a result the bowel above the narrowing becomes dilated owing to the accumulation of faeces within it. It is this dilatation which is responsible for the word **megacolon,** meaning "large colon", in the alternative name of the disease.

The condition is, however, more frequently referred to as Hirschsprung's disease, after H. Hirschsprung, who was a Danish physician.

The narrow segment is thought to result from a failure of development of certain nerve cells in the affected part of the colon. The narrowing usually commences just above the apex of the rectum and only involves a very short segment of pelvic colon. Rarely, however, it may affect the whole pelvic colon and extend into the descending colon. The dilatation above the narrow segment may be confined to the left half of the colon, or may involve the whole of the colon. It is to be noted that the rectum in this disease is of normal size.

Constipation from birth and increasing abdominal distention are the chief clinical features. Acute intestinal obstruction is a common complication.

The narrowed segment and the dilated bowel behind it may both be demonstrated by barium enema. B. C. H. Ward (2) has stressed the importance of screening and taking of films in a lateral projection, during this examination.

Treatment is surgical, the narrow segment and dilated portion of the colon being resected.

Congenital megacolon must be differentiated from another variety of colonic dilatation, called **idiopathic megacolon.** This latter disease, which is treated medically, is also characterized by chronic constipation and abdominal distension. There is, however, no narrowed segment of bowel and the rectum is dilated as well as the colon.

(*c*) **Imperforate anus**—this is a condition in which, as a result of developmental error, the rectum does not open normally into the anal canal. The two may merely be separated by a thin membrane, or the rectum may terminate blindly at some distance from the anus. The extent of the gap may often be shown by radiography. Films are taken with a metal marker placed at the anus and the child is held upside down, in order that gas in the bowel may rise and outline the terminal portion of the rectum.

Treatment is surgical.

(*d*) **Malrotation of the gut**—during foetal life the developing intestines undergo a considerable degree of rotation, in order to reach the positions in the abdomen which they normally occupy after birth. An upset in these processes constitutes malrotation of the gut, an uncommon condition comprising a group of major and minor abnormalities.

The most important major abnormality of this type is called **situs inversus partialis,** wherein the small bowel lies in the right side and the colon in the left side of the abdomen, the caecum being found near the midline.

Twisting of the intestine in the region of the duodeno-jejunal flexure and resultant duodenal obstruction is a not infrequent complication of malrotation.

(*e*) **Meconium Ileus**—this term indicates blockage of the small intestine by thick meconium, a disorder which occurs as a result of **muco-viscidosis** (see p. 140).

In a newly born infant the faeces are at first dark green in colour and at this stage are referred to as **meconium.** Any type of intestinal obstruction may be termed an **ileus.**

TRAUMATIC DISORDERS

The bowel may be contused or ruptured by injuries to the abdomen of non-penetrating type. Penetrating wounds may also cause contusion of the intestine, traumatic perforation, or sometimes complete division of a segment of bowel.

INFLAMMATORY DISEASES

It is to be noted that whilst **enteritis** means "inflammation of the intestine", it is sometimes used to indicate inflammation of the small bowel only.

Inflammation of the colon is called **colitis;** inflammation of the caecum, **typhlitis;** and inflammation of the rectum, **proctitis.**

Inflammation of the small bowel with concomitant inflammatory changes in the colon is sometimes described as **entero-colitis.**

Among the inflammatory disorders which occur in small and large bowel are:

(*a*) **Gastro-enteritis** due to food poisoning—see p. 117.

(*b*) **Regional enteritis** (Crohn's disease)—this is a chronic inflammatory disorder, so called as the changes affect one or more regions of bowel, rather than being generalized in distribution. It is, however, perhaps more widely referred to as **Crohn's disease,** after B. B. Crohn, an American physician. Its cause is unknown. Its maximum incidence is chiefly in young adults but is not of very common occurrence.

The disease affects principally the terminal portion of the ileum, but can occur elsewhere in the small or large bowel, (particularly in the ano-rectal region, where it is a frequent cause of **fistula-in-ano,)** and rarely in the stomach. When the lesions are confined to the ileum it is sometimes referred to as **regional ileitis.**

In an affected area the chronic inflammatory lesions cause considerable fibrosis with thickening of the bowel wall and consequent narrowing of its lumen. They also produce ulceration of the intestinal mucosa and perforation of ulcerated areas may lead to the formation of multiple small abscesses around the bowel. Such abscesses may ultimately produce internal fistulae, which communicate with other loops of bowel, or external fistulae which lead from the bowel and discharge faeces and pus through the abdominal wall. These latter, which discharge faecal matter externally, are called **faecal fistulae.**

Other complications include intestinal obstruction and malabsorption syndrome.

The principal clinical features of regional enteritis are pain and diarrhoea and a palpable abdominal swelling develops in many patients. There is usually loss of weight and general debility.

Narrowing of the small bowel may be shown radiologically by a small-bowel barium meal, and colonic changes, when present, by a barium enema.

Medical treatment is generally nowadays advised in the first instance in uncomplicated cases; surgical measures being usually reserved for certain of the complications of the disease.

(*c*) **Intestinal tuberculosis**—the intestine as noted in Part III may be the site of primary tuberculosis and infection in this site may lead to inflammatory changes in draining lymph glands in the mesentery, i.e. **tuberculous mesenteric adenitis.** Evidence of this latter infection, which is generally mild, may be seen subsequently on X-ray films in the form of pathological calcification in old healed infective foci within the glands.

Another form of tuberculosis of the intestine is **tuberculous ileitis,** a complication of advanced post-primary pulmonary tuberculosis. This condition causes the formation of tuberculous ulcers in the mucosa of the ileum and these may heal with much fibrosis and resultant formation of numerous strictures.

Tuberculous infection in the region of the anus is a rare cause of **fistula-in-ano,** a condition wherein a fistulous track leads from an opening in the skin, near the anus, to an internal opening in the anal canal.

(*d*) **Typhoid Fever** (Enteric Fever)—see p. 49.

(*e*) **Appendicitis**—this term means inflammation of the appendix and includes inflammatory conditions such as **acute appendicitis, recurrent appendicitis, sub-acute appendicitis, chronic appendicitis,** and **"grumbling appendix".**

Infection appears to be an important factor in provoking the inflammation. In the type of disorder termed **acute obstructive appendicitis,** the infection appears to be a secondary result of obstruction of the lumen of the appendix.

Obstructive appendicitis may result in **perforation of the appendix** with either the formation of a localized **appendix abscess** in the region of the perforated organ, or in the discharge of infective material into the peritoneal cavity producing a condition called **general peritonitis.**

The clinical features vary considerably with the type of inflammation present but, in most instances, pain and tenderness in the right iliac fossa are cardinal features of an attack of the disease.

The diagnosis is made on the clinical features but in the less acute forms of appendicitis, radiological investigations may be required to exclude other diseases which might produce similar signs and symptoms.

Treatment is by appendicectomy (removal of the appendix) but, according to the nature of the case, this may be required to be performed as an emergency operation or, in other instances, delayed until after the subsidence of an active phase of the disease.

When the disease is complicated by general peritonitis, drainage of the infected peritoneal cavity is required in addition to appendicectomy. This is effected by inserting a rubber tube, or strip of corrugated rubber, so that it provides a channel for the escape of infective material to the exterior. The outer end of the **drain** (i.e. the tube or corrugated rubber) is brought out through a small "stab" incision in the abdominal wall in order not to interfere with the main abdominal incision required for the appendicectomy. Some cases of appendix abscess also require surgical drainage.

(*f*) **Dysentery**—colitis caused by bacillary dysentery and amoebic dysentery will be referred to in Part V.

(*g*) **Ulcerative Colitis**—non-specific ulcerative colitis is an inflammatory disease of the large bowel which frequently leads to widespread ulceration of the colonic mucosa and fibrosis of the walls of the colon. The rectum is also usually involved by the disease and also, not infrequently, the caecum.

The cause is unknown and whilst the full name of the condition distinguishes it from other causes of colonic ulceration (e.g. amoebic and bacillary dysentery), it is generally referred to simply as "ulcerative colitis".

The inflammatory changes result in diarrhoea, often with blood and mucus in the stools. The disease pursues a chronic course but periodic remissions (i.e. periods during which the symptoms diminish in intensity or subside) are a common feature. Sometimes, however, the disease may present initially in acute form.

The early lesions are usually seen in the distal part of the pelvic colon and can be visualized through a sigmoidoscope.

Barium enema examination is useful to show the extent of the disease and to reveal complications such as stricture of the bowel and the development of a carcinoma in a diseased area of colon.

There is usually an accompanying anaemia requiring investigation by haemoglobin estimations and blood cell counts.

The development of a carcinoma in a diseased area of bowel is a not infrequent complication of ulcerative colitis.

A type of arthritis, resembling ankylosing spondylitis, occurs in some patients with the disease and is called **colitic arthritis.**

Medical treatment is extensively employed in ulcerative colitis, and this often serves to control the disease. A proportion of patients, however, sooner or later require surgery and in these it is now generally the practice to perform **total colectomy** (removal of the whole colon) with, or without, concomitant **proctectomy** (removal of the rectum).

(*h*) **Irritable Colon**—this is an ill-defined disorder, also called **spastic colon** or **colospasm.** In many cases the condition appears to be due to a mild inflammation of the colon, whilst in others it appears to be a functional disorder and one in which psychological factors play a part.

Clinical features include attacks of both diarrhoea and constipation and cramp-like abdominal pains.

(*i*) **Colonic Diverticulitis**—it has been already noted that pouches, called diverticula (singular: diverticulum) may be found in the pharynx, oesophagus, stomach and duodenum. They may also occur in the jejunum and less commonly in the ileum. The commonest site for their occurrence is, however, in the large bowel, especially in the sigmoid part of the colon.

The presence of diverticula constitutes **diverticulosis,** and if inflammatory changes develop in the walls of the pouches the condition is then referred to as **diverticulitis.** Used without a qualifying adjective, the term "diverticulitis" is generally taken to refer to **colonic diverticulitis.**

Diverticula may be congenital or acquired. In diverticulosis, the diverticula are, in the great majority of instances, of the acquired type and consist of small pouches of colonic mucosa which protrude through weak areas in the bowel wall (i.e. generally through areas where small blood vessels pierce the muscular layers of the colonic wall). It is not known exactly why such pouches develop, but raised pressure within the bowel, resulting from chronic constipation, is thought to be a factor in many patients.

Stagnation of faecal matter readily occurs within diverticula, resulting in infection and the resultant inflammatory changes of diverticulitis.

Diverticulitis is a common disease in middle-aged and elderly subjects of both sexes and produces a variety of clinical features according to whether the inflammation is acute or chronic in type.

Acute diverticulitis may resemble an attack of acute appendicitis, except that the signs are referable to the left iliac fossa. Perforation of an acutely inflamed diverticulum may result in the formation of a **paracolic abscess** or general peritonitis. An abscess may burst into the bladder or vagina, forming either a **vesico-colic fistula** or a **vagino-colic fistula** (*note:* **vesico-** means pertaining to the urinary bladder).

Chronic diverticulitis causes pain in the left iliac fossa and constipation, often interrupted by intermittent attacks of diarrhoea. The stools often contain blood. Intestinal obstruction may develop in severe cases.

Colonic diverticula and evidence of inflammatory changes, when present, are demonstrable by barium enema examination.

Treatment in mild and uncomplicated cases is by diet and laxatives. Complicated and severe cases frequently require surgical treatment.

(*j*) **Ischio-rectal Abscess**—this is the name given to an abscess which develops in the ischio-rectal fossa (i.e. an area in each side of the perineum, lying between the anal canal and the side wall of the bony pelvis). The initial cause of the infection is often not obvious but it is thought that in most instances pathogens gain access to this fossa through some lesion in the wall of the anal canal or lower part of the rectum.

An ischio-rectal abscess may burst so as to cause a fistula, communicating at one end with the anal canal, and, at the other end, opening on the surface of the skin near the anal margin. Such a fistula is termed a **fistula-in-ano.** As has been noted, it can occur as a result of tuberculous infection but it is much more frequently due to infection with bacteria such as *B. coli, staphylococci,* and *streptococci;* or to Crohn's disease.

NEOPLASMS

Benign and malignant neoplasms are rare in the small bowel, and with the exception of a tumour called a **solitary adenoma,** benign neoplasms are also rare in the large bowel. Carcinoma arising from the mucosa of the large bowel is, however, of fairly frequent occurrence in older subjects.

An adenoma in some instances grows so that its main part becomes rounded and is connected to the mucous membrane from which it arises by a stem-like process, referred to as a **pedicle.** It may then be referred to as a **polyp** or **polypoid adenoma.**

Some important types of neoplastic disease are:

(*a*) **Multiple Familial Polyposis (Polyposis coli)**—multiple adenomas, many with polypoid form, are found in this rare but interesting hereditary disease. The tumours are small but often widespread in the bowel and bleed very easily. Rectal haemorrhage is the cardinal feature of the disease, often appearing in childhood. Carcinomatous changes in polyps are of frequent occurrence and, accordingly, removal of the whole of the large bowel is frequently carried out in this disorder.

(*b*) **Carcinoid tumours**—this name describes certain uncommon tumours which occur in the appendix or more rarely, in the ileum. They are slow growing, but in the course of time some of them develop malignant properties; hence the name **carcinoid,** which means "cancer-like". They are also called **argentaffinomas** or **chromaffinomas** from the names given to the cells from which they arise.

(*c*) **Carcinoma of the large intestine**—the cause of carcinoma of the large intestine is unknown, but pre-existing polyps and changes due to ulcerative colitis may be predisposing factors in its development. Both sexes show an equal incidence of this disease. It may occur in any site between the tip of the caecum and the anal canal but is seen most frequently in the rectum and sigmoid colon.

The growth may produce a large mass which projects into the lumen of the bowel, or may infiltrate the bowel producing a localized area of narrowing of the lumen. Intestinal obstruction is a common complication of advanced growths.

Metastases in lymph-glands usually occurs much earlier than do blood-borne metastases. The liver is the commonest site for the latter.

The growth, when advanced, may spread through the bowel wall and involve organs such as the bladder, small intestine or stomach. Peritoneal involvement results in **malignant ascites** (i.e. effusion into the peritoneal cavity), and involvement of other hollow organs in fistula formation, e.g. **vesico-colic fistula** when the bladder is involved; and **gastro-colic fistula** when a growth of the colon extends through the wall of the stomach.

The clinical features vary considerably according to the site of the carcinoma. In the left half of the colon alteration in bowel habit is often an early symptom. In the right half of the colon pain is often an early feature. In the rectum, passage of blood in the stools may be the first sign of the disease. Not infrequently a colonic carcinoma produces little in the way of clinical signs and symptoms until those of intestinal obstruction develop.

In investigating a suspected case of carcinoma of the large intestine, radiology plays a major role except with growths of the rectum. In this latter situation digital examination and visual inspection through a **proctoscope** are the essential diagnostic methods. In the distal part of the pelvic colon, it is to be stressed that radiological examination is complementary to **sigmoidoscopy.** Barium enema is the radiological method of choice in the investigation of all patients who are fit enough to undergo this examination.

The treatment of carcinoma of the large bowel is surgical whenever practicable. Treatment by radiotherapy is of value in certain cases of carcinoma of the rectum employed either in combination with surgery, or by itself.

(*d*) **Intussusception**—In this condition a portion of the bowel wall invaginates into the lumen of the portion of the bowel immediately distal to it.

Cochrane Shanks (3) describes an intussusception as consisting of three concentric tubes, i.e. an entering tube, a returning tube and a receiving tube or sheath.

The invaginating process tends to be progressive once it has started, and the blood vessels which supply the bowel are dragged into the intussusception. As the condition advances, interference with the blood supply may be such as to cause gangrene of the affected parts of the bowel wall.

Intussusception occurs most commonly in the first two years of life but is occasionally seen in older children and adults.

The chief clinical features are intermittent attacks of colic and the passage of blood and mucus per rectum. A sausage-shaped tumour may be palpable in the abdomen. Later, there is a vomiting due to intestinal obstruction.

The diagnosis can usually be made clinically, but a barium enema may be required to demonstrate the nature of the condition when the clinical signs are not clear-cut. In some centres, reduction of intussusceptions by barium enema is practised as a therapeutic measure. In this country, however, surgical reduction is generally considered the treatment of choice.

VOLVULUS OF THE INTESTINE

This is a condition in which a segment of the intestine becomes twisted around its long axis. It can occur in either small or large intestine, but in the majority of instances it is seen in the pelvic colon of elderly subjects. The twisting of the bowel results in intestinal obstruction. Valuable evidence regarding the presence of volvulus may be obtained from plain radiographs, and barium enema examination may also be requested if the patient is fit enough.

Treatment is surgical.

INTESTINAL OBSTRUCTION

The nature of this condition is self-explanatory. In intestinal obstruction the normal onward passage of faeces and **flatus** (i.e. intestinal gas) is markedly delayed, or completely prevented, according to whether the lumen of the bowel is partially or totally blocked. The obstruction may result from disease of the intestinal wall, external pressure on the intestinal wall, or causes within the lumen of the bowel.

As regards the first cause: changes in the bowel wall resulting from diverticulitis, carcinoma, regional enteritis, tuberculosis of the small intestine may all result in intestinal obstruction. Fibrous strictures resulting from colitis may also be a cause of the condition and the twisting of the bowel wall which occurs in intestinal volvulus, inevitably causes obstruction.

Among the external causes of intestinal obstruction are constriction of the bowel wall by peritoneal adhesions, pressure from a pelvic tumour, and pressure on the bowel walls by the edges of a hernial orifice (see p. 130).

Impacted foreign bodies: impaction of a large gall-stone which has ulcerated through the gall-bladder wall into the bowel; and masses of inspissated faeces resulting from severe chronic constipation, are some of the factors within the actual lumen of the bowel which may cause blockage of the intestinal canal.

All the above causes of intestinal obstruction are mechanical in nature. There is also another important type of intestinal obstruction which is of nervous origin, and is due to paralysis of the musculature of the small bowel. This type is called **paralytic ileus,** and usually only affects the small bowel. It may occur as a complication following a major operation, in the course of **peritonitis** (inflammation of the peritoneum lining the abdominal cavity and covering the abdominal organs), as a sequel to injuries which cause haemorrhage into the retroperitoneal tissues, and following childbirth.

Intestinal obstruction may present as an acute or chronic condition. The chief clinical features are colicky pain, constipation, increasing distension of the abdomen and vomiting. There is also accompanying toxaemia due to absorption of toxins from the stagnant intestinal contents.

Plain radiography is often of great assistance in establishing the diagnosis of intestinal obstruction. In patients who are fit enough for contrast radiography the site of obstruction may be defined by a barium enema if it is in the large intestine, or by an opaque meal if in the small intestine. For this latter examination it is often advisable to use an iodine containing contrast medium, called gastrografin, instead of barium.

The treatment of intestinal obstruction is surgical.

10. MALABSORPTION SYNDROMES

The malabsorption syndromes comprise a large number of different disorders which possess the common characteristic of causing defective absorption of essential foodstuffs from the bowel into the blood stream.

The defective absorption may be due to damage to the mucosa of the small intestine, as occurs in certain intestinal diseases (e.g. coeliac disease, idiopathic steatorrhoea, tropical sprue); digestive disorder arising from disease of the biliary system or pancreas; and effects such as intestinal hurry which may sometimes result from certain operations on the alimentary canal (e.g. total or partial gastrectomy, small bowel resection).

Chronic diarrhoea is a usual feature of malabsorption syndromes and, in some, excessive amounts of fat are present in the stools. This latter condition is called **steatorrhoea.** It causes an abnormal appearance of the stools and biochemical testing of these will establish the presence of an abnormally high fat content.

Other common features of these syndromes are anaemia, debility and loss of weight and in some a bone disorder called **osteomalacia** (see p. 231) may develop owing to defective absorption of Vitamin D and calcium.

Radiological investigation is of help in many cases and biopsy of the jejunal mucosa may yield information of considerable value in patients in whom there is disease of the small bowel mucosa.

Coeliac disease is a disease of infancy and childhood in which there is steathorrhoea, anaemia and retardation of growth. Absorption of fats and carbohydrates is deficient and may result in a type of rickets called coeliac rickets.

5

Coeliac disease is thought to be due to an abnormal sensitivity to gluten, a substance found in wheat flour and other cereals.

Idiopathic steatorrhoea (Non-tropical sprue) is a condition allied to coeliac disease but occurring in adults. It is thought also to be due to gluten sensitivity.

Tropical Sprue—bears some similarity to idiopathic steatorrhoea but is believed to be caused by defective absorption of folic acid, a vitamin belonging to the Vitamin B complex. It is a disease of warm climates, and steatorrhoea is one of its main features.

Among the many other causes of malabsorption syndromes may be mentioned **blind loop syndrome**—a condition in which features of malabsorption develop as a result of the presence of a blind loop of bowel (in most instances due to surgery) in which there is stasis of bowel contents and infection; and **Whipple's disease**—a rare condition in which steatorrhoea is associated with chronic polyarthritis (inflammatory changes in many joints) and widespread enlargement of lymph glands.

11. HERNIAS

The term **hernia** describes a protrusion of any structure through the wall of the cavity in which it is normally contained.

The opening through which a hernia protrudes is known as a **hernial orifice** and may be:

(i) an opening which is normally present, e.g. hiatus hernia—a projection of stomach through the oesophageal hiatus in the diaphragm;

(ii) an opening due to developmental defect, e.g. hernia through a development defect in the diaphragm;

(iii) an acquired opening, e.g. an **incisional hernia** where the herniated structures protrude through an area of weakness caused by a surgical incision.

In the abdomen hernias which project through the walls of the abdominal cavity are called **external hernias,** and the most important of these are: (i) **inguinal hernia,** in which the hernia protrudes through the inguinal canal, or through part of this canal. An inguinal hernia may form a bulge in the groin, or in a male may descend into the scrotum (scrotal hernia) and in a female into the labium majus (labial hernia); (ii) **femoral hernia**—the hernia protrudes through the femoral canal in the upper part of the thigh; (iii) **umbilical hernia**—the hernia protrudes through the umbilicus or, in adults, just above or to the side of the umbilicus.

Abdominal hernias which protrude through some opening, congenital or acquired, in the interior of the abdominal cavity are called **internal** hernias. They are uncommon but may cause intestinal obstruction.

Hernias are described as **reducible** or **irreducible** according to whether, or not, the hernial contents can be returned back through the hernial orifice through which they are protruding. When, as is frequently the case, a portion of the small or large intestine is present in an irreducible hernia, pressure of the margins of the hernial orifice on the bowel frequently results in the development of intestinal obstruction. Such pressure may also deprive the hernial contents of their normal blood supply and eventually result in necrosis and gangrene. A hernia, in which there is such impairment of blood supply, is known as a **strangulated hernia.**

12. DISEASES OF THE LIVER

Congenital abnormalities are rare in the liver. One condition of interest is called **polycystic disease of the liver** and may be associated with a similar disorder known as congenital polycystic kidneys.

As regards traumatic disorders, **rupture of the liver** not infrequently occurs as a result of the more severe types of injury to the upper abdomen and lower thorax, especially in crush injuries. The liver being a very vascular organ, tears in its substance may cause much bleeding into the peritoneum. The presence of blood in the peritoneal cavity is termed **haemoperitoneum.**

The liver may be the site of certain infective diseases, of infestation with worms and other parasites and of primary and secondary neoplasms. Amongst its other disorders, of considerable interest are several types of disease associated with permanent damage to liver cells, resulting from infection, poisoning, and deficiencies in diet.

As the portal vein carries venous blood from the stomach, intestine, spleen and pancreas to the liver, it will also be convenient to refer here to certain terms relating to disorders of the portal circulation.

INFECTIVE DISEASES

(*a*) **Viral hepatitis**—this term indicates two distinct types of inflammation of the liver due to virus infection: i.e. (i) **infective hepatitis,** wherein sufferers and carriers of the disease excrete the causal virus in their faeces and spread of the disease occurs as a result of faecal contamination of food and water; and (ii) **serum hepatitis** (syringe hepatitis) which is transmitted only by injection of whole blood, serum or plasma containing the causal virus, or by use of syringes and needles which have been contaminated by infected blood and imperfectly sterilized.

Clinically, the two types of viral hepatitis show a marked similarity; although serum hepatitis has a longer incubation period, and infective hepatitis may produce large epidemics under conditions in which hygienic standards are low. Both take the form of a febrile illness accompanied in most cases by jaundice and hepatomegaly (enlargement of the liver).

Complete recovery occurs in most cases, but occasionally permanent damage to liver cells may result, causing some form of liver necrosis or cirrhosis (see later). Viral hepatitis may thus sometimes lead to chronic hepatic disorders.

There is no specific treatment for viral hepatitis.

(*b*) **Bacterial infections—multiple hepatic abscesses** may form, in the course of a general septicaemia, when pyogenic bacteria are present in the systemic circulation and reach the liver via the hepatic artery. They may also develop as a result of a disorder of the biliary system called **infective cholangitis.** This infection may develop in conditions in which there is some obstruction to the flow of bile and occurs most commonly as a sequel to impaction of a gall-stone in the common bile duct.

Thirdly, multiple abscesses may result from the carriage of pyogenic bacteria in the portal vein from a septic focus in the area of drainage of this vein (e.g. a suppurating appendix). The presence of pus-producing bacteria in the portal circulation, together with the production of multiple liver abscesses, constitutes the disorder known as **portal pyaemia.** This condition is often associated with septic inflammatory changes of spreading type in the veins of the portal system, associated with clot formation, i.e. a septic thrombophlebitis which is referred to as **septic pylephlebitis.** Inflammation of veins is called **phlebitis,** and the prefix **pyle-** means "pertaining to the portal vein".

(*c*) **Amoebic hepatitis (Hepatic amoebiasis)**—is a term describing inflammatory changes in the liver resulting from infection with *entamoeba histolytica,* a protozoon which is the causal pathogen of amoebic dysentery. This infection may lead to the formation of an abscess within the liver, known as an **amoebic liver abscess** or **tropical abscess.**

(*d*) **Other Hepatic Infections**—among these are: hepatitis due to (i) **actinomycosis**; (ii) **Weil's disease** (leptospirosis), a spirochaetal disease of world-wide distribution which is carried by infected rats, who excrete the causal spirochaetes in their urine. It is characterized by a febrile illness accompanied by jaundice in many patients and by a purpuric rash and various types of haemorrhage; (iii) **Yellow fever**—a virus disease of the tropics carried by a mosquito called the *Aedes aegypti.* The name of this disease derives from the jaundice resulting from the inflammatory changes in the liver; (iv) **Visceral Leishmaniasis**—(Kala-azar) an infection of the cells of the reticulo-endothelial system in which lesions occur in the liver, spleen, other organs and lymph glands. It is due to a protozoon called *Leishmania donovani,* and transmitted by sandflies.

DISEASES DUE TO PARASITIC WORMS AND FLUKES

These diseases are more properly referred to as **infestations** rather than infections, as they are caused by parasitic organisms which consist of more than one cell. (*Note:* infections are caused by pathogenic micro-organisms, i.e. bacteria, viruses, rickettsiae, fungi and protozoa; all of which are single celled organisms.)

Among the diseases of this type, in which clinical signs and symptoms result from infestations of the liver are: **hydatid (echinococcus) disease** of the liver; **clonorchiasis,** a tropical disease due to Chinese liver fluke, and infestation with the sheep liver fluke.

Hydatid disease (Echinococcus disease) — is due to *taenia echinococcus,* a small tapeworm which is a parasite of dogs, who excrete its ova in their faeces. If these ova are ingested by man they may develop into larvae and, after penetrating the intestinal wall, settle in some site such as the liver or less commonly in tissues such as the lungs, spleen, bone, etc. A larva that survives may then develop into a hydatid cyst.

Hydatid cysts occur most frequently in the liver, and in this organ usually only one cyst develops in any one individual. It may, however, attain a large size and require surgical treatment.

Suspected cases of hydatid disease are investigated by a blood test of the type called a complement fixation test and a skin test called the **Casoni intradermal test.** A blood count will frequently show an **eosinophilia,** i.e. increased numbers of circulating eosinophil leucocytes (white blood cells).

NEOPLASMS

The liver is a common site for metastases from primary carcinomas arising within the area of drainage of the portal vein (e.g. carcinomas of the stomach and large bowel) and metastases from other primary carcinomas (e.g. lung and breast) are also of frequent occurrence in this organ.

There is also a rare primary tumour of liver cells called a **malignant hepatoma.**

OTHER HEPATIC DISEASES

Included among these are a number of diseases, the clinical manifestations of which are the result of serious damage to liver cells. Such damage may be due to causes such as infective processes (e.g. viral hepatitis), to toxic agents of various types (e.g. certain drugs, chemical poisons, toxic substances present in the toxaemia of pregnancy called eclampsia), to deficiencies in diet and other factors.

The damage to the liver cells may be of rapid development and where extensive may produce a condition termed **acute massive liver necrosis,** which usually causes death from hepatic failure within a short period of time.

With less severe forms of acute liver necrosis, damaged cells may be replaced partly by regeneration of liver cells and partly by overgrowth of surrounding fibrous connective tissue, producing a type of disorder called **post-necrotic cirrhosis** (see later).

Damage to liver cells of a slower onset is also associated with the presence of fibrosis and areas of regenerated liver cells resulting in the development of certain other forms of cirrhosis of the liver. (*Note:* the liver is one of the organs whose specialized cells retain their powers of multiplication throughout life and can thus to some extent undergo the form of repair called regeneration).

Some of the clinical disorders occurring as a result of acute or chronic liver damage are:

(*a*) **Acute Massive Liver Necrosis** (Acute Yellow Atrophy)—this uncommon disease may follow hepatic infections or poisonings, or rarely develop as a complication of eclampsia.

It produces features such as jaundice, haemorrhages and mental changes which, in this condition, are manifestations of **hepatic failure.** The disease usually terminates fatally with a form of coma, termed **hepatic coma,** preceding death.

(*b*) **Cirrhosis of the liver**—this is a disorder caused by damage to hepatic cells, and fibrosis is one of its principal features. Excess of fibrous tissue gives the liver a harder consistency than normal, and the word "cirrhosis" has thus come to indicate "hardening" or "fibrosis", although its correct meaning is "yellowish red" from the colour the organ may acquire in some forms of this disorder.

(i) **Portal cirrhosis** (Laennec's cirrhosis) is the commonest form of hepatic cirrhosis and is so called because the fibrosis usually commences around small branches of the portal vein. Previous infective diseases of the liver, deficiencies in diet and chronic alcoholism are factors which can operate in its causation. When it occurs in chronic alcoholics it may be referred to as **alcoholic cirrhosis.**

The extensive and widespread fibrosis which develops in this disease causes narrowing of many of the intrahepatic branches of the portal venous system, causing a rise in venous pressure through this system spoken of as **portal hypertension.**

One effect of the obstruction to the passage of portal blood through the liver is to cause dilatation of anastomotic (communicating) channels which connect the portal and systemic veins. One site for such channels is the mucosa at the lower end of the oesophagus, where the dilated veins are called **oesophageal varices** and may be demonstrable by barium swallow. They frequently bleed, causing haematemesis and melaena, and leading to the development of anaemia. Another effect of portal hypertension is to cause **ascites** (exudation of fluid from the blood into the peritoneal cavity).

Other clinical features are seen in portal cirrhosis which are due to impairment of various liver functions and the disease leads slowly, but ultimately, to hepatic failure.

Portal vein thrombosis occasionally develops as a complication of cirrhosis and also of a number of other conditions (e.g. pylephlebitis, etc.). Its presence may be demonstrated by an X-ray investigation called portal venography.

There is no specific treatment for cirrhosis but medical measures (e.g. appropriate diet, administration of diuretics) may arrest deterioration of the disease for a long time. Emergency surgery may be required for haemorrhage and, in selected patients, surgical measures may be employed to reduce the portal venous pressure, e.g. portocaval anastomosis.

(ii) **Other types of hepatic cirrhosis**—these include **obstructive biliary cirrhosis,** associated with obstructive jaundice and resulting from long-standing obstruction to the biliary system; **haemachromatosis** (bronze diabetes), a disease in which there is an error of iron metabolism;

and **post-necrotic cirrhosis** which has already been mentioned as a sequel to the less severe forms of acute liver necrosis.

13. DISEASES OF THE BILIARY SYSTEM

The biliary system comprises the gall-bladder and the intrahepatic and extrahepatic bile ducts. Bile is formed in the liver and carried through the bile ducts into the duodenum, being concentrated in the gall-bladder on its way through the biliary system.

The pigment called **bilirubin,** is formed from the haemoglobin of red cells, whose life in the circulation is finished. It is carried to the liver and excreted by hepatic cells in the bile. If excessive amounts of bilirubin accumulate in the circulating blood, the skin and mucous membranes acquire a yellowish tinge and **jaundice** is then said to be present. Alternatively, but less commonly the condition may be called **icterus.**

The word "jaundice" derives from the French word "jaune", meaning yellow.

Excessive amounts of bilirubin in the blood can result from: (i) excessive breakdown of red cells as in **haemolytic jaundice**; (ii) failure of normal excretion of bilirubin in the bile as a result of damage to liver cells—**hepatic jaundice** (parenchymatous jaundice); (iii) obstruction to the flow of bile into the duodenum—**obstructive jaundice.**

The two commonest disorders affecting the biliary system are cholecystitis and gall-stones, and these often co-exist in the same patient.

CHOLECYSTITIS

Chole—means "bile", **"cyst"** means a bladder. The name of this condition thus indicates inflammation of the gall bladder. The word **gall** is a synonym of "bile".

Cholecystitis may present in acute or chronic form and either form is often associated with gall-stones.

The inflammatory changes are usually due to infection with a mixture of pathogenic microbes, i.e. a so-called **non-specific infection,** except in those uncommon instances when cholecystitis occurs as a complication of typhoid or paratyphoid fever, and is due to a **specific infection** with typhoid or paratyphoid bacilli.

The infection of **acute cholecystitis** frequently develops as a secondary result of blockage of the cystic duct (i.e. the duct which leads from the gall-bladder and joins the common hepatic duct to form the common bile duct), by an impacted gall-stone. A patient with **acute cholecystitis** is usually very ill with pain in the upper right side of the upper abdomen and sometimes also in the right shoulder-blade, or tip of the right shoulder; fever and increased pulse-rate. Cholecystography is contra-indicated in this condition, but plain X-rays are frequently requested to see if any opaque gall-stones are present.

Chronic cholecystitis may develop insidiously, or may be the sequel to an attack of acute cholecystitis. It is much commoner in females than in males, and uncommon before middle age is reached. Common symptoms are indigestion, flatulence, intolerance to fatty foods, pain in the right side of the upper abdomen and sometimes also in the right shoulder-blade, or tip of the right shoulder and periodic attacks of vomiting. Both oral and intravenous cholecystography are extensively used in the investigation of this disease.

Acute cholecystitis is usually treated medically until the acute inflammation has subsided. Surgical treatment is then carried out. Chronic cholecystitis may be treated either medically or surgically; surgical treatment is usually advised in patients who are suitable for operation.

GALL-STONES (CHOLELITHIASIS)

Gall-stones are formed as a result of precipitation from the bile of one or more of its main constituents. They are of three main types: (*a*) **cholesterol stones;** (*b*) **bile pigment stones;** (*c*) **mixed stones** consisting of a mixture of cholesterol, bile pigment and calcium. (*Note:* **cholesterol** is a fatty substance normally present in the bile.)

They are frequently found in association with cholecystitis, and are commoner in women than in men. Their maximum incidence occurs in middle age. They are occasionally seen in children who suffer from an uncommon blood disease known as **acholuric jaundice.**

Gall-stones which remain confined in the gall-bladder may be symptomless. If, however, one or more stones pass out of this organ and lodge in either the cystic or common bile ducts, severe cramp-like pains called **biliary colic** are caused.

Impaction of a stone in the common bile duct may block the duct and cause jaundice of the obstructive type. Persistence of this condition may in the course of time lead to the liver disease called **obstructive biliary cirrhosis.** Impaction of a stone in this site may also lead to an ascending infection of the bile ducts termed **infective cholangitis.** As has been noted when discussing hepatic infections, infective cholangitis can result in the formation of multiple liver abscesses.

As was noted when discussing intestinal obstruction, gall-stones occasionally ulcerate through the gall-bladder wall into the bowel. A large gall-stone may then cause obstruction of the lumen of the bowel.

Cases suspected of having gall-stones are investigated radiologically by plain films and oral or intravenous cholecystography.

Treatment of gall-stones which are causing symptoms is by surgery.

OTHER DISEASES OF THE BILIARY SYSTEM

Among these are the following:

(*a*) **Cholesterosis**—more commonly called **"strawberry gall-bladder"**, a condition in which multiple small deposits of cholesterol (a fatty substance, normally present in bile) are found in the mucosa lining the gall-bladder. Kerley (4) classifies this disease as a form of mild chronic inflammation of the gall-bladder.

(*b*) **Carcinoma of the gall-bladder**—an uncommon type of carcinoma. Irritation of the mucosa by gall-stones is thought to play a part in the causation of some cases.

(*c*) **Cholangitis**—this term means inflammation of the bile ducts. **Infective cholangitis** is a not uncommon complication when a gall-stone becomes impacted in the common bile duct.

(*d*) **Biliary fistula**—a fistula may develop in connection with the biliary system either as a result of disease, or following a surgical operation. Biliary fistulae, according to their cause, may open on the surface of the body or into the stomach, duodenum, small intestine or colon. E.g. **cholecysto-gastric fistula**—connecting the gall-bladder and stomach; **choledocho-duodenal fistula**—connecting the common bile duct and duodenum.

14. DISEASES OF THE PANCREAS

The pancreas contains cells, arranged in lobules, which produce digestive enzymes and collections of endocrine cells, the so-called islet cells, which constitute the islets of Langerhans and secrete the hormone insulin.

The digestive enzymes are discharged into the duodenum through the main and accessory pancreatic ducts, whilst insulin is secreted directly into the bloodstream.

Diseases of the pancreas are, with the exception of diabetes mellitus, uncommon and, apart from this disease, the most important are certain inflammations, pancreatic carcinoma, pancreatic cysts, and fibrocystic disease of the pancreas.

Diabetes mellitus is generally classified as an endocrine disorder, and thus will be discussed in Section I.

INFLAMMATIONS

(*a*) **Acute Pancreatitis** (Acute Haemorrhagic Pancreatitis, Acute Pancreatic Necrosis)—an acute inflammatory disorder, the cause of which is unknown. In a proportion of cases, there appears to be some association between this disorder and infection of the bile ducts. In others a blood-borne infection has been suggested as a likely cause of the inflammation.

The inflammatory changes are generally severe and may result in haemorrhages within the gland, necrosis of its cells, and digestion of pancreatic tissue by its own enzymes which are set free by the disease processes. Self-digestion of this type is called **autolysis** or **autodigestion.**

Acute pancreatitis rarely occurs before middle age. Its onset is usually sudden with severe abdominal pain, shock and vomiting. Mild jaundice develops in many patients, and in a few an appearance of bruising appears in the loins. This latter is due to extravasation of blood from the inflamed pancreas, and its spreading through the soft tissues. (*Note:* **extravasation** means an escape of fluid from the vessel, space or cavity in which it is normally contained).

The pancreatic enzyme concerned with carbohydrate digestion is called amylase and, in acute pancreatitis this substance may be demonstrated in greatly increased amounts in blood serum, during the early stages of the disease.

Acute pancreatitis is difficult to diagnose clinically, and the nature of the condition is frequently often first discovered at operation. If, however, a definite diagnosis of this condition can be made without diagnostic laparotomy (p. 145), conservative (i.e. non-operative treatment) is most usually advocated.

(*b*) **Subacute Pancreatitis**—a relatively mild form of inflammation which may sometimes complicate mumps and certain other infective diseases.

(*c*) **Chronic Pancreatitis**—a chronic inflammatory condition, which may occur as a sequel to acute pancreatitis or chronic alcoholism and, in many instances, is associated with the presence of gall-stones. It produces diffuse fibrosis and may cause abdominal pain and steatorrhoea; and also diabetes mellitus if the endocrine cells in the organ are involved by the disease processes.

Obstructive jaundice may be a serious complication as a result of compression, by fibrous tissue, of the lower part of the common bile duct where it lies in its groove on the posterior aspect of the head of the pancreas.

Various surgical procedures may be employed in treatment, e.g. partial pancreatectomy.

NEOPLASMS

(*a*) **Carcinoma of the Pancreas**—this is not a very common type of malignant neoplasm. The most usual site for its origin is in the head of the gland and here it may grow so as to cause blockage of the common bile duct and resultant obstructive jaundice.

Pain is a usual feature of the disease and signs of disordered pancreatic function such as glycosuria (sugar in the urine) and steatorrhoea (excess of fat in the stools) are not infrequent.

Pancreatic carcinomas often displace or infiltrate the stomach and those arising in the head of the pancreas may cause deformity of the duodenum, thus producing signs which may be detectable by appropriate forms of radiological investigation.

(*b*) **Islet Cell Tumour** (Insulinoma)—a name given to a rare and usually benign tumour of the endocrine cells of the islets of Langerhans. Tumours of this type, which may be either single or multiple, are associated with excessive secretion of insulin.

CYSTS

Various types of **true pancreatic cysts** may occur, e.g. retention cysts, neoplastic cysts, hydatids, etc., and may attain a large size. There also arise in connection with this gland what are called **pancreatic pseudocysts,** i.e. false cysts.

A pseudocyst usually forms within a recess in the peritoneal cavity, called the lesser sac, and contains fluid which has leaked from the pancreas as a result of traumatic injury or severe inflammation of the gland.

OTHER DISEASES

MUCO-VISCIDOSIS (FIBROCYSTIC DISEASE OF THE
PANCREAS)

This is a generalized disease of glands which secrete mucus throughout the body. These glands when affected by muco-viscidosis, for some unknown cause, produce an abnormally viscid secretion. This results in obstruction of ducts and secondary effects, of a serious nature, in the intestinal tract and the lungs.

Duct obstruction may lead to fibrosis and cyst formation in the pancreas, hence the name of **fibrocystic disease** or **cystic fibrosis of the pancreas.**

Clinical signs of muco-viscidosis may appear during the first few days after birth when absence of mucus from the stools may result in solidification of the intestinal contents, and resultant intestinal obstruction which is usually fatal. The intestinal contents of a newly born baby are known as **meconium,** and this manifestation of the disease is called **meconium ileus.**

In other older infants, the disease may take the form of a fatty diarrhoea. The stearrhoea results from a deficiency of digestive enzymes normally secreted by the pancreas and this type of the disease constitutes one variety of malabsorption syndrome.

Mucus secreting glands in the mucosa of the bronchi are frequently involved in muco-viscidosis, and many of the infants with fatty diarrhoea subsequently develop recurrent lung infections which lead eventually to permanent lung damage. The lung changes are demonstrable radiologically.

15. SUBPHRENIC ABSCESS

This condition is conveniently discussed here, as it is a not infrequent complication of certain diseases of the digestive system, and it may also follow certain abdominal operations.

The term **subphrenic** means "under the diaphragm" and **subdiaphragmatic abscess** is another name for this condition. A subphrenic abscess can be caused by a blood-borne infection. It is usually due, however, to infective material reaching the area below the diaphragm from some intra-abdominal lesion, such as a perforated peptic ulcer, or perforated appendix: or as a result of certain surgical operations on the stomach, duodenum, intestine or biliary tract.

Pleural effusion or pneumonitis (inflammation of lung tissue), or a mixture of both, frequently develop in the region of the base of the lung on the affected side when a subphrenic abscess is present.

A subphrenic abscess causes fever, increased pulse rate and general malaise, together with pain in the region of the abscess, and often pain in the shoulder blade on the affected side. Examination of the blood shows a marked increase in the numbers of circulating polymorphs.

Radiological examination frequently gives considerable help in diagnosis, particularly if the abscess cavity contains a fluid level or, if on screening, restriction or absence of diaphragmatic movement is demonstrated on the side of the suspected abscess.

16. PNEUMOPERITONEUM

The presence of air or other gas in the peritoneal cavity is called **pneumoperitoneum.**

This condition occurs as a result of **laparotomy** (i.e. the surgical operation of making an opening into the abdominal cavity). It is also produced by perforation of the stomach or intestine as a result of disease or trauma. Perforation of a peptic ulcer is a common cause.

SOME OPERATIONS ON THE DIGESTIVE SYSTEM

A. MOUTH AND PHARYNX

(*a*) **Glossectomy**—Excision of the tongue, total or partial.

(*b*) **Pharyngectomy**—Excision of part of the pharynx.

B. OESOPHAGUS

(*a*) **Heller's operation**—An operation performed for relief of achalasia of the cardia; a longitudinal incision being made in the muscles around the narrow area at the lower end of the oesophagus and the mucous membrane being allowed to bulge through the gap.

(*b*) **Oesophagectomy**—Partial or complete removal of the oesophagus.

(*c*) **Oesophago-duodenostomy and oesophago-jejunostomy**—See under "total gastrectomy".

C. STOMACH AND DUODENUM

(*a*) **Gastrectomy**

(i) **Partial gastrectomy**—removal of part of the stomach. This operation is mainly performed for peptic ulceration and for early carcinoma in the distal part of the stomach. The gastric remnant is made to open into either the duodenum, as in the **Billroth I** type of operation; or into the upper jejunum, as in the **Billroth II** and **Polya** types of partial gastrectomy. The new opening is termed a **stoma.**

(**Stomal ulceration,** i.e. peptic ulceration at the stoma is a rare sequel to partial gastrectomy but occurs rather more frequently after gastro-jejunostomy (see later). Other undesirable sequelae which may some-times follow partial gastrectomy are referred to as **post-gastrectomy syndromes.**)

(ii) **Total gastrectomy**—in this operation which is mainly performed for carcinoma of the stomach, the whole of the stomach is removed. The oesophagus is then made to open into the duodenum—**oesophago-duodenostomy** or, the cut end of the duodenum is closed and the oesophagus is made to open into the side of a loop of upper jejunum—**oesophago-jejunostomy.**

(*b*) **Vagotomy**—In this operation the lower parts of the right and left vagus nerves are divided, with the object of removing vagal nerve influences from the stomach and so reducing the secretion of acid.

As the vagus supplies motor fibres to the stomach, some form of drainage operation, in the form of gastro-jejunostomy or pyloroplasty (see below), is generally performed at the same time as the vagotomy to facilitate gastric emptying. Vagotomy together with a drainage operation is widely employed in the surgical treatment of chronic peptic ulcers, especially those occurring in the duodenum.

(*c*) **Gastro-jejunostomy (Gastro-enterostomy)**—In this operation no tissue is removed, but an opening is made between the stomach and one of the upper loops of the jejunum. A short circuit is thus provided whereby food can pass direct from the stomach into the upper part of the small intestine, without passing through the pylorus and duodenum. This operation is extensively used in cases of pyloric obstruction, due to either peptic ulceration or carcinoma. As in a partial gastrectomy, the new opening between the stomach and the intestine is called a **stoma.**

Gastro-jejunostomy may also be employed, as an alternative to partial gastrectomy, in certain cases of peptic ulceration uncomplicated by pyloric stenosis. It is then often combined with vagotomy (see above).

(*d*) **Pyloroplasty**—This is a reconstructive operation designed to enlarge the pylorus and facilitate emptying of the gastric contents into the duodenum. It is most often performed in association with vagotomy (see above).

(*e*) **Rammstedt's operation**—An operation, for the relief of congenital pyloric stenosis in infants, wherein the thickened muscles around the narrowed pyloric canal are incised longitudinally and the mucosa of the pyloric canal allowed to bulge through the gap.

D. INTESTINE

(*a*) **Appendicectomy**—Removal of the vermiform appendix.

(*b*) **Intestinal resection**—This term means removal of a portion of the intestine and includes:

(i) **Partial enterectomy**—removal of part of the small bowel.

(ii) **Partial colectomy**—removal of part of the colon.

(iii) **Total colectomy**—removal of the whole of the colon.

(iv) **Proctectomy**—excision of the rectum. This operation is usually performed through incisions made both into the abdominal cavity and perineum and is then termed **abdomino-perineal resection of the rectum.**

Following intestinal resection, **intestinal anastomosis** or alternatively **ileostomy** or **colostomy** are performed (see below).

(*c*) **Intestinal Anastomosis**—An operation of joining one portion of the bowel to another. It may be employed to join the cut ends of the intestine immediately after an intestinal resection; or at a later stage, when it is desired to close a temporary colostomy, or ileostomy, which has been made in conjunction with an intestinal resection. Alternatively, it may be used to short circuit an inoperable lesion which is causing obstruction of the bowel.

According to the manner in which the two portions of the bowel are joined, an anastomosis may be described as an **end-to-end, end-to-side,** or **lateral anastomosis.**

Examples of intestinal anastomosis are: (i) **ileo-colic anastomosis,** wherein the terminal ileum is joined to the left half of the transverse colon after removal of the right half of the colon and the caecum, and (ii) **ileo-rectal anastomosis** following total colectomy.

(*d*) **Colostomy and Ileostomy**—These are two types of operation wherein a portion of bowel is made to open on the anterior abdominal wall, thus providing a permanent or temporary artificial anus through which the faeces are discharged. If the portion of bowel employed in this manner is part of the colon, the operation is called **colostomy;** or if part of the ileum, **ileostomy.**

Operations of this type are chiefly performed in cases of intestinal obstruction. Ileostomy may be also used to rest the inflamed bowel in ulcerative colitis.

E. PORTAL VEIN

Porto-caval Anastomosis—An operation for the relief of portal hypertension wherein the distal part of the portal vein is made to open into the inferior vena cava.

F. BILIARY TRACT

(*a*) **Cholecystectomy**—Removal of the gall-bladder.

Symptoms of biliary disease, occurring after removal of the gall bladder, are referred to as **post-cholecystectomy symptoms** and may be investigated by intravenous cholangiography. Laws (5) states that the commonest cause of such symptoms is the presence of stones within the common bile duct.

(*b*) **Cholecystostomy**—Opening and drainage of the gall-bladder.

(*c*) **Choledochotomy**—Opening of the common bile duct. Usually employed in order that the interior of the duct may be explored for the presence of gall-stones.

(*d*) **Choledochostomy**—Drainage of the common bile duct. Post-operative cholangiography is performed by injection of contrast medium through the drainage tube inserted at this operation.

(*e*) **Cholecysto-gastrostomy**—The making of an opening, between the gall-bladder and stomach, to short-circuit a lesion which is causing obstruction of the common bile duct.

(*f*) **Cholecysto-duodenostomy**—The making of an opening between the gall-bladder and duodenum. Used for the same purpose as cholecysto-gastrostomy.

G. PANCREAS

Pancreatectomy—Total or partial removal of the pancreas.

H. DIAGNOSTIC LAPAROTOMY

An operation wherein the abdominal cavity is opened in order to inspect the organs of the digestive system or other structures. This operation is frequently indicated when other investigations have failed to establish a cause for abdominal symptoms.

REFERENCES

(1) Illingworth, Sir Charles. *A Short Textbook of Surgery.* J. and A. Churchill, 1965.
(2) Bodian, M., Stephens, F. D. and Ward, B. C. H. *Lancet* 1948, No. 6.
(3) Shanks, S. Cochrane. *A Textbook of X-ray Diagnosis* (British Authors). H. K. Lewis, 1958.
(4) Kerley, Peter. *A Textbook of X-ray Diagnosis* (British Authors). H. K. Lewis, 1958.
(5) Laws, J. W. *Recent Advances in Radiology* (Ed. T. Lodge). J. and A. Churchill, 1964.

Section D. THE URINARY SYSTEM AND MALE REPRODUCTIVE SYSTEM

1. SOME ANATOMICAL AND PHYSIOLOGICAL CONSIDERATIONS

The **urinary system** consists of the *kidneys, ureters,* the *urinary bladder* and the *urethra. Urine* is secreted by the kidneys, these organs being concerned with the excretion of the waste products of metabolism and of foreign substances from the body, the maintenance of a normal water balance and normal balance of *electrolytes* (i.e. inorganic ions such as sodium, potassium, calcium, bicarbonate, chloride, phosphate, etc.) in the blood and tissue fluids. In the exercise of this latter function the kidneys are thus concerned with the maintenance of a normal reaction (*acid-base balance*) in the blood and tissue fluids.

The **male reproductive system** comprises the *testes* and *epididymes*: the *vasa deferentia,* the *seminal vesicles* and *ejaculatory ducts*: the *prostate gland:* and the greater part of the *urethra.* This last-named structure is, in the male, common during most of its length, to both the reproductive system and to the urinary system. (Note: in the female the two systems are entirely separate as far as the point where the lower end of the urethra opens into the vulva).

The testes are the reproductive glands of the male and produce the male germ cells, called *spermatozoa,* and secrete the male sex hormone, *testosterone.* The testes occupy the *scrotum.* The distal part of the urethra is contained within the penis.

The prefixes **reno-** and **nephro-** both mean "pertaining to the kidney", **pyelo-** "pertaining to the pelvis of the kidney, and **cysto-** and **vesico** "pertaining to the bladder". **Orchi-** and **orchid-** mean "pertaining to the testis".

2. SOME GENERAL ASPECTS OF DISEASES OF THE URINARY AND MALE REPRODUCTIVE SYSTEMS

Both these systems may be affected by congenital abnormalities, traumatic conditions, infective and other inflammatory conditions, neoplasms and other types of acquired disease.

Among the clinical signs and symptoms of these diseases may be mentioned **albuminuria** (the passage of the protein called albumen in the urine), **dysuria** (difficulty in passing urine), **haematuria** (blood in the urine), **pyuria** (pus in the urine), **retention** (inability to void urine from the bladder, **anuria** (suppression of the excretion of urine from the kidneys), **incontinence of urine** (inability to control the emptying of urine from the bladder), **oliguria** (passing of urine in amounts which are much less and more concentrated than the normal), **polyuria** (passing excessive amounts of dilute urine), painful micturition (i.e. pain on passing urine), scalding micturition; palpable swellings of the kidney, prostate gland, testes and epididymis; pain in the loin, bladder region or testis; pain of the type termed **renal colic** (see p. 156).

It is also to be noted that high blood pressure may be a sign of kidney disease (see "hypertension of renal origin").

The branch of medicine concerned with diseases of the urinary system is called **urology.**

Surgical disorders of the urinary system in both sexes and the male reproductive system fall within the province of the branch of surgery called **genito-urinary surgery,** whereas surgical disorders of the female reproductive system are the concern of the gynaecologist.

Certain of the infective diseases which affect the male reproductive system are of venereal origin and reference has already been made to these in Part III. (See "Venereal Diseases).

3. SPECIAL METHODS OF INVESTIGATION

(*a*) **Urine Examination**—investigations under this heading include naked eye examination of the urine for abnormal colouration, presence of threads, etc.; determination of reaction and specific gravity of the urine; microscopic examination for blood cells, pus cells, crystals, and abnormal structures formed under certain disease conditions in the kidney tubules and called **urinary casts** (renal casts); bacteriological examination and culture to determine the nature of infective organisms excreted in the urine; and chemical tests to investigate the presence of abnormal substances such as albumen and blood in the urine. Chemical examination of the urine may also be employed in certain tests of renal function (see later) and quantitative examinations may be carried out to determine whether normal urinary constituents such as chlorides, calcium, etc., are present in normal or abnormal amounts.

(*b*) **Blood Examinations**—in a number of types of urinary disease, damage to renal cells may diminish the ability of the kidneys to excrete waste products of metabolism. Substances such as urea and creatinine, which are breakdown products of protein metabolism, may then be show to be present in the circulating blood in amounts above the normal, by various forms of quantitative chemical tests. The best known of such tests is the **blood urea estimation.**

(*c*) **Renal Function Tests**—reference was made to the various functions of the kidneys on p. 146.

Urine is formed in these organs by filtration through capillary tufts called **renal glomeruli.** This filtrate then passes through structures in the solid part of the kidney called **renal tubules** before being collected in the renal pelvis and calyces and passed down the ureters. In the tubules, according to the current needs of the body, the urine is concentrated by reabsorption of water and electrolytes (e.g. sodium, potassium, calcium, etc.) and various other substances (e.g. glucose, urea, etc.) are also reabsorbed. These processes are referred to as **selective tubular reabsorption.**

Renal function tests may be designed to investigate either the function of the glomeruli (e.g. blood urea estimation, urea clearance test, creatinine clearance test) or of the tubules (e.g. urine concentration test, estimation of amounts of various electrolytes in the blood plasma or urine, etc.).

(*d*) **Radiological Investigations**—certain information regarding the urinary system can be obtained from plain X-rays but many patients with suspected urinary disease require some form of **contrast urography.** This term includes the examination generally described as **intravenous pyelography** (I.V.P.), but more correctly termed **intravenous urography** as the investigation is not confined to demonstration of the renal pelvis, but also comprises the taking of films to show the ureters and bladder. Radiological investigation also includes the examinations of **retrograde urography** (retrograde pyelography), **conventional and micturating cystography** (contrast-radiography of the bladder) and **urethrography** (contrast-radiography of the urethra).

In selected cases it may be desirable to demonstrate the renal blood vessels by performing **aortography** or **selective renal angiography.**

Radioactive isotopes may be employed in **radioactive renography** to investigate renal function and may also be utilized to demonstrate renal tumours.

(*e*) **Visual Inspection by Special Instruments**—the interior of the urethra may be inspected by a panendoscope and that of the bladder by a cystoscope, these procedures being termed respectively **urethroscopy** and **cystoscopy.**

Biopsy of lesions in the bladder may be carried out during cystoscopy.

(*f*) **Renal biopsy**—the taking of a minute fragment of renal tissue for microscopic examination.

4. DISEASES OF THE KIDNEYS AND URETERS. CONGENITAL ABNORMALITIES

A large number of developmental abnormalities may occur in the kidneys and ureters. Many are of a minor nature and the more marked of them are not very common. They include:—

(*a*) **Congenital Absence of one Kidney**—a serious disability if the patient's only kidney becomes diseased.

(*b*) **Ectopic Kidney**—the term **ectopic** means "abnormally placed" or "displaced". As a result of developmental error an ectopic kidney lies in the pelvic cavity or lower abdomen.

(*c*) **Congenital Hypoplastic Kidney**—a kidney which fails to develop normally both as regards size and in the development of its internal structure.

(*d*) **Horseshoe Kidney**—a condition of which there is a partial fusion of the two kidneys. The fusion is usually between the lower poles, which are joined by a band of renal tissue which lies in front of the spine.

(*e*) **Duplex Kidney** (Duplication of the Renal Pelvis)—in this anomaly, which may be present on one or both sides, the renal pelvis consists of two partial or complete divisions. In the latter instance there is usually an associated partial or complete duplication of the ureter.

(*f*) **Congenital Polycystic Kidneys**—in this condition the kidneys are enlarged and contain numerous thin-walled cysts. It is due to developmental error and, although present at birth, symptoms do not appear until adult life is reached. Haematuria is a common symptom. Hypertension (high blood pressure) may develop as a complication of the disease.

The cysts cause deformity of the renal pelves and calyces, which is demonstrable by urography.

(*g*) **"Sponge Kidney"**—a congenital abnormality of the kidneys in which there is widespread dilatation of renal tubules and associated cyst formation. There is often some accompanying degree of **nephrocalcinosis** i.e. deposition of calcium salts in the solid part of the kidneys.

TRAUMATIC CONDITIONS

Injuries in the region of the loin (e.g. blows, kicks, crushing injuries) may result in (i) bruising referred to as **contusion of the kidney;** (ii) tearing of kidney substance when the condition is referred to as **ruptured kidney**; or, rarely, (iii) tearing through of the renal pedicle with separation of the kidney from its ureter and renal artery and veins. This is termed **total avulsion of the kidney,** the word "avulsion" meaning "tearing off" and being sometimes also employed in the description of fractures and injuries elsewhere in the body.

Haematuria is a usual feature of renal trauma. Intravenous urography is indicated in all suspected cases, not only to try and obtain information regarding kidney damage but also to assess the state of the uninjured kidney; this being of considerable importance if the case is one in which surgical treatment is required.

INFECTIVE DISEASES

Pathogenic micro-organisms may reach the kidney by the blood stream or by ascending up the ureter from the lower part of the urinary tract.

Hodson and Edwards (1) have shown that, in a high proportion of patients with chronic kidney infection, **vesico-ureteric reflux,** i.e. reflux of urine from the bladder, back into the ureter, occurs on one or both sides. Such reflux can be demonstrated by a form of contrast radiography termed **micturating cystography** and it is thought to afford a ready means by which infection may be carried by infected urine from the bladder up to the kidney.

In the urinary system any condition which produces any degree of obstruction to the normal flow of urine, through the system to the exterior, predisposes to infection above the site of the obstruction. Abnormal delay in the passage of urine through the urinary system is referred to as **urinary stasis.**

The principal infective diseases found in the kidney are:

(*a*) **Pyelonephritis**—this term indicates that both the renal pelvis and its calyces (i.e. the hollow part of the kidney) together with the solid part of the kidney are affected by inflammatory changes resulting from an infection (other than a tuberculous infection), i.e. there is **pyelitis** (inflammation of the renal pelvis and calyces) plus **nephritis** (inflammation of the renal substance).

The use of the term "pyelitis" alone seems to be falling into disuse with general acceptance of the view that in practically all cases of the infection of renal pelvis, the kidney substance is also involved to some extent.

Acute pyelonephritis is predominantly a disease of females. Pregnancy appears to be a predisposing factor but this infection can occur at any age. It sometimes occurs in males, generally as a complication in disorders causing urinary stasis.

The most frequent causal pathogen is a bacterium called the *escherichia coli* or *bacillus coli*, which is a normal inhabitant of the human instestinal tract.

The infection usually affects only one kidney but may be bilateral. Common symptoms are pain in the loin, frequent and painful micturition, pyrexia, tachycardia and **rigors**, i.e. shivering attacks.

The infecting micro-organisms may be cultured from the urine and, when the acute attack has subsided, radiological investigation may be requested to exclude associated abnormalities in the urinary system.

Chronic Pyelonephritis—this disease, which may also be unilateral or bilateral, may develop as a sequel to acute pyelonephritis or may be of chronic nature from its outset. It is often associated with some pre-existing disease, congenital or acquired, in the urinary system and with vesico-ureteric reflux (see p. 150). Radiological examination is thus an important procedure and may not infrequently show evidence of an obstructive lesion in the lower urinary tract, as well as changes in the kidneys typical of the disease.

Common long term results of chronic pyelonephritis are scarring of affected kidneys, the development of hypertension (high blood pressure) and renal failure.

Treatment is by sulphonamides or antibiotics.

(*b*) **Pyonephrosis**—a condition in which the renal pelvis and its calyces are dilated and filled with pus (cf. hydronephrosis in which the dilated pelvis and calyces are filled with urine). The dilatation is caused by some form of obstruction to the outflow of urine from the renal pelvis, e.g. by a calculus (stone) impacted in the ureter, and the pus is produced as a result of supervening infection with pyogenic bacteria.

(*c*) **Renal Carbuncle** (Carbuncle of the Kidney)—a carbuncle is an inflammatory mass that breaks down to form multiple small abscess cavities. Renal carbuncle is usually due to a blood-borne infection with *staphylococci* derived from some other focus of infection such as a boil in the skin.

(*d*) **Perinephric Abscess** (Perirenal Abscess)—this is an abscess which forms in the fatty tissues around the kidney. It may be due to blood-borne infection or direct spread of infection from a lesion within the kidney.

(*e*) **Renal Tuberculosis**—tuberculosis infection of the kidney is due to blood-borne infection. The causative *tubercle bacilli* may be derived from an active or a reactivated primary tuberculous lesion in a site such as the lung, hilar or mesenteric lymph glands, or less commonly from the lesions of post-primary tuberculosis. It is thus classified as a form of metastatic tuberculosis.

Robinson (2) states "bilateral renal involvement is probably invariable". Fortunately renal tuberculosis is nowadays of less frequent occurrence than formerly. When it does develop, its highest incidence is in young adults.

The infection first causes inflammatory lesions in the cortices of the kidneys, which may heal or may progress so as to spread both within the solid part of the kidney and into the renal pelvis. *Tubercle bacilli* are discharged in the urine and foci of infection may, as a result, develop in the ureters and bladder. In males spread of disease to the reproductive organs may occur resulting in tuberculous infection in sites such as the prostate, seminal vescicles, epidydimis and testis.

Among the clinical features of chronic renal tuberculosis are general ill-health, loss of weight, frequency of micturition, pyuria, haematuria and pain in the loin.

Radiological examination is of value in showing evidence of the disease but the diagnosis is established by demonstration (using bacteriological methods) of the causative *tubercle bacilli* in the urine.

Associated bladder lesions may be demonstrated at cystoscopy.

Treatment is by antituberculous drugs and measures to improve the general condition of the patient. Surgery is required in certain types of kidney lesion and for some of the complications of the disease.

GLOMERULONEPHRITIS (NEPHRITIS)

A number of diseases, the majority of which are of inflammatory origin and all of which are non-suppurative and affect glomeruli in both kidneys, fall in the group or disorders referred to as **glomerulonephritis** or, more shortly, as **nephritis.**

Miller, Slade and Leather (3) describe three main types of glomerulonephritis, namely:— **Acute poststreptococcal glomerulonephritis, membranous glomerulonephritis** and **focal nephritis.** They also emphasize that mixed types occur.

The first of these types is frequently referred to briefly as **acute nephritis** and is widely thought to be a manifestation of hypersensitivity to streptococcal infection. It often follows a streptococcal tonsillitis and takes the form of an acute illness, among the characteristic features of which are albuminuria, haematuria, oedema (often affecting the face as well as the dependant parts of the body), pleural effusions, ascites and high blood pressure. This disease may clear up completely or may undergo slow progression to a chronic condition called **chronic nephritis** or **chronic glomerulonephritis,** which ultimately leads to **chronic renal failure,** i.e. failure of normal kidney function.

In **membranous glomerulonephritis** there is no acute phase, the condition being chronic from the outset, and associated with the development of the so-called **nephrotic syndrome.** This latter comprises the excretion of large amounts of protein in the urine, the presence of diminished amounts of protein in the blood, and the presence of oedema.

(*Note:* Certain forms of kidney disease in which there is damage to the renal tubules may develop features with a resemblance to the nephrotic syndrome and are called **nephroses).**

Like acute nephritis, membranous glomerulonephritis progresses ultimately to chronic glomerulonephritis and eventual chronic renal failure.

Focal nephritis differs from the types of nephritis described above in that its lesions are scattered instead of diffuse. It is not generally of itself, a serious disease but may occur as a complication of severe diseases such as subacute bacterial endocarditis and certain collagen diseases.

Renal function tests are of great importance in the diagnosis and assessment of progress in patients with various types of glomerulonephritis. Renal biopsy is employed in some cases to establish the diagnosis.

There are no curative treatments for patients with nephritis but dietetic measures with special reference to the intake of fluids, protein and salt are of great importance. Diuretics, i.e. drugs which increase the secretion of urine, are often required in chronic cases with oedema. Cases of membranous glomerulonephritis may benefit considerably from steroid therapy.

NEOPLASMS

Neoplasms may arise in the solid part of the kidney and in the renal pelvis and ureter. The most important are:

(*a*) **Adenocarcinoma,** (Hypernephroma)—a carcinomatous growth of the solid part of the kidney which occurs in adult life, most usually in middle age and is of fairly common incidence. It is frequently referred to as a **hypernephroma,** owing to a formerly held belief that it derived from misplaced suprarenal tissue. (The suprarenal glands lie above the kidneys—hyper—above; nephr—kidney; -oma—tumour).

The growth may remain confined to the kidney for a considerable time in some patients. In others early blood-borne metastases may occur in sites such as the lungs and bones.

Haematuria is often the first sign of the disease. Pain in the loin tends to be a fairly late feature, as does the development of a palpable mass due to the tumour. Occasionally a metastatic deposit may produce the first evidence of the disease in the form of a haemoptysis or a pathological fracture of bone. In such instances the primary tumour may be difficult to detect and be referred to as a **"hidden primary tumour".**

Blood and occasionally malignant cells may be demonstrable in the urine. Radiological investigation with contrast urography, and sometimes renal angiography are important diagnostic measures. Radioactive isotopes may also be useful in demonstrating the presence of a hypernephroma and are also helpful in differentiating between renal neoplasms and cysts.

(*b*) **Embryoma** (Wilms' tumour, nephroblastoma, adenosarcoma)— this is a rare neoplasm of the solid part of the kidney, which occurs in infants and young children. It is believed to originate in remants of embryonic tissue which persist in the kidney, and to be of sarcomatous type. In clinical practice it is usually known by its old name of **Wilms' tumour,** after M. Wilms, a German surgeon.

The neoplasm is usually unilateral, but cases have been reported in which tumours have been found in both kidneys.

Growth of a Wilms' tumour is usually very rapid and produces a very large abdominal swelling. Haematuria, usually a common feature of renal neoplasms, is rare. Widespread early metastases are common, the lungs being one of the principal sites for their occurrence.

Plain radiographs, intravenous urography and sometimes renal angiography are of considerable help in diagnosis.

Surgical removal of the kidney, combined with radiotherapy, is the usual treatment, if the disease is diagnosed before there is evidence of metastatic spread. Metastases are treated by radiotherapy.

(*c*) **Carcinoma of the renal pelvis**—this tumour of the hollow part of the kidney may take the form of a **malignant papilloma,** or less commonly of a neoplasm called an **epidermoid carcinoma.** Haematuria is the cardinal symptom. The growth may produce a filling defect in the renal pelvis, demonstrable by ascending or descending pyelography. Treatment is surgical, in all suitable cases.

CYST FORMATION

Renal cysts are not very common but when they do occur, it is important to differentiate them from renal neoplasms. The occurrence of multiple cysts in the disorder called **congenital polycystic kidneys** has already been mentioned. **Solitary cysts** of the kidney are thought, usually, to develop as a result of acquired abnormality.

RENAL CALCULUS (STONE IN THE KIDNEY, RENAL LITHIASIS)

Chemical salts may be precipitated from the urine to form solid bodies known as calculi. Calculus formation in the kidney usually commences in a calyx. From this site the calculus may migrate into the renal pelvis. Here it may remain and may gradually increase in size, as a result of further precipitation of urinary constituents. Alternatively, it may migrate into the ureter and pass through the bladder and urethra, being ultimately voided in the urine. Sometimes a calculus, which has entered the ureter, may become lodged in this structure, when it is described as an **impacted ureteric calculus.**

Renal calculi usually consist of a mixture of chemical substances but are named according to their principal constituents, e.g. **phosphate calculi, calcium oxalate calculi, uric acid** and **urate calculi.**

A large number of factors may operate in the production of calculi. Among these may be mentioned urinary stasis resulting from obstructive lesions, congenital or acquired, within the urinary system; urinary stasis from prolonged lying in bed as a result of operation or illness; diseases in which there is marked loss of calcium from the bones with consequent increase in the amounts of calcium in the blood and urine (e.g. hyperparathyroidism, see p. 213); excessive sweating, such as occurs in hot countries and leads to the passage of unduly concentrated urine.

It is to be noted that calculus formation, in the urinary system, is not confined to the kidney but may also occur in the bladder, and occasionally in the urethra. In the male reproductive system calculi may form within the prostate gland.

Renal calculi may form in one or both kidneys; and may be single or multiple. They occur in childhood and adult life, and are found in both sexes. In some cases they are symptomless, but in most instances they cause pain in the loin and not infrequently haematuria.

Passage of a stone down the ureter causes colicky pains of a type called **renal colic.** These pains are felt in the abdomen and often radiate into the groin or external genital organs.

The majority of renal calculi contain sufficient calcium salts to render them visible on plain radiographs, but contrast radiography is generally necessary to differentiate them from other calcified opacities which can be found in the abdomen or cavity of the pelvis, e.g. opaque gallstones, calcified mesenteric glands, **phleboliths** (i.e. small calcified thrombi in pelvic veins).

A calculus may cause a partial obstruction of the pelviureteric junction resulting in the development of a hydronephrosis or a partial obstruction of a ureter, causing hydroureter and hydronephrosis (see later).

Urinary stasis, urinary infection and calculus formation are not infrequently found in association, and it may be difficult, or impossible, to determine which of these abnormal conditions was the first to develop.

Operative treatment is necessary in a high proportion of patients with renal calculus and may also be required in cases of impacted ureteric calculus, when the stone fails to pass onwards into the bladder after a reasonable period of observation.

HYDRONEPHROSIS AND HYDROURETER

The term **hydronephrosis** indicates a condition of dilatation of the renal pelvis and its calyces, and **hydroureter,** dilation of the ureter.

Dilation of the renal calyces is termed **hydrocalycosis.**

It is generally only a partial or intermittent obstruction that will lead to hydronephrosis. Complete obstruction of a ureter generally results in cessation of secretion of urine, i.e. **anuria,** from the kidney above it and, if the obstruction is not relieved, eventually to atrophy of the affected kidney.

Hydronephrosis may, or may not, be accompanied by hydroureter, and may develop on one or both sides according to the site of the obstructing lesion, or lesions, e.g. bilateral hydronephrosis and hydroureters may occur as a result of obstructive lesions at the bladder neck or in the urethra, whereas a partial obstruction of the pelviureteric junction on one side only will produce a unilateral hydronephrosis.

In many cases of hydronephrosis, no mechanical cause for the condition can be discovered and it is widely considered that these are due to **neuromuscular inco-ordination;** this term meaning that the muscles do not react normally in response to impulses from the nerves which supply them. The obstruction in this type of hydronephrosis is thought to be due to a failure of normal relaxation of muscular tissue at either the pelviureteric junction or lower end of the ureter, on one or both sides; or at the bladder neck. In the latter two sites there will be ureteric dilatation as well as hydronephrosis.

Badenoch (4) refers to the type of hydronephrosis considered to be due to neuromuscular incoordination as **idiopathic hydronephrosis.**

Unilateral hydronephrosis is most commonly idiopathic in type and due to neuro-muscular inco-ordination. Among the many other causes of this condition are: (*a*) impaction of a calculus in the ureter or at the pelviureteric junction; (*b*) partial blockage of the ureteric junction by a renal neoplasm; (*c*) kinking of the upper end of the ureter by an **aberrant renal artery** (i.e. a renal artery which, as a result of developmental error, is abnormal in position); (*d*) pressure on the lower end of one ureter by a pelvic neoplasm (e.g. an advanced carcinoma of the uterine cervix); (*e*) an uncommon condition, called **periureteric fibrosis** or **retroperitoneal fibrosis,** wherein ureteric compression, by surrounding inflammatory fibrosis in the retroperitoneal tissues, leads to partial obstruction and medial displacement of the ureter on one or both sides. Treatment is surgical. It is not possible to determine the cause of development of the fibrous tissue in the majority of cases.

Bilateral hydronephrosis may be due to neuro-muscular inco-ordination at the bladder neck. Among its other causes are: (*a*) congenital strictures and valves in the urethra; (*b*) obstruction of the urethra by an enlarged prostate gland; (*c*) acquired urethral stricture; (*d*) lesions which cause obstruction of both ureters, e.g. bilateral calculi, extensive pelvic neoplasms, periureteric fibrosis.

Slight and moderate degrees of hydronephrosis can be readily demonstrated by intravenous urography. With a large hydronephrosis, however, destruction of renal tissue may be of such a degree that no concentration of the dye occurs on the affected side. Retrograde pyelography is then necessary to demonstrate the condition.

Hydronephrosis in its early stages is often a reversible condition and a return to normal may follow removal of its cause, when this is possible. **Nephrectomy** (surgical removal of the kidney) is frequently required in advanced degrees of unilateral hydronephrosis.

It is to be noted that during pregnancy some dilatation of the upper part of the ureter and renal pelvis and calyces occurs on both sides. Such changes are greater on the right side than on the left. As described by Rohan Williams (5), these, and certain other accompanying changes, are due to altered physiology consequent upon the pregnancy and are transitory in nature.

RENAL FAILURE

This term describes a condition wherein, as a result of severe kidney disease or other factors, the kidneys are unable adequately to carry out their normal functions. Accordingly, waste products accumulate in the blood, the normal water and electrolyte balances are upset, and alterations occur in the reaction of the blood.

Accumulation of acid waste products in the circulating blood results in a condition termed **acidosis.** Accumulation of waste products generally, including urea, a protein breakdown product, causes a clinical picture with features such as headache, drowsiness, mental confusion, convulsions, coma, and sometimes accompanying haemorrhages, which are referred to as being due to **uraemia.**

According to the factors responsible, renal failure may present in acute or chronic form. In the acute type excretion of urine is either scanty **(oliguria)** or ceases altogether **(anuria)** in the early phase of the disorder. In chronic renal failure, however, there is characteristically **polyuria,** i.e. the passage of excessive amounts of urine.

Long-standing chronic renal failure may result in a secondary overgrowth of the parathyroid glands and resultant secondary hyperparathyroidism, with associated bone lesions. It may also lead to bone changes due to osteomalacia (see p. 232).

Appropriate chemical tests may be employed to demonstrate abnormalities in the blood and urine arising from renal failure, e.g. estimation of blood urea, plasma bicarbonate, plasma potassium and sodium, urine concentration tests, etc.

There are many factors that can operate in the production of renal failure. These include severe kidney diseases (e.g. acute and chronic glomerulonephritis, chronic pyelonephritis, etc.); conditions which produce a sustained diminution of blood supply to the kidneys (e.g. severe haemorrhages, loss of blood plasma due to severe burns, crush injuries of the kidney, transfusion of incompatible blood—all of which factors may sometimes produce a widespread destruction of the renal tubules known as **acute tubular necrosis);** severe generalized infections; and conditions causing obstruction of the ureters or lower urinary tract leading to secondary atrophy of renal tissue.

The treatment of renal failure is directed to treating its cause when practicable, correcting abnormalities of blood reaction and water and electrolyte balance, administering a suitable diet, and preventing the development of intercurrent infections.

In suitable cases a method of treatment called **extracorporeal dialysis** may be employed to remove accumulated waste products. This is carried out in special centres and involves passing the whole of the circulating blood through a semi-permeable membrane contained within a machine referred to as an **artificial kidney.** (*Note:* "extracorporeal" means "outside the body".)

Renal transplantation is sometimes carried out in patients suffering from failing kidneys due to severe irreversible bilateral renal damage.

HYPERTENSION OF RENAL ORIGIN

This expression is self-explanatory, indicating high blood pressure which develops as a result of kidney disease.

Hodson (6) lists among the common types of renal diseases associated with hypertension, certain forms of nephritis, chronic pyelonephritis, and certain lesions in the renal arterial tree which result in a decreased blood flow.

These latter cause **renal ischaemia,** i.e. a localized deficiency of blood in affected areas. The extent of the ischaemia varies according to the distribution of the arterial lesions. Loss of renal substance, and other abnormalities due to chronic pyelonephritis or renal ischaemia, may be shown by intravenous urography and the distribution of vascular changes in the latter condition by renal angiography.

Radiological studies play a very important role in the investigation of many cases of hypertension as, when unilateral renal disease can be shown to be the cause of the high blood pressure, surgical removal of the affected kidney may produce very beneficial results.

(*Note:* One cause of ischaemia is narrowing of the main trunk of one or both renal arteries, constituting unilateral or bilateral **renal artery stenosis.**)

SOME OTHER TERMS REFERRING TO KIDNEY DISEASES

(*a*) **Referring to renal tubular defects** (i.e. disorders in which the renal tubules are unable to carry out their normal functions with respect to the reabsorption of certain of the substances excreted by the glomeruli).

(i) **Renal Tubular Acidosis** (Lightwood-Albright syndrome)—a disorder in which acid substances are retained in the blood. The type described as **idiopathic renal acidosis of infancy** and also the type that occurs in older children and adults are both frequently associated with **nephrocalcinosis,** i.e. the deposition of calcium salts in the solid part of the kidney.

Osteomalacia is also a common feature in the latter type.

Idiopathic hyperchloraemia is an alternative name for renal tubular acidosis, the term hyperchloraemia indicating an excess of chloride ions in the blood which is a feature of the disease.

(ii) **Fanconi syndrome**—a congenital disorder of the renal tubules.

(b) **Referring to vascular disorders of the kidney** (i.e. disorders in the renal blood supply).

(i) **Acute Tubular Necrosis**—see p. 158.

(ii) **Atheroma of the renal arteries**—this arterial disease may lead to localized or diffuse renal ischaemia according to its distribution, and result in a condition referred to as **atheromatous nephrosclerosis.**

Nephrosclerosis means "hardening of the kidneys" and indicates the hardening which occurs when damaged renal tissue is replaced by fibrous tissue.

Renal artery stenosis (see p. 159) is usually due to atheroma.

(c) **Referring to other diseases which may produce kidney lesions.**

The following are among the other diseases which may produce kidney lesions, and are referred to in other parts of the book:—essential hypertension, causing hypertensive nephrosclerosis; diabetes mellitus, causing **"diabetic kidney";** primary hyperparathyroidism causing calculus formation and nephrocalcinosis; amyloid disease; myelomatosis causing **myeloma kidney** with which is associated passage in the urine of protein, referred to as **Bence-Jones protein,** polyarteritis nodosa, a collagen disease.

RENAL OSTEODYSTROPHY

This term indicates metabolic bone disease which occurs as a secondary result of renal disease.

Among the kidney diseases which may give rise to osteodystrophy are renal tubular acidosis (Lightwood-Albright syndrome) and Fanconi syndrome. The bone changes usually take the form of a type of osteomalacia referred to as **renal rickets.** (See under "Metabolic Bone Diseases").

5. DISEASES OF THE URINARY BLADDER.

CONGENITAL ABNORMALITIES

(a) **Congenital bladder neck obstruction** this is a fairly common condition. The obstruction is due to hypertrophy of muscle fibres around the bladder neck (i.e. the region where the urethra leaves the bladder). It may produce obstructive symptoms in childhood but frequently produces no symptoms until adult life is reached.

(*b*) **Ectopia vesicae** (exstrophy of the bladder, extraversion of the bladder)—a rare anomaly in which, as a result of developmental failure, the anterior wall of the bladder and part of the anterior abdominal wall are absent. The two pubic bones are widely separated at the symphysis pubis, and the posterior wall of the bladder and the urethral orifices lie on the anterior surface of the lower abdomen.

(*c*) **Patent urachus**—this condition results from partial or complete failure of obliteration of the lumen of a structure called the urachus, which is connected with the bladder and normally patent only during certain stages of foetal life. Such failure results in a condition called **patent urachus** which may present as:—

> (i) **a vesico-umbilical fistula,** i.e. a patent track connecting the bladder and umbilicus; (ii) a type of cyst termed a **urachal cyst,** or (iii) a congenital pouch arising from the superior surface of the bladder termed a **urachal diverticulum.**

TRAUMATIC CONDITIONS

The bladder may be torn as a result of injury and, according to the site of the tear in its wall, the injury is termed **intraperitoneal rupture** or **extraperitoneal rupture of the bladder.** The former condition results in leakage of urine into the peritoneal cavity and consequent peritonitis. In extraperitoneal rupture, urine is extravasated into the soft tissues behind and above the pubis. Both injuries are frequently associated with fractures of the pelvis.

INFECTIVE DISEASES

Infection of the bladder wall results in a condition of inflammation termed **cystitis** which may develop in acute or chronic form. Such infection may be caused by pathogens reaching the organ via either the ureter or the urethra. In the latter instance infection may ascend from the bladder so as to involve the kidney pelvis and solid part of the kidney, the organisms being carried up through the ureter as a result of reflux of urine from the bladder back through one or both ureteric orifices. Such reflux is called **vesico-ureteric reflux** and its occurrence may be demonstrated by a form of contrast radiology called micturating cystography.

6

Cystitis is commoner in females than in males. In the former, pregnancy is one of the common predisposing factors, whilst in males the disease often develops as a secondary result of some obstructive lesion (e.g. enlarged prostate, urethral stricture) in the lower urinary tract.

Among other conditions associated with cystitis are vesical calculi, diverticula of the bladder, carcinoma of the bladder, neurogenic bladder disorders and foreign body in the bladder.

In the tropics and semitropics, cystitis may be caused by parasitic worms in the disease called schistosomiasis (bilharziasis).

Passage of a catheter into the bladder always carries some risk of introducing infective organisms and thus causing a cystitis; hence the need for strict asepsis during this procedure.

The causal pathogens of a cystitis may be demonstrated in specimens of urine by bacteriological methods. The commonest infecting microorganism to be thus found is the *bacillus coli,* but in other cases the infection may be staphylococcal or streptococcal in nature or due to various other types of bacteria including the *bacillus proteus* and a bacillus called *pseudomonas pyocyanea.* (Note the *bacillus coli* is also referred to as the *bacterium coli* or *escherichia coli*).

A small proportion of bladder infections are due to tuberculous infection and are secondary to tuberculous infection in the kidneys.

Sulphonamides, antibiotics, and certain other drugs are employed in the treatment of simple cystitis.

NEOPLASMS

Two types of neoplasm are fairly common in the bladder:

(*a*) **Papilloma of the Bladder**—the word **papilla** means "a nipple" and strictly speaking, **papilloma** means "a nipple-like tumour". The term is however used to describe a class of benign tumours of epithelium which are raised above normal surrounding epithelium but are of varying sizes and shapes.

A bladder papilloma arises in the epithelial lining of the organ and gives rise to painless haematuria. In the majority of instances it is single, but sometimes multiple growths may occur. The diagnosis is usually made by cystoscopy and biopsy.

The tumour may be destroyed by **diathermy,** i.e. a method in which a high frequency current is used to generate heat in an area of body tissue. In surgical diathermy the heat is such as to cause death of tissues touched by the operating electrode. When dealing with bladder growths, the electrode is introduced into the interior of the organ through a cystoscope.

Malignant change may develop in a papilloma, the condition then developing into one of **papillary carcinoma.**

(*b*) **Carcinoma of the Bladder**—a carcinomatous growth arising in the epithelial lining of the bladder may be of the papillary type described above or arise *de novo* in a bladder without papillomata.

The condition is more common in males than in females.

Haematuria and frequency of micturition are common early features of the disease and cystitis often develops as a complication.

Both lymphatic and blood-borne metastases may occur and the latter may be found in lungs and bone.

The diagnosis of bladder carcinoma is usually made at cystoscopy and confirmed by biopsy. Local complications of the disease include bladder neck obstruction; involvement of a ureteric orifice leading to hydroureter and hydronephrosis, or a non-functioning kidney; and spread to neighbouring organs with fistula formation, e.g. vesico-colic fistula.

Treatment is by surgery or radiotherapy, used singly or in combination.

NEUROGENIC BLADDER DISORDERS

These are a group of disorders in which there is interference with normal nervous control of the bladder. They may be congenital in origin or result from various types of diseases and injuries of the spinal cord. Such disorders may cause bladder neck obstruction with retention of urine. Resulting from such retention urine may overflow from the full bladder down the urethra; a state of affairs termed **retention with overflow** and giving rise to **overflow incontinence** (false incontinence).

In other neurogenic bladder disorders there may be no bladder neck obstruction and inability of the bladder to hold urine may result in a continual leakage of this fluid into the urethra, producing what is known as **true incontinence.**

OTHER BLADDER DISORDERS

(*a*) **Vesical Calculus**—calculi (stones) found in the urinary bladder may have formed therein, or migrated there from the kidney. Small calculi may be voided through the urethra. Calculi which remain in the bladder frequently show a gradual increase in size owing to repeated deposition of urinary constituents on their external surfaces.

Vesical calculi may be single or multiple; the majority are radio-opaque. They are similar in composition to renal calculi and similar factors operate in their production (see p. 155). Urinary obstruction (e.g. due to an enlarged prostate or urethral stricture) is often a pre-disposing factor in their formation.

Painful and frequent micturition, often associated with haematuria, is the chief clinical feature. Treatment is surgical.

(*b*) **Bladder Diverticula**—diverticula, or pouches, of the bladder may be congenital or acquired, and single or multiple. They consist of protrusions of mucosa through the muscular wall of the organ. The acquired variety tend to develop as a secondary result of some obstruction to the outflow of urine from the bladder (e.g. due to an enlarged prostate or urethral stricture).

Stasis of urine, with subsequent infection, is common in diverticula, and calculi and neoplasms may form within them.

Diverticula are readily demonstrated by descending or ascending cystograms.

(*c*) **Vesical Fistulae**—fistulae of the bladder may be congenital, or may form between the bladder and adjacent organs as a result of disease, or injury, e.g. **vesico-vaginal fistula, vesico-colic fistula.** Contrast radiography may be employed to demonstrate such fistulae.

Vesico-colic fistula may occur as a complication of diverticulitis of the colon, or a carcinoma of the colon. The condition results in cystitis and the passage of intestinal gas in the urine. This latter symptom is called **pneumaturia.**

6. DISEASES OF THE MALE URETHRA

CONGENITAL ABNORMALITIES

These include:

(*a*) **Congenital urethral stenosis** (congenital stricture)—this mal-formation usually takes the form of a localized stenosis (narrowing) at some point during the course of the urethra. If it occurs at the external urinary meatus (external urethral orifice) it produces a con-dition referred to as **pin-hole meatus.**

Congenital urethral stenosis is one of the causes of obstruction of the lower urinary system and may lead to bilateral hydroureter and hydronephrosis.

(*b*) **Congenital Urethral Valves**—these are abnormal folds of mucous membrane which exert a valve-like action causing obstruction to the flow of urine through the urethra. They are found only in males and occur predominantly in the posterior urethra (i.e. the part of the urethra comprised by its prostatic and membranous portions).

(c) **Hypospadias**—a rare condition in which the external opening of the urethra lies on the under surface of the penis, or in the perineum. The name of the anomaly means "drawn beneath".

(d) **Epispadias**—this is the opposite of hypospadias being a condition in which the external urethral orifice is situated on the dorsal surface of the penis. It is extremely rare.

TRAUMATIC CONDITIONS

(a) **Traumatic Rupture of the Urethra** is a not uncommon injury in males, the membranous portion being especially liable to damage. It may be associated with a fracture of the pelvis. Urethral stricture is a frequent sequel to urethral injury.

(b) **Foreign body in the urethra**—a variety of types of foreign body may be inserted into the urethra. X-ray investigation is often of value in suspected cases.

INFLAMMATORY CONDITIONS

Inflammation of the urethra is called **urethritis.** A high proportion of cases of this condition are due to gonococcal infection. Of the remainder the majority fall into a group referred to as being due to non-specific urethritis.

Urethral stricture is a not uncommon sequel in both the gonococcal and non-specific forms of urethritis.

It has already been noted that urethritis is sometimes associated with arthritis and conjunctivitis in a condition called **Reiter's syndrome** (see p. 57).

URETHRAL STRICTURE

A stricture (stenosis) of the urethra may be congenital, traumatic or inflammatory in origin.

The cardinal symptom of this lesion is difficulty in passing urine, which may progress to a condition in which the patient is unable to pass hardly any urine, or no urine at all. This is referred to as a condition of **retention of urine,** or more simply spoken of as **retention.** Valuable information regarding the condition of a urethral stricture may be obtained by performing ascending and descending urethrography.

Urethral stricture may lead to distension of the bladder and bilateral hydronephrosis and hydroureter. Intravenous urography is thus generally requested for patients with this condition. Cystitis is also a common complication, and the formation of vesical calculi and diverticula may also occur.

Treatment is usually by dilatation of the stricture by instruments called **bougies,** but surgical operations may be performed in selected cases.

URETHRAL CALCULUS

A calculus which has been voided from the bladder may lodge in the urethra. It is then referred to as a urethral calculus. Calculi may also form in the urethra in patients who have some pre-existing abnormality in this structure, e.g. urethral stricture.

NEOPLASMS OF THE URETHRA

These are very rare. **Carcinoma of the urethra** is treated by radio-therapy.

7. DISEASES OF THE FEMALE URETHRA

The female urethra is very much less liable to disease or injury than that of the male. Among the disorders which may uncommonly affect this structure are injury to the urethra during childbirth or surgical operations, urethritis, carcinoma and urethral diverticulum. Lesions in the female urethra may cause urinary obstruction and urethral abnormalities in women are among the causes of a type of incontinence of urine called **stress incontinence.** This is defined by Baynes (7) as a condition in which urine is passed involuntarily when intra-abdominal pressure is raised, as when the patient coughs, laughs or strains.

The displacement of the urethra and bladder neck which may occur in genital prolapse (p. 180) is an important cause of stress incontinence.

8. DISEASES OF THE PENIS

These include:—

(*a*) **Balanitis**—inflammation of the glans penis and foreskin.

(*b*) **Phimosis**—constriction of the distal end of the foreskin preventing its normal retraction so as to completely uncover the glans penis. This condition is treated by the surgical operation of **circumcision,** i.e. excision of the prepuce (i.e. the foreskin).

(*c*) **Paraphimosis**—a condition wherein the prepuce having been retracted, cannot be replaced and causes a constriction at the distal part of the penis just below the glans with resultant marked swelling of the glans.

(*d*) **Priapism**—a condition of persistent erection of the penis, usually the result of venous thrombosis within the organ.

(*e*) **Carcinoma of the penis**—an uncommon type of neoplasm which is practically confined to uncircumcised subjects and occurs in the glans. Radiotherapy is the treatment of choice.

9. DISEASES OF THE PROSTATE GLAND

The prostate gland lies below the base of the bladder and the prostatic urethra runs through its substance.

Compression of the urethra, with resultant urinary obstruction, is a common secondary feature of diseases which cause prostatic enlargement. The most important of these are benign enlargement and carcinoma. Among the other conditions which may affect the gland are **prostatitis** (inflammation of the prostate), which is of infective origin and may be acute or chronic in type, and **prostatic calculi** which are usually symptomless but show as well defined opacities on X-ray films.

BENIGN ENLARGEMENT OF THE PROSTATE GLAND (SIMPLE PROSTATIC ENLARGEMENT, SENILE HYPERPLASIA OF THE PROSTATE, ADENOMA OF THE PROSTATE)

This is a common disease as, in many males, some degree of enlargement of the prostate occurs as old age approaches and this is frequently such as to cause some degree of compression of the prostatic urethra and consequent interference with normal micturition.

Miller, Slade and Leather (8) who refer to the condition as **senile prostatic hypertrophy** state that the enlargement is thought to be a degenerative change due to hormonal imbalance.

Urinary symptoms may be slight and non-progressive. In other instances the disease may result in a degree of obstruction that prevents the bladder from achieving complete expulsion of its contents. This organ then always contains some residual urine after micturition. Cystitis is a common complication. Acute retention may supervene. Other complications which may develop, consequent upon the urinary obstruction, are bilateral hydronephrosis and hydroureter; calculus and diverticulum formation in the bladder; and disordered renal function which may progress to renal failure.

In most instances the enlarged prostate gland can be felt at rectal examination. Renal function tests, including blood urea estimation, are important in assessing whether there is any secondary renal damage and intravenous urography is important to assess the condition of the upper part of the urinary system, and also to show the amount of residual urine in the bladder.

Operative treatment is frequently indicated for benign enlargement of the prostate, prostatectomy being performed. In patients with retention a period of catheter drainage of the bladder may be necessary as a pre-operative measure.

CARCINOMA OF THE PROSTATE GLAND

Like benign enlargement of the prostate, prostatic carcinoma also occurs in elderly men but is much less common than the former condition.

The growth causes disturbances of micturition and leads to urethral compression which in turn results in complications such as cystitis and bilateral hydronephrosis and hydroureter.

Bony metastases are often an early feature in the disease and may cause pain in the back. Pulmonary metastases may occur as a late feature.

The growth may be palpable on rectal examination. Radiological investigation is valuable in showing changes produced in the urinary system and metastases in bones.

Blood examination may show increased amounts of an enzyme called **serum acid phosphatase** and, when bony metastases are present, another enzyme called **serum alkaline phosphatase** may also show increased blood levels.

Radical surgery may be employed in very early cases but, in the majority, palliative treatment is used and comprises administration of female hormes (oestrogens). This is frequently successful in relieving pain and producing temporary regression of both the primary growth and any metastases present. The operation of bilateral **orchidectomy** (removal of the testes) may be employed in conjunction with hormone therapy.

10. DISEASES OF THE TESTIS, EPIDIDYMIS, AND SCROTUM

IMPERFECT DESCENT OF THE TESTIS

The testes develop during foetal life in the retroperitoneal tissues in the region of the kidneys and descend into the scrotum shortly before birth. Upset of the normal processes of descent may result in the testis remaining in the abdomen, or being arrested at some point along its normal route of descent. This constitutes the condition known as **undescended testis.** Alternatively, such upset may result in the testis descending to some abnormal position when the condition is referred to as **ectopic testis,** the word **ectopic** meaning abnormally placed.

Undescended testis and ectopic testis may both occur as unilateral or bilateral abnormalities.

Spontaneous descent of undescended testes may occur during childhood in many patients. Others with this disorder will require treatment with hormones or surgery. Ectopic testes invariably require surgical treatment.

TORSION OF THE TESTIS

A condition in which, as a result of imperfect fixation of the testis within the scrotum, the spermatic cord (i.e. the structure which suspends the testis within the scrotum and is formed by the distal part of the vas deferens and the blood vessels and nerves of the testis) becomes twisted, compressing the veins draining blood from the testis. As a result the testis becomes swollen and tender and there is severe pain. Unless the condition is speedily relieved, permanent damage to the tissues of the testis will result.

An undescended testis is more liable to torsion than a normal testis.

INFLAMMATORY DISEASES

Acute inflammatory changes in the testis are practically always accompanied by similar changes in the epididymis, the condition being called **epididymo-orchitis.**

Acute epididymo-orchitis may occur as a complication of infections in the urethra and prostate gland and during the course of mumps.

Chronic inflammatory changes may often affect only the epididymis as is frequent in **tuberculous epididymitis,** or only the testis as is common in **syphilic orchitis.**

Tuberculous epididymitis is usually secondary to renal tuberculosis and is often accompanied by **tuberculous vesiculitis** (i.e. inflammation of the seminal vesicles).

NEOPLASMS

(*a*) **Neoplasms of the testis** are rare, but those that develop usually show a high degree of malignancy with early glandular spread and subsequent blood-borne metastases in the lungs. Lymphangiography (contrast radiography of the lymphatic system) is of great value in demonstrating metastases in the iliac and para-aortic lymph glands.

Malignant tumours of the testis are of three main types:—

  (*i*) **Seminoma** (spermatocytoma)—a carcinomatous tumour, the name of which derives from its origin from epithelial cells lining the seminiferous tubules, i.e. the structures in which spermatozoa are produced.

  (ii) **Teratoma**—thought to arise from embryonic cells which persist into adult life. A very rare type of teratoma is called a **chorion-carcinoma** or **chorion-epithelioma of the testis.** This tumour is of considerable interest as, although in this instance arising in the male, it produces cells resembling those normally only found in chorionic epithelium formed within the uterus during pregnancy. (*Note:* the **chorion** is the outer of the foetal membranes).

  The usual treatment of testicular neoplasms is by **orchidectomy** (removal of the testis) followed by post-operative radiotherapy to the iliac and para-aortic lymph glands.

(*b*) **Carcinoma of the Scrotum**—a malignant tumour arising from the skin of the scrotum. It is nowadays seldom seen but formerly was common in chimney sweeps.

OTHER DISORDERS

These include:

(*a*) **Hydrocele**—used without qualification this term indicates a collection of fluid contained in a structure in the scrotum, called the tunica vaginalis.

Hydro- means "water" or "fluid", and -**cele** a "tumour" or "swelling". This latter suffix is usually only applied to swellings other than those due to neoplasms.

A hydrocele of tunica vaginalis may develop as a result of inflammatory or other diseases of the testis and epididymis, or be due to trauma or of unknown causation.

(*b*) **Haematocele**—a collection of blood in the tunica vaginalis (see above) resulting from trauma or other cause.

(*c*) **Varicocele**—a swelling produced by varicosity of the veins of the pampiniform plexus, i.e. a plexus of veins which lie in the spermatic cord anterior to the vas deferens.

(*d*) **Spermatocele**—a cyst arising in the epididymis or in close relation to this structure.

SOME GENITO-URINARY OPERATIONS

A. KIDNEY AND URETER

Nephrectomy—removal of a kidney.

Nephrostomy—surgical drainage of the renal pelvis.

Nephro-Ureterectomy—removal of a kidney and its ureter.

Plastic Operations on the Renal Pelvis—these are employed in certain cases of hydronephrosis to relieve obstruction at the pelvi-ureteric junction. One of the best known is called the **Anderson-Hynes operation** and involves excising the pelviureteric junction and anastomosing (i.e. making a communication between) the residual part of of the renal pelvis and the upper end of the ureter.

Renal Transplantation—transplantation of a kindey, from a living donor, or from a donor within about two hours of death, to another individual. This operation is used in certain selected cases as a form of treatment for severe bilateral and irreversible kidney damage.

B. BLADDER AND URETHRA

Cystectomy—removal of the urinary bladder. This may take the form of partial or total removal of the organ.

When total cystectomy is performed, some operative procedure must also be carried out to effect satisfactory drainage of urine. This is termed **urinary diversion** and at the present time the most favoured method is by the construction of an **ileal conduit.** This involves transplanting the lower ends of the ureters into a segment of ileum which is isolated from the rest of the small bowel, and made to open on to the anterior abdominal wall. Another method is called **uretero-colostomy** and involves transplantation of the ureters into the colon.

Cystotomy—opening the bladder by a surgical incision.

Lithotomy—this term means the opening of an organ to remove a calculus. Used without qualification, it denotes surgical opening of the bladder to remove a vesical calculus.

Suprapubic Cystostomy—surgical drainage of the bladder through an incision made through the anterior part of the lower abdominal wall just above the pubis.

Urethrotomy—an operation in which an incision is made in order to widen or excise a urethral stricture.

Urethroplasty—a plastic operation for relief of a urethral stricture.

C. PROSTATE

Prostatectomy—removal of the prostate gland.

According to the route employed to gain access to the gland the operation may be referred as a **suprapubic** or **retropubic prostatectomy** or **trans-urethral resection of the prostate.** (T.U.R.)

D. TESTIS AND EPIDIDYMIS

Epididymo-Orchidectomy—removal of the testis and epididymis.
Orchidectomy—removal of the testis.
Orchiopexy—an operation to fix the testis in the scrotum, employed in certain cases of undescended testis.

REFERENCES

(1) Hodson, C. J. and Edwards, D. *Clin. Radiol.* II, 219, 1960.
(2) Robinson, J. O. *Surgery.* Longmans, 1965.
(3) (8) Miller, A. Slade N. and Leather, H. M. *A Synopsis of Renal Diseases and Urology.* John Wright & Sons Ltd., 1966.
(4) Badenoch, A. W. *Manual of Urology.* Wm. Heinemann Medical Books Ltd., 1953.
(5) Rohan Williams, E. *A Textbook of X-ray Diagnosis* (British Authors). H. K. Lewis, 1958.
(6) Hodson, C. J. *Modern Trends in Diagnostic Radiology* (Ed. J. W. McLaren). Butterworths, 1960.
(7) Baynes, T. L. S. *Handbook of Gynaecology.* Sylviro Publications, 1951.

Section E. THE FEMALE REPRODUCTIVE SYSTEM

1. SOME ANATOMICAL AND PHYSIOLOGICAL CONSIDERATIONS

The **female reproductive system** comprises (*a*) the *internal genital organs,* namely the two *ovaries,* the *uterus* and the two *uterine* (*Fallopian*) *tubes* and the *vagina,* (*b*) *the external genital organs,* which collectively constitute the *vulva.*

The female *breasts* are accessory organs of this system but terminology related to diseases of the breast will be dealt with more conveniently in a separate section. (See Section G).

The ovaries are the reproductive glands of the female and produce the female germ cells which are called *ova* (singular: *ovum*).

The processes of reproduction commence when following **coitus** (sexual intercourse) an ovum is fertilized by a spermatozoon, a process described as **conception. Pregnancy** is a condition which exists from the time of conception until the commencement of labour (childbirth) and has an average duration of forty weeks as reckoned from the last menstrual period.

The active phase of reproductive life in both sexes commences at a period referred to as **puberty.** In the female this period is marked by the onset of menstruation, enlargement of the breasts and other changes.

The end of reproductive activity in the female is characterized by cessation of menstruation and is called the **menopause.** It is sometimes also termed the **climacteric.**

The prefixes **utero-** and **hystero-** both refer to the uterus, whilst **salpingo-** refers to the uterine tubes, and both **vagino-** and **colpo-** refer to the vagina.

The prefix **metro-** also means pertaining to the uterus, e.g. metritis means "inflammation of the uterus".

2. SOME GENERAL ASPECTS OF DISEASES OF THE FEMALE REPRODUCTIVE SYSTEM

Diseases of this system may be congenital, traumatic, inflammatory, neoplastic or due to other causes.

The branch of medicine concerned with diseases of the female reproductive organs is called **gynaecology** and is closely allied with the speciality of **obstetrics** which deals with the management of pregnancy, labour and the puerperium. Terms relating more specifically to the practice of obstetrics will be discussed in the next section (see Section F.)

Among the principal signs and symptoms of gynaecological disorders are disorders of menstruation; vaginal discharge, which may take the form of a blood-stained discharge, or a discharge without blood known as **leucorrhoea;** abnormal bleeding from the vagina; pain in the pelvis, lower abdomen and back; **dyspareunia** i.e. difficulty or pain on sexual intercourse, **sterility** (see p. 180).

3. SPECIAL METHODS OF INVESTIGATION

These include (i) microscopic examination of **curettings** from the uterus, i.e. specimens of the lining mucosa of the uterus obtained during a procedure called **dilatation and curettage.** (D. & C.), wherein the cervix of the uterus is dilated and the mucosa of the cavity of the uterus is scraped with an instrument called a uterine **curette.** (ii) demonstration of the interior of the uterus and uterine tubes by a form of contrast radiography called **hystero-salpingography.** (iii) demonstration of the ovaries by another form of contrast radiography called **pelvic pneumography.** (iv) **utero-tubal insufflation** i.e. testing of the patency of the uterine tubes by attempting to blow carbon dioxide through them under pressure. (v) biopsy of suspected neoplasms— (vi) **cervical cytology**—see p. 179. (vii) **peritoneoscopy**—visual examination of the pelvic organs with an instrument inserted into the peritoneal cavity through a small incision in the lower abdominal wall or posterior fornix of the vagina.

It is to be noted that care must be taken when using ionizing radiations in females, below or of reproductive age, for diagnostic or therapeutic purposes, to limit as far as practicable the dose of radiation to the ovaries and thus minimise not only somatic but also genetic hazards (see p. 309). Especial care, moreover, must be taken with regard to the use of such radiations during pregnancy on account of the fact that foetal tissues are more sensitive to the effects of radiation than are adult tissues.

4. CONGENITAL ABNORMALITIES

There are a variety of congenital abnormalities of the female reproductive system but none of them are common. The names of a few of them are as follows:—**ovarian agenesis** (failure of development of the ovaries); **hypoplasia of the uterus** (underdevelopment of the uterus); **double uterus** (the body of the uterus consists of two portions; the neck of the uterus is often also double and the vagina is **septate,** i.e. divided by a partition of tissue called a **septum**); **bicornuate uterus** (the uterus is incompletely divided so as its upper parts consists of two structures resembling horns in shape); **atresia of the vagina** (failure of the development of the normal lumen of the vagina, usually in its lower part)—a condition which may lead after puberty to retention of menstrual blood in the vagina and uterus—conditions called respectively **haematocolpos** and **haematometra.**

It is to be noted that certain congenital abnormalities of female and male reproductive organs may be associated with a condition termed **hermaphroditism.** A true **hermaphrodite** is an individual possessing tissue of the sex glands of both sexes (i.e. ovaries and testes). Certain other congenital abnormalities may be associated with **pseudo-hermaphroditism** or with a condition termed **intersex.** In patients with disorders of these types studies of their chromosomes are employed to determine their true sex.

(*Note:* **Chromosomes** are thread-like protein bodies which occur in the nuclei of all cells and carry the **genes**, i.e. units of hereditary material. A normal human being possesses 46 chromosomes. Two of these are sex chromosomes being termed XX in the female and XY in the male).

5. INFLAMMATORY DISEASES

(*a*) **Salpingitis**—this term means inflammation of the uterine tubes. Such inflammation is frequently accompanied by inflammation of the ovaries, when the condition is more correctly called **salpingo-oophoritis.**

Salpingitis may be seen as a result of an acute or chronic infection. Infection may reach the tubes via the uterus or bloodstream, or as a result of direct spread from an infective process in the peritoneal cavity. Among the causes of infection are gonorrhoea; infection following childbirth or abortion; and chronic infection due to tuberculosis. Acute salpingitis may result in a development of a **pyosalpix** (a tube distended with pus) or an abscess involving both tube and ovary and termed a **tubo-ovarian abscess.** Chronic salpingitis may result in a tube becoming distended with clear fluid; a condition termed a **hydrosalpinx.**

In either type of salpingitis, infection may spread from the tubes to the connective tissues of the pelvis causing **pelvic cellulitis.**

Salpingitis, salpingo-oophoritis, and pelvic cellulitis and other infections in the region of the pelvis (e.g. acute appendicitis etc.), when due to pyogenic organisms, may result in the formation of a **pelvic abscess.** Such an abscess may burst and drain into the rectum or vagina or be drained surgically through the posterior fornix of the vagina, but, should it burst into the general peritoneal cavity, it will cause a generalized infection termed **general peritonitis.**

(*b*) **Endometritis**—a condition of inflammation of the **endometrium** i.e. the mucous membrane lining the interior of the uterus. In its acute form it may occur as a result of gonococcal infection, or of infection following on childbirth or abortion. Spread of infection readily occurs from the endometrium to the uterine tubes and ovaries. The chronic form of endometritis is usually due to tuberculosis.

(*c*) **Cervicitis**—a term used to denote inflammation of the cervix or neck of the uterus. The causes of acute cervicitis include those described above as also being causes of acute endometritis.

An important type of chronic inflammation of the cervix occurs in the condition termed **cervical erosion.** (An **erosion** is a localized area which has lost it normal epithelial covering and thus appears raw and tends to bleed easily).

Erosions of the cervix may be congenital or acquired as a result of trauma during childbirth, or infection. Both types cause vaginal discharge and sometimes bleeding.

The majority of cervical erosions are treated by cauterization, using a high frequency electric current. It is, however, important to exclude carcinoma by cervical smear examination or biopsy before such treatment is given.

(*d*) **Vaginitis**—inflammation of the vagina which may result from a variety of infections including gonorrhoea in infants; infection with a protozoan organism called the *trichomonas vaginalis*: and infection with a fungus called *monilia albicans*. Trichomonas vaginitis is a fairly common disease and is generally transmitted by sexual intercourse.

Inflammatory changes in the vagina are often accompanied by similar changes in the vulva and the condition is then described as **vulvo-vaginitis.**

(*e*) **Puerperal infections**—(see "Puerperal Sepsis" p. 188).

6. NEOPLASMS

(*a*) OVARIAN NEOPLASMS

A large variety of cystic and solid tumours may arise in the ovaries, and a number of them may be of sufficient size to produce a soft-tissue swelling demonstrable by plain radiography. The type known as a **cystadenoma** may attain a tremendous size and occupy a considerable portion of the pelvis and abdomen, causing marked displacement of other viscera and elevation of the diaphragm.

Calcification may sometimes be shown radiologically in ovarian tumours and of particular interest is the **ovarian dermoid cyst,** which may contain imperfectly formed teeth.

In so-called **Meigs' syndrome** the presence of a benign ovarian tumour is associated with presence of bilateral pleural effusions and ascites.

Endocrine disturbances are found in some uncommon types of ovarian tumour.

The ovaries may be the site of metastases from carcinoma of other organs. The so-called **Krukenberg tumours** are metastatic growths from primary carcinomas of the stomach, breast or colon.

The following is a list of some of the main types of primary ovarian neoplasm:

(*a*) **Benign**—pseudo mucinous cystadenoma, papillary cystadenoma, fibroma, dermoid cyst, endometrioma, follicular cyst, luteal cyst, serous cyst.

(*b*) **Malignant**—carcinoma, papillary adenocarcinoma, granulosa cell tumour, arrhenoblastoma, dysgerminoma, malignant teratoma.

Speaking generally, the commonest form of spread of malignant ovarian neoplasms is by direct extension into the peritoneum, with resultant ascites. Blood-borne metastases are also common but lymphatic spread occurs infrequently.

Benign ovarian tumours are treated surgically. Radiotherapy is extensively employed in the treatment of malignant ovarian neoplasms either singly or in combination with surgery.

(*b*) UTERINE NEOPLASMS

These most frequently encountered are:

(*a*) **Leiomyoma** (Fibromyoma)—this is a benign tumour, which consists of a mixture of fibrous and muscle tissue, as indicated by its name. In clinical practice it is more usually referred to as a **fibroid.** Fibroids are usually multiple. They are common tumours, which develop in women of child-bearing age. They are generally of slow growth, and usually undergo atrophy after the menopause has been reached.

Fibroids are, in many instances, symptomless, but in others, may cause ill-effects through pressure on adjacent organs, e.g. bladder or pelvic colon, or as a result of changes in the tumours themselves (e.g. degeneration). The presence of fibroids may be also associated with certain forms of menstrual disorder, e.g. menorrhagia and dysmenorrhoea. Malignant change can occur in a fibroid but this is extremely rare. Among other conditions which may also be attributed to fibroids are certain cases of sterility and abortion. Large fibroids may also obstruct the birth canal, in cases when pregnancy has otherwise proceeded normally. Their presence may then necessitate Caesarean section.

Fibroids which are causing symptoms, in most instances, require surgical removal. Removal of one or more tumour masses is called **myomectomy.** In some cases this operation will suffice. In others hysterectomy (removal of the uterus) must be performed.

(*b*) **Polyp**—a benign tumour with a stem-like process termed a pedicle. Uterine polyps may be single or multiple and may arise within the cervical canal (**cervical polypus**), or within the cavity of the uterus. They may sometimes undergo malignant change. Those arising from the mucous membrane lining the uterus are called **endometrial polyps.**

(*c*) **Carcinoma of the Body of the Uterus**—(Carcinoma Corpus uteri, Endometrial Carcinoma)—a fairly common form of carcinoma arising from the mucous membrane lining the cavity of the uterus and occurring more frequently in women who have never borne children. It usually arises after the menopause.

The chief clinical features are post-menopausal bleeding from the uterus, offensive vaginal discharge and later pain in the pelvis.

Diagnosis is made by microscopic examination of curettings obtained from the uterine mucosa.

Spread of growth outside the uterus is relatively slow in some cases but in others, lymphatic metastases may occur relatively early in the disease. Blood-borne metastases are usually a late feature and are found most commonly in the lungs.

Suitable cases are treated by a combination of surgery, radiotherapy and hormone treatment; and advanced cases by radio-therapy alone.

(*d*) **Carcinoma of the Cervix Uteri.** (Cervical Carcinoma)—a common type of carcinoma arising from the mucuous membrane on the vaginal surface of the cervix uteri, or within the cervical canal. It is usually referred to more shortly as **carcinoma of the cervix** or **cervical carcinoma.**

In contradistinction to carcinoma of the body of the uterus, carcinoma of the crevix occurs more frequently in women who have borne children.

While the growth is confined to the epithelium of the cervix, it is termed **carcinoma-in-situ** (intra-epithelial carcinoma) and when it starts to spread outside this epithelium it is described as **invasive carcinoma of the cervix.** Direct spread of the growth may occur in any direction and may eventually lead to involvement of the rectum, bladder or lower ends of one or both ureters.

Spread to the rectum may cause the formation of a fistula between this organ and the vagina, i.e. a **recto-vaginal fistula,** whereas bladder involvement may result in a **vesico-vaginal fistula.** Pressure on a ureter may cause some degree of urinary obstruction on the affected side with resultant hydroureter and hydronephrosis.

As in carcinoma of the breast, the extent of the growth as assessed by clinical examination can be indicated by a type of classification called **clinical staging,** Stages 0, 1, 2, 3 and 4 being described. Carcinoma-in-situ is classified as Stage 0. A growth which has distant metastases or has involved the rectum or bladder falls into Stage 4.

The cardinal symptoms caused by the neoplasm are irregular vaginal bleeding and blood-stained vaginal discharge.

Early diagnosis of cervical carcinoma, in its pre-invasive stages, has been greatly facilitated by the extended use of **cervical cytology,** an investigation wherein smears taken from the uterine cervix are examined microscopically for malignant cells.

(*Note:* **Cytology** is a branch of science concerned with the study of cells).

In cases which give positive findings by this method, and in other clinically suspected cases, the diagnosis may be confirmed by microscopic examination of curettings from the cervix or by a type of biopsy called **cone biopsy.** The treatment of the disease may be by surgery and radiotherapy combined or, in advanced cases, by radiotherapy alone.

(*c*) OTHER NEOPLASMS

These include carcinomas of the uterine tubes, vagina and vulva, all of which are uncommon.

7. DISORDERS OF MENSTRUATION

The following terms are among those used in the description of menstrual disorders:

(*a*) **Amenorrhoea**—a term indicating absence of menstruation.

Amenorrhoea is a normal condition before puberty, during and shortly after pregnancy, and also after the menopause. In all other circumstances it is abnormal and may be due to one or other of a variety of causes. These include disorders of the pituitary, adrenal and thyroid glands and abnormal conditions of the ovaries and uterus.

As described by Barnes (1) a type of this disorder called variously **psychogenic, hypothalmic** or **environmental amenorrhoea** may follow emotional shock, or a change of environment or climate.

(*b*) **Cryptomenorrhoea**—a rare condition in which menstruation occurs but blood is retained within the vagina **(haematocolpos)** and sometimes also within the uterus **(haematometra)** as a result of an imperforate hymen, atresia, of the vagina, etc. Cryptomenorrhoea means "hidden menstruation".

(*c*) **Dysmenorrhoea**—painful menstruation.

(*d*) **Menorrhagia**—excessive loss of blood during menstruation.

(*e*) **Metrorrhagia**—bleeding from the uterus other than that due to menstruation.

(*f*) **Dysfunctional uterine bleeding**—this name indicates abnormal bleeding which occurs in the absence of any evidence of organic cause (e.g. trauma, infection, neoplasm, etc.), and is thus ascribed to disordered function.

One common type of dysfunctional bleeding is associated with changes in the endometrium described as being due to **metropathia haemorrhagica.** This condition is due to endocrine disorder.

Dysfunctional bleeding from the uterus occurs most frequently at or near the time of the menopause.

(*g*) **Polymenorrhoea**—menstruation occuring more frequently than normal.

8. STERILITY (Infertility)

This term is defined in "Diseases of Women" by Ten Teachers (2) as meaning that "there have been unsuccessful attempts to initiate the reproductive process'. Barnes (3) states that "infertility or sterility may be said to occur when pregnancy does not occur after one year during which coitus takes place at regular intervals".

Failure of conception may result from factors affecting either or both the male and female partner.

Female sterility may result from a number of local or general causes. Among the former are various congenital and acquired disorders of the reproductive system, e.g. congenital malformations such as atresia of the vagina, double uterus, etc.; inflammatory diseases of the reproductive system such as salpingitis; uterine tumours; acquired displacements of the uterus such as **retroversion** (i.e. a condition in which the uterus is tilted backwards).

General causes include various debilitating and systemic diseases and endocrine disorders.

The investigation of sterility involves the taking of histories and clinical examination of both wife and husband. In many instances special investigations are required, e.g. utero-tubal insufflation, hystero-salpingography in the female spouse; analysis of the seminal fluid in the male spouse.

9. PROLAPSE

In gynaecology, this means a protrusion of one or more pelvic organs into the vagina or through the pelvic floor. Prolapse is most commonly due to injury to the pelvic floor during childbirth. It is an important cause of stress incontinence (see p. 166).

A prolapse of the bladder is called a **cystocele** and a prolapse of the rectum, a **rectocele.**

Prolapse may be treated surgically by one of the types of operation, which are known collectively as **repair operations.** Alternatively, when surgery is not deemed advisable it may be treated by a supporting instrument, called a **pessary,** which is inserted into the vagina.

10. ENDOMETRIOSIS

Endometrium is the name given to the mucous membrane lining the uterine cavity. The presence of endometrial tissue in other sites constitutes a disorder termed **endometriosis.** This disorder may occur in the form of **uterine endometriosis,** also called **uterine adenomyosis,** when endometrial deposits are found in the muscular wall of the uterus, and **external endometriosis,** when deposits occur in other sites such as the ovaries, uterine tubes, intestine, peritoneum, umbilicus, etc.

Endometrial deposits undergo premenstrual changes and bleed at the time of the menstrual periods. They thus cause pain which begins with a menstrual period and reaches its peak on the second or third day of the period.

Uterine endometriosis is associated with menorrhagia. Ovarian endometriosis produces blood containing cysts which may be of a type termed **"chocolate cysts".**

Surgery is often required in the treatment of endometriosis but some patients respond to treatment with hormones.

11. OTHER DISORDERS

(*a*) **Pruritus vulvae**—the word **pruritus** means "itching". Pruritus vulvae may be due to one of a great many different causes. Among these are certain skin diseases, infective conditions of the vulva and vagina, external irritants and psychogenic causes.

(*b*) **Leucoplakia vulvae**—a condition of unknown origin in which there is thickening of the skin of the vulva associated with the development of the white patches which give the disease its name. Malignant changes may supervene.

(*c*) **Kraurosis vulvae**—a degenerative post-menopausal condition in which there is atrophy of the tissues of the vulva.

(*d*) **Vaginismus**—a term describing a condition of spasm of the muscles of the pelvic floor.

(*e*) **Diseases of Bartholin's glands**—Bartholin's glands (greater vestibular glands) lie, one on either side of the opening of the vagina. They may sometimes be the site of infection and abscess formation, cyst formation, and very rarely of a carcimona.

Inflammation of these glands is called **bartholinitis.**

SOME GYNAECOLOGICAL OPERATIONS

(*a*) **Colpoplasty**—a plastic operation on the vagina.

(*b*) **Dilatation of the Cervix and Uterine Curettage.** ("D. & C").
(See p. (173).

(*c*) **Hysterectomy**—removal of the uterus.

In **total hysterectomy** the whole of the uterus is removed.

In **subtotal hysterectomy** the cervix uteri is left in situ, the remainder of the organ being removed.

Pan-hysterectomy comprises total removal of the uterus together with the uterine tubes and ovaries. **Wertheim's hysterectomy** involves removal of the whole of the uterus together with the tubes, ovaries, pelvic cellular tissues, pelvic lymph glands and upper part of the vagina.

(*d*) **Myomectomy**—removal of a leiomyoma (fibroid).

(*e*) **Oophorectomy**—removal of an ovary.

(*f*) **Salpingectomy**—removal of a uterine tube. The operation of bilateral partial salpingectomy may be employed as a method of **sterilisation,** i.e. rendering the subject incapable of reproduction.

(*g*) **Salpingostomy**—making a new opening from a uterine tube into either the peritoneal cavity or the cavity of the uterus. This operation is undertaken in certain cases of sterility caused by tubal occlusion.

(*h*) **Repair operations**—a group of operations undertaken for genital prolapse.

(*i*) **Vulvectomy**—excision of the vulva.

REFERENCES

(1), (3) Barnes, Josephine. *Lecture Notes on Gynaecology*. Blackwell Scientific Publications, 1966.

(2) Ten Teachers. *Diseases of Women*. Edward Arnold Ltd., 1964.

Section F. OBSTETRIC CONDITIONS
(Normal and Abnormal)

The branch of medicine concerned with the management of pregnancy, labour and the puerperium is termed **obstetrics,** or alternatively, **midwifery.**

Pregnancy is a condition which exists from the time of **conception** (fertilization of an ovum by a spermatozoon) until the end of labour.
The normal duration of pregnancy is forty weeks. A woman in her first pregnancy is called a **primipara,** and in a second and any subsequent

pregnancies, a **multipara.** (*Note:* **parous** means "bearing or having borne offspring").

The processes which result in the expulsion of the foetus and subsequently the **afterbirth** (i.e. the placenta and foetal membranes) form the uterus constitute **labour** and may also be referred to as **childbirth** or **parturition.** The birth of a child is often referred to as a **delivery,** the mother being set free of, i.e. delivered of the child.

The period immediately following upon labour, during which the uterus returns gradually to its non-pregnant size and **lactation** (secretion of milk by the breasts) commences, is termed the **puerperium.** This period lasts about six weeks and the early part is sometimes also referred to as the **lying-in period.**

Fertilization of an ovum occurs usually in one of the Fallopian tubes. Subsequently the fertilized ovum makes its way into the uterus and imbeds itself in the uterine wall forming an **embryo** which as it develops is referred to as **foetus.** The meaning of the word "foetus" is an "offspring".

Also developed together with the growing foetus are the placenta to which the foetus is connected by the umbilical cord and foetal membranes.

The **placenta** is a vascular structure which is firmly attached to the uterine wall during pregnancy but, after the birth of the child, becomes separated and is then, together with the membranes, expelled from the uterus. The **foetal membranes** are structures which develop within the uterus so as to enclose the foetus. They are two in number, the outer being called the **chorion** and the inner, the **amnion.** The amnion bounds the **amniotic cavity** in which the foetus lies surrounded by the **amniotic fluid,** (liquor amnii). This fluid permits movement of the foetus during pregnancy and also serves as a protection against external injury.

Signs and Symptoms of Pregnancy:—these include: symptoms: amenorrhoea, nausea, morning sickness, feeling of foetal movements (18th–20th weeks) and abdominal swelling (16th–18th weeks); signs: palpable uterine enlargement, swelling of the breasts, audible foetal heart sounds (24th week onwards).

Pregnancy tests—these depend on the fact that a pregnant woman, from an early stage of her pregnancy, excretes increased amounts of a particular hormone (called chorionic gonadotrophin) in her urine. Such increased amounts may be demonstrated in various ways, e.g. by injecting a small amount of urine into a female xenopus toad as in the **Hogben test**; or by demonstrating a reaction between the urine and certain specially prepared types of antibody as in the **Pregnosticon** and **Prepuerin** tests.

Some important terms related to the practice of obstetrics are:

VIABILITY AND MATURITY

The normal duration of pregnancy is forty weeks—but at the twenty-eighth week the foetus is considered to have reached a state of development which renders it capable of survival, should premature labour take place. During and after the twenty-eighth week of uterine life, therefore, the foetus is said to be **viable.** A forty-week-old foetus is stated to be **mature** or **"at term".**

A living baby born before the fortieth week of pregnancy is stated to be **immature,** and if it weighs less than $5\frac{1}{2}$ pounds it is described as **premature.**

A dead baby born during or after the twenty-eighth week of pregnancy is called a **stillbirth.**

Expulsion of the uterine contents before the twenty-eighth week of pregnancy is known as **abortion,** or **miscarriage.**

A baby born after the fortieth week of pregnancy is described as being **postmature.**

ECTOPIC PREGNANCY (ECTOPIC GESTATION, EXTRA-UTERINE PREGNANCY)

This term indicates that the fertilised ovum has become imbedded in some site other than the cavity of the uterus. The term **ectopic** means "abnormally placed" or displaced.

The commonest form of ectopic pregnancy is **tubal pregnancy** (i.e. the ovum becomes imbedded in the wall of one of the Fallopian tubes). This condition usually terminates with rupture of the affected tube, accompanied by severe haemorrhage into the peritoneal cavity and marked shock.

MULTIPLE PREGNANCY

This term indicates the presence of more than one foetus, e.g. twins, triplets, etc.

FOETAL PRESENTATION

The part of the foetus which lies in the lowermost portion of the body of the uterus is termed the **presenting part. A normal presentation** is one in which the vertex of the foetal skull forms the presenting part, as in normal labour the foetus enters the birth canal head first.

Any form of presentation other than a vertex presentation constitutes a **malpresentation.** The commonest form of malpresentation is a **breech presentation,** when the buttocks form the presenting part.

FOETAL ABNORMALITY

This term is used to describe abnormalities which may affect the foetus as a result of developmental errors, or due to disease acquired during intra-uterine life.

A large variety of developmental errors may occur during foetal life. In many, the causes are completely unknown but in some, hereditary factors are known to play a part. As noted, when discussing diseases of the heart an association has been shown, in some cases, between the occurrence of rubella in the mother during early pregnancy and the birth of child with abnormalities such as congenital heart disease, congenital deafness and congenital cataract.

Serious congenital malformations were also noted to develop in the offspring of mothers who had taken a drug called thalidomide in early pregnancy, e.g. amelia and phocomelia (see p. 237).

Certain types of severe foetal abnormality may be demonstrated on ante-natal X-ray films. Among these are:

(*a*) **Anencephaly**—a rare developmental abnormality, the name of which means "absence of the brain". The brain fails to develop and as a result there is associated failure of development of the bones of the vault of the foetal skull and deformity of the bones of the skull base.

(*b*) **Hydrocephalus**—a condition of excessive accumulation of cerebrospinal fluid within the cranium, which may occur as a result of developmental error in foetal life or be due to acquired disease in post-natal life. The former type is called **foetal hydrocephalus** and leads to enlargement of the skull. Such enlargement may be marked and render normal delivery of the foetus impossible.

(*c*) **Foetal Death**—this is often referred to as **intrauterine death** and referred to by the initials **I.U.D.** (*Note:* this abbreviation is, however, confusing as it is also applied to certain contraceptive appliances which are collectively known as intra-uterine devices, e.g. Lippes loop, etc. Such appliances are better designated by the letters I.U.C.D.)

Prior to the onset of labour, suggestive evidence of foetal death is given by demonstrating overlapping of the bones of the cranial vault of the foetus on an antenatal radiograph of the maternal abdomen. This appearance is known as **Spalding's sign.**

(*d*) **Hydrops foetalis** (see under "Erythroblastosis foetalis—Haemolytic Disease of the Newborn").

ERYTHROBLASTOSIS FOETALIS—HAEMOLYTIC DISEASE OF THE NEWBORN

These terms are both used to indicate a group of diseases which are characterised by anaemia developing in intra-uterine life as a result of **haemolysis** (destruction of red blood cells with setting free of their haemoglobin in the blood stream). The term **erythroblastosis** indicates another feature of the disease; the presence of primitive red blood cells called **erythroblasts** in the circulation. Unlike mature red blood cells, i.e. **erythrocytes,** erythroblasts possess nuclei.

Erythroblastosis foetalis is usually caused by a condition termed **rhesus incompatibility,** and may result when a mother whose blood is of a relatively uncommon type called **Rh-negative** (rhesus negative) produces a foetus whose blood is **Rh-positive** (rhesus positive). Under such circumstances the mother may produce antigenic substances in her blood, which gaining admittance to the foetal blood stream via the placenta, set up a reaction in the blood of the foetus. This reaction causes haemolysis of foetal blood cells and resultant anaemia of varying degrees of severity.

If the reaction is not too severe, a living infant with a **haemolytic anaemia** may be born. A more marked reaction may result in a condition termed **icterus gravis neonatorum** and meaning "severe jaundice of newborn". Babies with severe jaundice may develop cerebral damage associated with pathological condition affecting the brain called **kernicterus.**

More serious forms of the disease, which are uncommon, result in a disorder called **hydrops foetalis,** in which, together with marked anaemia there is oedema of foetal tissues and ascites; or in death and maceration of the foetus and resultant stillbirth.

The blood of an infant born with haemolytic disease of the newborn will give a positive result to a test called a **direct Coombs' test.** Such an infant may require a type of blood transfusion called an **exchange transfusion,** further untoward reactions being prevented by replacing its Rh-positive red cells by Rh-negative cells from a donor with a compatible blood group.

A recent advance in the treatment of this disease is the development of a technique of **intra-uterine foetal blood transfusion.**

Medical Terms Referring to Diseases

The determination of the rhesus and ABO (see p. 198) blood groups is nowadays an important procedure in antenatal care.

ASPHYXIA NEONATORUM

A condition in which **asphyxia** i.e. a failure of normal, in respiratory function occurs immediately after birth.

A **neonate** is a newly born infant.

DISPROPORTION

This term refers to a condition in which the relative sizes of the foetus and the maternal pelvis are such as to render passage of the former through the birth canal difficult, or impossible. It may arise from the presence of a large foetus or abnormality of shape or size of the pelvis; or a combination of these factors.

In suspected disproportion valuable information regarding the internal measurements of the bony pelvis and the shape of this structure may be obtained from a radiological investigation termed **X-ray pelvimetry.**

Disproportion may necessitate forceps delivery of the child or, in severe cases, Caesarean section.

HYDRAMNIOS

A condition in which amniotic fluid forms in excessive amount. It is frequently associated with uniovular twin pregnancy; some foetal disorder in which there is difficulty in swallowing e.g. oesophageal atresia, anencephaly; erythroblastosis foetalis; or maternal diabetes. (*Note:* the opposite condition to hydramnios in which there is deficiency of amniotic fluid is called **oligohydramnios**).

ANTE-PARTUM HAEMORRHAGE

"**Ante-partum**" means before the birth of the child. **Ante-partum haemorrhage** is the name given to bleeding from the genital tract before delivery. The two commonest types of ante-partum haemorrhage are:

(*a*) **Accidental haemorrhage**—in this condition the placenta is normally situated in the upper uterine segment but becomes partially or completely separated from the uterine wall before delivery.

(*b*) **Unavoidable haemorrhage**—in this condition either the whole or part of the placenta is attached to the wall of the lower segment of the uterus. A placenta with such an abnormal site of attachment is termed a **placenta praevia.**

Ante-partum haemorrhage is a serious condition, and it is of prime importance to the obstetrician to determine whether it is of the accidental or unavoidable variety, as the treatment of the two types and the subsequent management of labour follows different lines. Considerable help in their differentiation may be obtained from soft-tissue placentography or placental angiography.

HYDATIDIFORM MOLE

This is a benign tumour of chorionic tissue and is sometimes referred to as a **chorion adenoma** (the chorion is the outer of the foetal membranes and is derived from the developing ovum).

The term **mole** means a mass, and this tumour consists of masses of small cysts which have been likened to the cysts which can occur as a result of hydatid infection.

Hydatidiform mole is an uncommon complication of pregnancy and results in enlargement of the uterus, uterine haemorrhage, and usually failure of development of the foetus. It is occasionally associated with severe pre-eclampsia.

Following the ending of a pregnancy by the formation of a hydatidiform mole, another rare complication of pregnancy may ensue. This is the development of a chorionepithelioma in the uterus (see below).

CHORIONEPITHELIOMA (CHORION CARCINOMA)

This is a malignant tumour of chorionic tissue which may develop either after: (*a*) a pregnancy which has ended with the formation of a hydatidiform mole; (*b*) a pregnancy which has ended in abortion; or (*c*) more uncommonly after the conclusion of a normal pregnancy. This neoplasm is usually highly malignant and early metastases in the lungs are frequent.

The curious fact that a chorionepithelioma may in rare instances develop in the male testis has already been noted (see p. 170).

Modern treatment of both primary growth and metastases is by administration of cytotoxic drugs.

PUERPERAL SEPSIS

Puerperal sepsis is defined by Gibberd (1) as "an infection which has entered the birth canal during or after labour or abortion". Such infection may be due to streptococci, staphylococci, or various other pathogenic bacteria. Fever (**puerperal pyrexia**) together with increased pulse rate are important clinical features, and signs and symptoms due to the localized effects of the infection in the birth canal may be present.

TOXAEMIAS OF PREGNANCY

A group of diseases of unknown causation are commonly referred to as toxaemias of pregnancy, although as pointed out by Gibberd (2) the term "toxaemia" may be a misnomer. (*Note;* **toxaemia** means the presence of poisonous substances, i.e. **toxins** in the blood).

Included in this group are:—

(*a*) **Hyperemesis gravidarum**—a condition of excessive vomiting occurring during pregnancy.

(*b*) **Pre-eclamptic toxaemia** (albuminuria of pregnancy)—a condition in which there is a raised blood pressure and the protein albumen is passed in the urine, and in which eclampsia may develop.

(*c*) **Eclampsia**—a condition in which a raised blood pressure and albuminuria are accompanied by convulsions referred to as **eclamptic fits.**

This disease is associated with lesions in the kidneys and liver, which usually appear to resolve completely after the conclusion of the pregnancy, although occasionally the liver lesions may lead to permanent liver damage and eventual hepatic failure. Intrauterine death of the foetus is common in the more severe types of eclampsia. Induction of labour is frequently necessary to avoid this complication of the disease.

POST PARTUM HAEMORRHAGE

This term indicates excessive bleeding from the uterus during the process of separation of the placenta during the last stage of labour, or shortly after the conclusion of labour.

SOME OBSTETRIC PROCEDURES AND OPERATIONS

(*a*) **Version**—a manipulative procedure employed to remedy an unfavourable foetal presentation.

Altering a malpresentation into a normal vertex presentation is called **cephalic version**; whereas turning some other type of malpresentation into a breech presentation (the type of malpresentation least unfavourable to delivery of the foetus per vaginam) is termed **podalic version.** According to the method employed version may be described as **external** or **internal version.**

(*b*) **Forceps Delivery**—delivery of the foetus per vaginam by traction on its skull with instruments called **obstetric forceps.** This procedure is employed in certain cases when labour has failed to progress normally as a result of the more minor degrees of disproportion, in certain cases of malpresentation, and in **uterine inertia** (i.e. a condition in which the uterine contractions are inadequate to expel the foetus), etc.

(*c*) **Induction of Labour**—the employment of various procedures, medical or surgical, with the object of starting the processes of labour.

(*d*) **Caesarean Section**—the delivery of the foetus through a surgical incision made through the abdominal wall and the wall of the uterus. This operation is employed in patients with marked disproportion, and in some cases of malpresentation, placenta praevia, etc.

(*e*) **Medical Termination of Pregnancy**—this term is used to indicate procedures such as induction of abortion, induction of labour and Caesarean section which may be employed when medical reasons indicate the artificial termination of a pregnancy.

(*f*) **Episiotomy** (Perineotomy)—the making of an incision in the perineum when this latter is unduly rigid and interferes with the normal passage of the foetus through the vulva to the exterior. This operation thus prevents severe perineal tearing during childbirth.

(*g*) **Vacuum Extraction**—a method employed in certain circumstances, to assist delivery of the foetus by applying suction to the foetal skull with an instrument termed a vacuum extractor.

REFERENCE

(1), (2) Gibberd, G. F. *A Short Textbook of Midwifery*. J. and A. Churchill, 1965.

Section G. THE BREAST

The two *breasts* or *mammae* (mammary glands) are, in the female, accessory organs of the reproductive system. They undergo considerable changes at puberty and further development occurs during pregnancy in preparation for lactation (milk secretion) subsequent to childbirth. Later, at the time of the menopause, they are the subject of certain atrophic changes referred to as being due to **involution** of breast tissue.

Contained in the female breast are glandular structures called *alveoli* which are composed of epithelium. Clusters of *alveoli* are grouped together to form *lobules* and these communicate with a system of ducts called *lactiferous* (*milk-carrying*) ducts. The main ducts open to the exterior on the surface of each *nipple*.

In the male, the breasts are rudimentary in nature.

The breast may be the site of congenital abnormality, traumatic disorder, infection, neoplasm, cyst formation, or be affected by endocrine disorder or idiopathic disease.

Some of the diseases that occur in the female breast can also occur in the rudimentary breast tissue of the male. Abnormal endocrine influences or the administration of oestrogens (e.g. in the hormone treatment of prostatic carcinoma) may sometimes result in enlargement of the breasts in male subjects. This disorder is called **gynaecomastia.**

Among the signs of breast disease are **mastodynia,** i.e. pain in the breast; enlargement of the breast; tenderness in the breast; the presence of a palpable tumour; discharge from the nipple; and nipple retraction.

Special methods of investigation of breast disease include a form of soft-tissue radiography called **mammography,** and also **thermography,** an investigation in which recordings of emission of infra-red rays are made at different points over the surface of the breast.

The prefixes **mammo-** and **masto-** both mean "referring to the breast". The prefix **mazo-** is also sometimes used with reference to the breast, especially in American literature.

CONGENITAL ABNORMALITIES

Congenital abnormalities of the breast are not common. They include the development of **supernumerary nipples.**

INFLAMMATORY DISEASES

Inflammation of the breast is termed **mastitis. Acute mastitis** of infective origin may result in the formation of a **breast abscess** (mammary abscess), a not uncommon condition during lactation.

NEOPLASMS

Neoplasms of the breast are common and may be benign or malignant.

The most important are:

(*a*) **Benign Neoplasms**

  (i) **Fibroadenoma**—a common tumour in young women composed of glandular epithelium and fibrous tissue.

  (ii) **Duct papilloma**—an epithelial tumour usually arising in a main lactiferous duct. This tumour frequently causes bleeding from the nipple.

(*b*) Malignant Neoplasms

Carcinoma of the Breast. (Mammary Carcinoma)—this condition is the most common form of malignant disease in the female sex and shows its highest incidence in middle age.

The tumour may arise either in the epithelium of the alveoli or of the lactiferous ducts and may be of slow or rapid growth. Metastatic spread of disease, by the lymphatics or blood stream, may be either an early or late feature of the disease but lymphatic spread is usually earlier than is spread by the blood stream.

Lymphatic metastases may be found in glands in the axilla and supraclavicular region, and later in the mediastinum and opposite breast. The principal sites for blood-borne metastases are the lungs, pleural membranes, bones and liver.

Rarely carcinoma of the breast may occur in pregnancy or during lactation and it may then show rapid progression. It may rarely develop in the male sex, when it usually also shows a high degree of malignancy.

Another uncommon form of breast carcinoma occurs in association with an eczematous condition of the nipple called **Paget's disease of the nipple.**

Breast carcinomas may, according to their pathological type, be referred to as **scirrhous carcinomas, adenocarcinomas, encephaloid carcinomas, anaplastic carcinomas, intraduct carcinomas, acute carcinomas of pregnancy or lactation,** etc., the commonest type being the scirrhous carcinomas. The extent of the disease may be indicated by a procedure termed **clinical staging.** There are four stages of mammary carcinoma. In Stage 1 the tumour is a localised growth, whereas in Stage 4, the tumour is associated with metastases in distant organs.

The cardinal clinical sign of breast carcinoma is the presence of a palpable lump in the breast. It is however, to be noted that a lump in the breast can be due to a variety of other causes, e.g. inflammation, benign neoplasm, cyst formation, fibroadenosis, etc. Mammography and thermography are often helpful in the making of a differentiation between these conditions and, in cases which come to operation, immediate microscopic examination of a **frozen section** of tissue taken from the tumour is frequently of the highest value in deciding the correct line of operative treatment.

The following methods of treatment may be employed for carcinoma of the breast, and two or more of them are often employed in combination:

(i) *Surgical*—**mastectomy,** i.e. removal of the breast. This may be described as radical, or simple (conservative), according to the amount of tissue removed.

(ii) *Radiotherapy*—treatment with ionizing radiations.

(iii) *Hormone therapy*—certain malignant neoplasms are referred to as being "hormone dependent" and progress of growth in both the primary tumour and metastases may be temporarily controlled by giving hormones (e.g. testosterone) by mouth or, in other instances by diminishing the secretion of hormones by surgical operations such as bilateral **oophorectomy** (removal of the ovaries), bilateral **adrenalectomy** (removal of the adrenal glands) and **hypophysectomy** (removal of the pituitary gland).

As an alternative to performing a surgical operation the activities of adrenal cortex can be suppressed by the administration of the suprarenal hormone cortisone. Robinson (1) refers to this form of treatment as a **"medical" adrenalectomy.** It is also possible to abolish pituitary function by implantation of radioactive yttrium, a radioactive isotope, into the pituitary gland.

(iv) *Treatment with cytotoxic drug*s e.g. thiotepa.

CYSTS OF THE BREAST

These are of several varieties. They may be found in connection with simple or malignant tumours but are most commonly seen as a feature of fibroadenosis (see later).

One type of cyst which occurs during lactation is known as a **galactocele** or **milk cyst,** and is due to blockage of a main lactiferous duct.

OTHER DISEASES

Included among these are:

(*a*) **Dysplasia of the Breast** (Mammary Dysplasia)—this is a most important condition on account of the difficulty that frequently arises in differentiating its clinical manifestations from those that can be caused by carcinoma of the breast.

Dysplasia of the breast is a term which includes the disorders referred to as **fibroadenosis, cystic hyperplasia of the breast,** and **fibrocystic disease of the breast.** These conditions used to be referred

193

7

to as **chronic mastitis,** as result of a former belief that they were conditions of inflammatory origin. It now, however, is widely thought that some abnormality of the hormones acting on breast tissue is likely to be responsible for their development.

The principal pathological features of breast dysplasia are overgrowth of fibrous tissue (fibrosis), overgrowth of glandular epithelium (adenosis), and cyst formation of varying degree in one or both breasts. Such changes may be diffuse and affect both breasts, or be localised to a relatively small area in one breast.

Hormonal treatment may sometimes be employed in the diffuse form of the disease. In the localised form surgery is often advocated as the disease often results in a lump indistinguishable clinically from a carcinoma.

Mammography is often of great value in the investigation of this disorder.

(*b*) **Traumatic Fat Necrosis**—in this condition a hard lump develops in the breast as a result of injury. Marked pathological calcification frequently occurs within the lump.

REFERENCE

(1) Robinson, J. O. *Surgery*. Longmans, 1965.

Section H. THE LYMPHATIC AND RETICULO-ENDOTHELIAL SYSTEMS

1. GENERAL CONSIDERATIONS

(*a*) **The Lymphatic System**—this system consists of *lymph glands* (*lymph nodes*), which contain *lymphoid tissue,* and *lymphatic vessels* and is concerned with draining fluid from the tissue spaces and returning it to the blood. (*Note:* the tissue spaces contain *tissue fluid,* which carries nourishment to tissue cells and is formed from the blood by continuous diffusion from the capillaries. Some of this fluid returns direct to the blood. The remainder returns to the blood via the lymphatic system).

The fluid circulating in the lymphatic system is called *lymph*. The lymph glands through which the lymph passes contain *reticuloendothelial cells* (see later) which remove foreign matter (e.g. infective bacteria, tumour cells, etc.) and thus act like filters within the system. They also contain lymphatic tissue and in this tissue are produced the white blood cells called *lymphocytes*. These cells have already been noted as carriers of antibodies and they play an important role in many chronic inflammatory processes.

Lymph which comes from the small intestine is called *chyle*. All the lymph from the body ultimately enters one of two main lymph vessels which then return it into the blood stream. These main vessels are known as the *thoracic duct* and the *right lymph duct*.

(*b*) **The Reticulo-endothelial System**—the cells of this system are disseminated widely within tissues belonging to other systems of the body and are of two types: *static* (*fixed*) and *mobile*. Both types are *phagocytic*, i.e. they are able to take up into their cytoplasm foreign matter (e.g. infective bacteria, fragments of dead tissue, tumour cells, etc.).

The fixed cells of the reticulo-endothelial system are found in great numbers in sites such as lymph glands, liver, spleen, and bone marrow, and their phagocytic properties enable them to remove foreign substances from lymph and blood. The mobile cells are found in the tissue spaces, where they are referred to as *macrophages,* and in the circulating blood when they are called *monocytes*.

Reticulo-endothelial cells play an important role in the defence of the body against infection and, in addition to being phagocytic, they appear to play some incompletely understood role in the creation of immunity against various infective diseases. They also destroy worn-out red cells, setting free their haemoglobin into the blood, and they store fatty substances called *lipoids*.

2. SOME GENERAL ASPECTS OF DISEASES OF THE LYMPHATIC AND RETICULO-ENDOTHELIAL SYSTEMS

Diseases of these two systems are conveniently considered together. In addition to lymphoid tissue, lymph glands contain much reticulo-endothelial tissue and glandular enlargement of varying degree is a common feature in the disorders of both systems. Plentiful amounts of both these types of tissue are also present in the spleen and **splenomegaly** (splenic enlargement) is often another common feature of such disorders.

Biopsy of an enlarged superficial lymph gland is frequently an important diagnostic investigation in both lymphatic and reticulo-endothelial diseases.

Evidence of disease in some parts of the lymphatic system may be demonstrated by a type of contrast radiography called **lymphangiography** (lymphography).

Any disease of lymph glands may be called a **lymphadenopathy.** Infection and carcinomatous metastases are common causes of lymphadenopathy. All other diseases affecting lymphatic and reticuloendothelial tissue are rare.

Inflammation of lymph glands is termed **lymphadenitis** (or often more simply, **adenitis**) and of lymphatic vessels, **lymphangitis.** A **lymphoma** is a tumour of lymphoid tissue and a **lymphangioma,** a tumour consisting of lymphatic vessels.

Any disease causing overgrowth of reticulo-endothelial tissue is termed a **reticulosis.** Reticuloses are described as being benign or malignant but authorities often differ as to what conditions should be classified as reticuloses.

The following are some of the diseases which are widely regarded as **malignant reticuloses**:—

(*a*) **Hodgkin's Disease** (Lymphadenoma)—this disease was so-called after Thomas Hodgkin, a nineteenth century English Physician. Its alternative name of **lymphadenoma** indicates that many authorities regard it as being a type of neoplasm. The basic pathological feature is overgrowth of reticulo-endothelial tissue, firstly in lymph glands and later in the liver and spleen and other sites such as the bone marrow, lungs, pleura and intestine.

As the disease advances, fever, wasting and anaemia develop, together with symptoms caused by pressure of enlarged glands on various internal structures, e.g. jaundice owing to pressure of glands on the bile ducts in the porta hepatis.

Treatment is usually by a combination of radiotherapy and cytotoxic drugs. Surgical excision is sometimes combined with radiotherapy when the disease is localized to a single group of glands.

(*b*) **Lymphosarcoma**—this condition as its name indicates, is a sarcomatous neoplasm arising within the lymphatic system. In contradistinction to most forms of malignant disease (carcinomatous and sarcomatous) which originate as a single primary growth, in lymphosarcoma a number of foci of malignant growth arise simultaneously in different sites. It is therefore described as being a neoplasm of **multicentric,** or **polycentric origin.**

Like Hodgkin's disease, lymphosarcoma gives rise to widespread glandular enlargement, splenic enlargement, wasting and anaemia. The clinical features of the two diseases are very similar and they can only be differentiated by biopsy of an affected lymph gland.

Radiotherapy and cytotoxic drugs are both employed in lympho-sarcoma.

(*c*) **Other malignant reticuloses**—these include the conditions called **reticulum-celled sarcoma, Ewings tumour of bone, giant follicular lymphoma,** and **Burkitts tumour,** a malignant disorder of the reticulo-endothelial system which occurs in Tropical Africa.

(*d*) Another group of reticuloses are characterised by the accumulation of excessive amounts of lipoid in cells of the reticulo-endothelial system and are thus termed **lipoid reticuloses** (lipoid storage diseases).

Lipoid reticuloses are rare. The one seen most commonly in the United Kingdom is called **xanthomatosis** (Hand-Schüller-Christian disease). The conditions called **eosinophil granuloma of bone** and **Letterer-Siwe disease** are closely related to **xanthomatosis;** all three disorders being classified as different forms of a condition called **histiocytosis X.**

Gaucher's disease and **Niemann-Pick disease** are other types of lipoid reticuloses.

Section I. THE BLOOD

1. SOME ANATOMICAL AND PHYSIOLOGICAL CONSIDERATIONS

Blood is composed of a fluid called *plasma* in which are suspended *red corpuscles, white cells* and *platelets.*

A. **Red corpuscles,** or **erythrocytes**—are formed in red bone marrow, which in childhood is found in all bones, but in the adult is limited mainly to the vertebrae, sternum, ribs, pelvic bones, and the upper-ends of the femora and humeri. The red corpuscles contain haemo-globin (an iron-containing substance which combines readily with oxygen), and their function is the carriage of oxygen to the tissues.

B. **White cells,** or **leucocytes,** are of two main types:

(*a*) **Granulocytes** (neutrocytes) which have a granular cytoplasm and are divided into:
  - (i) *Polymorphonuclear leucocytes*—often referred to more simply as **polymorphs.**
  - (ii) *Eosinophil leucocytes.*
  - (iii) *Basophil leucocytes.*

(*b*) **Hyalines** which have a clear cytoplasm and are divided into:
  - (i) *Lymphocytes.*
  - (ii) *Monocytes* (large mononuclears).

The granulocytes are formed in red bone marrow. It is generally believed that the hyalines are formed in the lymphatic system.

Polymorphs, eosinophils and monocytes possess the property of **phagocytosis,** i.e. the ability to take up foreign matter (e.g. infective bacteria, fragments of dead tissue, etc.) into their cytoplasm.

The important role of the polymorphs in inflammatory reactions was noted on p. 35. In many types of acute infection there is an increase in the numbers of polymorphs in the circulating blood. An increase in the circulating white cells is called a **leucocytosis.** When such increase affects the polymorphs it is termed a **polymorphonuclear leucocytosis,** and when it affects the lymphocytes, it is called a **lymphocytosis.**

Lymphocytes are thought to play some role in the formation of antibodies.

(*Note:* **Antibodies** are substances formed within the body which react against pathogenic microbes and other foreign substances containing protein, which may be introduced into the body. They play an important role in protection against infection.

Substances which provoke antibody formation are known as **antigens.**)

A deficiency of white cells in the circulation is called **leucopaenia.** When such deficiency is due to a diminution in the numbers of granulocytes it is called **granulopaenia,** and when due to a diminution in the lymphocytes, **lymphocytopaenia.**

C. **Platelets,** or **thrombocytes,** play an important part in the process of clotting of the blood. An increase above the normal of the numbers of platelets in the circulating blood is called **thrombocytosis,** and a deficiency of patelets is known as **thrombocytopaenia.**

All human blood belongs to one of four main types known as **blood groups,** and these, under what is termed the A B O blood group system, are described as A, B, AB, and O. The majority of individuals possess an antigen in their red blood corpuscles termed the **rhesus factor,** on account of the same factor being present in the red cells of rhesus monkeys. Such individuals are said to be **Rhesus positive** (Rh +), whilst those lacking this factor (i.e. about 15% of individuals) are said to be **Rhesus negative** (Rh-ve).

The blood contains circulating substances, which when it is shed, cause it to **coagulate,** i.e. to form a clot. The platelets are involved in this process of blood coagulation together with a soluble protein called *fibrinogen* and other substances. The actual clot consists of blood cells and platelets entangled in a mesh of *fibrin* which is an insoluble form of *fibrinogen*. Also circulating in the blood are substances such as heparin, which prevent clot formation and are termed **anticoagulants.**

The fluid part of a quantity of blood in which clot formation has occurred is called *blood serum.*

The prefix **haem-** means "referring to the blood" and the branch of medicine concerned with the study of the blood and its diseases is called **haematology.**

The process of formation of red blood corpuscles is termed **haemopoiesis** and of white blood cells, **leucopoiesis.**

(*Note:* "haemopoiesis" may also be used in a wider sense to indicate formation of both red and white cells).

2. SOME GENERAL ASPECTS OF DISEASES OF THE BLOOD

Blood diseases may be associated with either excessive or deficient production of various cells of the blood and the blood platelets; deficiency of factors essential for the production of red cells (e.g. iron); abnormal destruction of red cells; hereditary factors; defects in coagulation; structural defects in the blood capillaries, etc.

Some important diseases of the blood are: anaemias, haemophilia, polycythaemia vera, agranulocytosis, leukaemias, thrombocytopaenic purpura, infective mononucleosis (glandular fever), and reactions due to transfusion of incompatible blood.

3. SPECIAL METHODS OF INVESTIGATION

(*a*) **Blood Examinations**—these comprise a variety of laboratory investigations employed on specimens of circulating blood taken from the patient. Among these are the following:

   (i) **Haemoglobin estimation**—the haemoglobin content being expressed as a percentage of the normal, or in grammes of haemoglobin per 100 millilitres of blood (g. per 100 ml.).
   (ii) **Blood Counts**—i.e. the counting of the numbers of red cells, white cells and platelets per cubic millimetre (c.mm.) of blood. In addition to the counting of the total numbers of white cells, the numbers of each type of white cell (e.g. polymorphs, lymphocytes, etc.) may be counted; a procedure known as a **differential white cell count.**
   (iii) Investigations such as estimations of the **P.C.V.** (Packed cell volume—also known as the **haematocrit value**); **M.C.V.**

(Mean corpusular volume); **M.C.D.** (Mean cell diameter); **M.C.H.** (Mean corpuscular haemoglobin).

(iv) **Estimation of bleeding time** and **clotting time.**

(v) **Estimation of the serum bilirubin**—to indicate degree of blood destruction (haemoglobin liberated by destruction of red cells is converted into bilirubin).

(b) **Bone Marrow biopsy**—microscopic examination of a small quantity of bone marrow obtained by instrumental puncture of some superficial bone such as the sternum.

(c) **Blood Grouping**—examination of a specimen of blood to determine its A B O and Rhesus groups.

Blood transfusion, a procedure involving transference of blood from one individual (the donor) to another (the recipient) is a frequently employed form of treatment for patients suffering from anaemia due to loss of blood or other causes.

It is to be noted that, when blood is transfused, it must first be ensured that the blood of the donor and of the recipient belong to compatible blood groups. It must then be further ascertained, in each separate transfusion, that no incompatibility exists between the cells of the donor and the serum of the intended individual recipient. This is done by carrying out a procedure called **cross-matching** prior to the transfusion.

The giving of a transfusion of incompatible blood will cause a reaction within the circulation of the recipient, resulting from the destruction of the transfused red cells. Such a reaction may result in circulatory collapse which may be fatal. In reactions of lesser severity the patient may suffer liver and kidney damage.

4. ANAEMIAS

The anaemias are a group of diseases in which the blood is lacking in either, or both, a normal content of haemoglobin in its red corpuscles or normal numbers of red cells.

Anaemias may be due to haemorrhage, due to interference with red cell production, or due to excessive destruction of red cells within the circulation (see later).

The presence of anaemia is revealed by performing a haemoglobin estimation and a red cell count on a specimen of blood.

Some forms of anaemia are characterised by the red cells generally being of greater or lesser size than normal. In the former instance, the cells are termed **macrocytes** (i.e. large cells) and the anaemia is called a **macrocytic anaemia**. Red cells which are smaller than normal are called **microcytes** and those of normal size, **normocytes.**

Red corpuscles, whose haemoglobin content is less than normal, stain more faintly than is normal in blood films. They are thus described as being **hypochromic** (i.e. deficient in colour). Hypochromic cells are frequently below normal size i.e. they are **microcytes.**

In all types of anaemia the oxygen-carrying capacity of the blood is diminished.

Common clinical features of anaemia are tiredness, shortness of breath on exertion, and a characteristic pallor of the mucous membranes and skin. If the condition is of marked degree, the heart rate may be also increased and dilatation of heart may occur in severe cases. Splenic enlargment occurs in many types of anaemia and enlargement of the liver may also occur.

There are many different forms of anaemia and descriptions by different authorities frequently show a differing use of nomenclature. It will only be possible here to indicate the names and nature of a limited number of these disorders, the majority of which, as stated by Dible (1), fall into three main groups which he describes as being due to loss of blood, due to defective blood formation, and due to excessive intravascular destruction of blood.

(*a*) **Post-haemorrhagic anaemias**—this term indicates anaemias resulting from loss of blood due to either injuries to blood vessels or diseases which cause bleeding, e.g. bleeding peptic ulcer, bleeding haemorrhoids, menorrhagia, bleeding due to the group of diseases called the **haemorrhagic diseases,** e.g. **haemophilia** and **Christmas disease** (see p. 205), **thrombocytopaenic purpura** (see p. 207).

(*b*) **Anaemias due to defective production of red blood cells**—these are frequently referred to as **dyshaemopoietic anaemias,** the term **dyshaemopoiesis** meaning "defective formation of red cells".

A large number of factors may interfere with normal production, by the bone marrow, of mature red blood corpuscles. Among these may be mentioned deficiency of essential factors in the diet, (e.g. iron, Vitamin B.12, folic acid, Vitamin C. etc), and failure of absorption of such factors from the food into the body (e.g. in malabsorption syndromes); deficiency of "intrinsic factor" (see p. 202); replacement of red-cell-producing bone marrow tissue by neoplastic tissue (e.g. secondary carcinomatous deposits, leukaemic deposits, multiple myelomata); depression of the activity of red bone marrow by serious diseases in other organs and tissues (e.g. chronic suppurative infections, malignant neoplasms, nephritis, etc); damage to the red marrow by toxic agents (e.g. cytotoxic drugs and certain other drugs) and by ionizing radiations.

Factors which interfere with normal red cell production may also cause depression of the activity of cells which produce white blood cells of the granulocyte variety and, also, cells which make blood platelets. Thus leucopaenia and thrombocytopaenia are also features of a number of the dyshaemopoietic anaemias.

Among the anaemias of this type are:—

(i) **Iron deficiency anaemias**—due to either a deficiency of iron in the diet or inadequate absorption of iron from the food. Anaemias of this type include the conditions called **chronic nutritional hypochromic anaemia, chronic microcytic anaemia,** and **hypochromic anaemia of pregnancy.**

Iron-deficiency anaemias are treated by the administration of iron by mouth or parenteral administration. (*Note:* the term **parenteral** means "external to the intestine" and this implies some form of injection. Certain preparations of iron are suitable for intravenous or intramuscular injection).

Female subjects with certain types of iron-deficiency anaemia may suffer from **Plummer-Vinson syndrome,** i.e. a combination of dysphagia (difficulty in swallowing), glossitis (inflammation of the tongue) and anaemia. In these, barium swallow examination may demonstrate a thin web in the lower pharynx, known as a **sideropenic web.** (*Note:* **sideropenic** means "iron-deficient").

(ii) **Pernicious Anaemia**—also called **Addison's anaemia,** after Thomas Addison, a nineteenth century English physician. (*Note:* Addison's disease of the suprarenal medulla was also so-called after this physician).

Pernicious anaemia is due to deficient absorption of vitamin B.12 (cyanocobalamin), a substance essential for normal red cell and also white cell production. Such deficient absorption results from changes in the lining mucosa of the stomach, which cause a failure of production by this organ of **Castles "intrinsic factor",** a substance whose presence is essential for the assimilation of Vitamin B.12 from the food into the body.

The disease has its maximum incidence in middle age. In addition to the general clinical features of a severe anaemia, there is often soreness of the tongue, and gastric disorder. Neurological symptoms, due to a complicating disease of the spinal cord called **combined subacute degeneration of the cord,** develop in about 10% of cases.

Pernicious anaemia is a macrocytic type of anaemia, the average size of the erythrocytes being greater than normal in this condition. The bone marrow in this disease shows an abnormally high percentage of primitive forms of red cells known as **megaloblasts** and of other forms of immature red cells. It is thus also referred to as a **megaloblastic anaemia.** In addition to the interference with normal red cell production, the deficiency of Vitamin B.12 also has the effect of interfering with the production of white cells of the granulocyte type, and also of blood platelets. There is thus also accompanying leucopaenia and thrombocytopaenia.

Treatment was formerly by injection of specially prepared extracts of liver, this organ being a rich source of Vitamin B.12. Nowadays, however, its treatment is by preparations of Vitamin B.12 administered by intramuscular injection.

It is to be noted that in addition to pernicious anaemia there are a number of other forms of megaloblastic anaemias that develop as a result of deficiency of Vitamin B.12 or of **folic acid** (a vitamin belonging to the Vitamin B complex), e.g. certain anaemias associated with **malabsorption syndromes,** the anaemia of **tropical sprue** and **macrocytic anaemia of pregnancy.**

(iii) **Aplastic and Hypoplastic Anaemias**—anaemias in which red cell production is brought to a stop, or depressed, as a result of a varying degree of disappearance of red-cell-forming tissue from the bone marrow; or absence or depression of the normal functional activity of such tissue. These anaemias may be due to unknown causes, or result from damage to the bone marrow from drugs and other clinical agents, infections, damage from ionizing radiations etc.

The formation of granulocytic white cells and platelets may also be depressed in these disorders.

(iv) **Leuco-erythroblastic anaemia**—this type of anaemia develops as a result of the replacement of blood-forming bone marrow tissue as a result of certain disease processes (e.g. multiple carcinomatous metastases in bone, multiple myelomata, fibrous tissue formation in a rare disorder called **myelosclerosis,** etc).

(*c*) **Anaemias due to excessive destruction of red cells**—these are known collectively as **haemolytic anaemias.**

Haemolysis means destruction of red cells and in haemolytic anaemias an excessive premature destruction of these cells takes place, either within phagocytic cells of the reticulo-endothelial system, or within the circulating blood; the rate of destruction being such that the red cells cannot be replaced by the production of new red cells by the bone marrow.

(*Note:* At the end of their normal life span, which is about four months, red cells are normally destroyed by the action of reticulo-endothelias cells; the site of such destruction being mainly in the liver and spleen).

Although these anaemias are uncommon, they are of a variety of types and a variety of different factors operate in their production; e.g. rhesus incompatibility (see "erythroblastosis foetalis"), inherited fragility of red cells (see "acholuric jaundice"); inherited defects in the manufacture of haemoglobin (see later); transfusion with blood of incompatible type; malarial infection; blackwater fever; certain severe bacterial and viral infections; certain chemical substances; sensitivity to certain drugs, etc.

Excessive destruction of red corpuscles within reticulo-endothelial cells leads to raised amounts of bilirubin (an iron-free breakdown product of haemoglobin) in the blood and, if the disorder is severe, clinical jaundice may thus develop as well as anaemia (see p. 136). When, however, such destruction occurs in the circulating blood, haemoglobin is set free in the plasma, and **haemoglobinaemia** is then said to be present. This condition results in **haemoglobinuria,** i.e. passage of haemoglobin in the urine.

Inherited defects in the manufacture of haemoglobin, referred to above and occurring principally in natives of countries with warm climates, are found in a group of disorders called **haemoglobinopathies,** and also in a form of anaemia called **thalassaemia** (also known as Cooley's anaemia or Mediterranean anaemia).

Sickle-celled anaemia is one form of haemoglobinopathy and its name derives from an appearance of "sickling" of the red cells which can be demonstrated on examination of blood films taken from patients with this disease.

Another uncommon but interesting type of haemolytic anaemia occurs in the disease called **acholuric jaundice,** in which excessive breakdown of red cells develops in childhood as a result of inherited abnormal fragility of the red corpuscles. Increased amounts of bilirubin are present in the blood leading to jaundice. Splenic enlargement is a common feature of the disease and the development of gallstones, composed of bile pigment, is a common complication.

Important blood examinations in the diagnosis of haemolytic anaemias include: **estimation of the serum bilirubin** (a pigment liberated by breakdown of haemoglobin); **Van den Bergh reaction** (a test which distinguishes excess bilirubin in the serum, resulting from breakdown of red cells, from that due to failure of excretion of bilirubin in the bile resulting from obstructive jaundice), **Coombs test** (a test for antibodies associated with destruction of red cells).

5. HAEMOPHILIA

This is a rare hereditary disease which belongs to the group of blood disorders called haemorrhagic disease and is due to a defect in the coaguability of the blood. It normally only affects males but can be transmitted by females in affected families.

The condition is characterised by severe attacks of bleeding which may occur without apparent cause or result from minor injuries, tooth extraction, etc. Common sites in which haemorrhage occurs include the skin and subcutaneous tissues, the nose, the joints, and the urinary tract.

Another rare hereditary haemorrhagic disease closely allied to haemophilia is called **Christmas disease.**

6. POLYCYTHAEMIA

The prefix **poly-** means "many" and the term **polycythaemia** is used to indicate that the circulating blood contains many more red blood cells than normal.

Increased numbers of red cells may be produced as a physiological response to residence at high altitudes in order to increase the oxygen-carrying capacity of the blood and thus offset the effects of lowered atmospheric pressure. This is referred to as **physiological polycythaemia.**

Secondary polycythaemia may develop as a compensatory mechanism in certain diseases of the heart and lungs which cause interference with the oxygenation of the blood.

Primary polycythaemia occurs as a result of a primary disease of the bone marrow in which there is overgrowth of tissue producing red cells, accompanied also by proliferation of tissue producing white cells and platelets. This disorder is more commonly termed **poly-cythaemia rubra vera** but may also be referred to as **erythraemia** or **Vaquez-Osler disease.** It is predominantly a disorder of middle age, characterised by headaches, thrombus (clot) formation in blood vessels, and bleeding from sites such as the nose, alimentary and urinary tracts. Thrombi may form in the vessels of the limbs, heart or brain. Death from heart failure, or the effects of cerebral thrombosis, is a common ending to the disease. In some cases there is associated renal disease, sometimes in the form of a hypernephroma (adeno-carcinoma of the kidney).

Treatment with radioactive phosphorus is often of considerable benefit in polycythaemia vera.

7. GRANULOCYTOPAENIA AND AGRANULOCYTOSIS

A deficiency in the total number of white blood cells is termed **leucopaenia.** The leucopaenia may be due to **lymphocytopaenia**—deficiency of lymphocytes, or to **granulocytopaenia**—deficiency of granulocytes. In most instances of the latter condition the deficiency affects principally the polymorphonuclear leucocytes and, as these cells may be also described as neutrophil granulocytes, the condition may then be termed **neutropaenia.**

Deficiency of granulocytes may be due to various infections, certain drugs (e.g. amidopyrine, cytotoxic drugs), ionizing radiations, etc., or may be of unknown causation. Granulocytes, like red cells, are formed in red bone marrow. Many of the causes which produce a deficiency of granulocytes in the blood may also depress red cell formation and thus granulocytopaenia is often seen as a concomitant of anaemia.

A marked degree of granulocytopaenia is referred to as **agranulocytosis** and may result in clinical features such as fever and infective lesions in the mouth and throat, often proceeding to severe ulceration. Infective lesions may also occur elsewhere in mucous membranes and in the skin.

8. LEUKAEMIAS

The literal meaning of the name **"leukaemia"** is "white blood".

The leukaemias are diseases in which there is an overgrowth of tissue responsible for producing white blood cells. This overgrowth, moreover, does not remain confined to sites of normal leucocyte production, but is found in the form of widely scattered deposits in various internal organs, and sometimes also in the skin. Such deposits are termed **leukaemic infiltrations.** They may occur in the lungs, bones and hilar and mediastinal lymph glands, and then be deomonstrable on X-ray films.

The presence of leukaemia, is, in the vast majority of cases, associated with a considerable increase in the numbers of leucocytes in the circulating blood. In most instances the diagnosis may be readily established by performing a white blood cell count. In some cases, however, marrow puncture is necessary to determine the nature of the condition.

Anaemia is an invariable accompaniment of leukaemia owing to interference with red corpuscle formation. Haemorrhages are also common owing to reduced production of blood platelets.

Leukaemias may develop in either acute or chronic form. In any single case there is only over-production of one type of leucocyte, or its parent cells. Thus according to whether granulocytes, lymphocytes, or monocytes, or their parent cells are involved, the leukaemias are classified as being **myeloid, lymphatic** or **monocytic** type.

Splenic enlargement is a common feature in the leukaemias, being especially marked in chronic myeloid leukaemia. Generalised enlargement of lymph glands and lymphoid tissue is seen in lymphatic leukaemia.

The cause of leukaemia is unknown. There is, however, evidence to suggest exposure to high doses of ionizing radiations has played a part in the genesis of some cases.

In the treatment of leukaemias, the anaemia is combated by blood transfusion. Acute leukaemias are treated by chemotherapy, and chronic leukaemias usually by a combination of chemotherapy and radiotherapy.

9. ESSENTIAL THROMBOCYTOPAENIA

This is a rare disease, which as indicated by the term thrombocytopaenia, has as its basic pathological feature a deficiency of blood platelets (thrombocytes). The cause of this deficiency is unknown and, as the disease is characterised by **purpura,** i.e. spontaneous haemorrhage into the skin and subcutaneous tissues, it is often referred to as **idiopathic thrombocytopaenic purpura.**

In addition to the skin haemorrhages, bleeding occurs from mucous membranes and may cause haematemesis, melaena or haematuria.

(*Note:* Purpura may also occur in other diseases in which there is a deficiency of platelets due to disease of the bone marrow, e.g. leukaemias, some anaemias; and also in diseases in which there is some abnormality of the capillary blood vessels, e.g. scurvy. It may also be seen as a manifestation of hypersensitivity to various agents as in the condition called **Henoch-Schonlein purpura** or **anaphylactoid purpura.**)

10. INFECTIVE MONONUCLEOSIS (GLANDULAR FEVER)

This is an infective disorder, thought to be due to a virus and characterized by fever, glandular enlargement of varying degree, and a **mononuclear leucocytosis,** i.e. a rise in the circulating blood of hyaline white cells of the type called monocytes. There is often soreness of the throat and sometimes a rash. Enlargement of the spleen is common.

A blood test called the **Paul-Bunnell test** is positive in many cases.

There is no specific treatment but spontaneous recovery occurs, usually in a few weeks.

11. DISEASES OF THE SPLEEN

The spleen acts as a reservoir for blood, manufactures red and white blood cells during foetal life, and white cells of the lymphocyte variety during adult life. It contains much lymphoid and reticulo-endothelial tissue and its phagocytic reticulo-endothelial cells destroy worn out red blood cells.

Splenomegaly, i.e. enlargement of the spleen is a common feature in many diseases of the blood and of the lymphatic and reticulo-endothelial systems. It also occurs frequently in a number of infective disorders, (e.g. malaria, typhoid fever, glandular fever). Among its other causes are chronic right-sided heart failure and portal hypertension.

Primary disorders of the spleen are uncommon and malignant neoplasms hardly ever develop in this organ.

Traumatic rupture of the spleen is a not uncommon abdominal injury and often results in severe haemorrhage.

Spontaneous rupture of the spleen—is a condition which occasionally occurs in some disorders associated with enlargement of this organ, e.g. glandular fever.

REFERENCE

(1) Dible, J. H. *Dible and Davie's Pathology*. J. and A. Churchill, 1950.

Section J. THE ENDOCRINE SYSTEM

The endocrine system consists of a number of ductless glands, i.e. the *pituitary, pineal, thyroid, parathyroid, adrenal* (suprarenal) glands, and also certain cells within the *pancreas, ovaries* and *testes*. All its components possess the common property of elaborating secretions called *hormones*. These latter pass from the endocrine cells into the blood stream and produce effects of various kinds in other organs and tissues.

The anterior lobe of the pituitary gland exercises a general control over many of the activities of the other components of the endocrine system.

The branch of medicine which deals specifically with diseases of the endocrine system is called **endocrinology.** There are a great many disorders resulting from hyperfunction (over activity) or hypofunction (underactivity) of endocrine organs. These range from minor disorders to severe and disabling diseases.

Certain complex relationships exist between a number of the endocrine glands and, accordingly, some of the diseases of this system are highly complex in nature. In general, it is only proposed here to refer to terms which describe some of the more clearly defined endocrine diseases.

1. DISEASES OF THE PITUITARY GLAND

The pituitary gland, or hypophysis, lies in the pituitary fossa (sella turcica) of the sphenoid bone, being connected to the base of the brain by the pituitary stalk. It consists of two lobes which differ in both structure and function:

(*a*) **The anterior pituitary lobe** develops from the buccal (mouth) cavity of the embryo and secretes hormones connected with growth and lactation, and other hormones which affect the activity of the thyroid, and suprarenal glands and the activities of endocrine cells in the ovaries and testes.

Overactivity of the anterior lobe is called **hyperpituitarism** and underactivity **hypopituitarism.**

Tumours of glandular tissue, called **pituitary adenomas** may develop in the anterior pituitary. These are of three types called **eosinophil, basophil** and **chromophobe adenomas;** being so-called according to the staining properties, with certain dyes, of the cells which compose the tumours (e.g. the cells of an eosinophil adenoma have an affinity for an acid dye called **eosin**).

Eosinophil adenoma is associated with over-production of growth hormone and, if it develops before growth of the skeleton is complete, leads to **pituitary gigantism.** After growth has ceased, however, such a tumour causes a condition called **acromegaly,** the name of which means "large extremities". Sufferers from acromegaly show overgrowth of certain bony structures and generalized overgrowth of soft tissues. They have large hands and feet and prominence of the lower jaw. Enlargement of the pituitary fossa also occurs and can be shown on X-ray films of the skull. Severe headaches are common and, if the tumour extends outside the pituitary fossa, it frequently causes disturbances of vision, ultimately resulting in blindness.

Basophil adenoma is very rare. It is usually small and thus does not enlarge the pituitary fossa. It may be associated with a disorder of the adrenal glands called **Cushing's syndrome** (see "Diseases of the Suprarenal Glands").

Chromophobe adenoma is the most frequently seen type of pituitary tumour. It often attains a large size resulting in enlargement of the pituitary fossa and destruction of its bony walls. It causes headaches, vomiting and blindness. There is often also amenorrhoea in females and **impotence** (i.e. inability to perform the sexual act) in males, as a result of deficient hormone secretion.

Other disorders of the anterior lobe of the pituitary gland include the following conditions which develop as a result of factors causing hypopituitarism:

(i) **Pituitary Dwarfism,** the main types of which are called **Lorain dwarfism** (pituitary infantilism) and **Fröhlich's syndrome** (dystrophia adiposo-genitalis).

(ii) **Simmonds' disease**—a condition of severe hypopituitarism seen most frequently in women, in whom it occurs as a result of destruction of the anterior lobe following upon childbirth. It is associated with amenorrhoea, wasting and premature senility.

(*b*) **The posterior pituitary lobe** develops as a downgrowth from the brain and thus consists of nervous tissue. Its hormones are secreted by cells in the base of the brain and stored by the posterior lobe and then released into the blood stream. These hormones can raise the blood pressure; stimulate contraction of the muscles of the uterus during and after labour; and exercise what is termed an **anti-diuretic effect** on the kidneys, i.e. prevent secretion of greater than normal amounts of urine.

(*Note:* **diuresis** means "secretion of increased amounts of urine".)

As a result of disease affecting the posterior lobe of the pituitary gland, pituitary stalk or certain structures in the base of the brain, secretion of the anti-diuretic hormone may be impaired causing **diabetes insipidus,** a disease characterized by severe thirst and **polyuria,** i.e. the passage of excessive amounts of urine.

Surgical removal of the pituitary gland is termed **hypophysectomy.**

2. DISEASES OF THE THYROID GLAND

The thyroid gland lies in the lower part of the neck. It consists of two lateral lobes, joined by an isthmus which lies in front of the upper part of the trachea. Its activities are subject to the control of the anterior lobe of the pituitary gland. It secretes an iodine containing hormone called **thyroxin** which exerts a considerable influence on the metabolism of tissues throughout the body. **Metabolism** is a term used to describe the processes whereby absorbed foodstuffs are modified for tissue building and repair; and whereby waste products are broken down into forms which can be excreted from the body.

Warwick (1) states that "too much or too little thyroxin in circulation results in a metabolic rate which is incorrectly balanced to the needs of the body".

The activity of the thyroid gland can be assessed by a procedure known as **estimation of the basal metabolic rate** (B.M.R. estimation) and also by tests which measure its uptake of radioactive iodine.

Overactivity of thyroid secretion is known as **hyperthyroidism,** and underactivity as **hypothyroidism.**

Enlargement of thyroid gland, diffuse or localized, is a feature of many thyroid diseases and any enlargement of thyroid tissue is termed a **goitre.**

Goitres may exert pressure effects on the trachea causing dyspnoea (difficulty in breathing) and on the oesophagus causing dysphagia (difficulty in swallowing).

Enlarged thyroid tissue may sometimes extend behind the sternum into the upper thorax. Such an extension is termed a **retrosternal goitre** and may be demonstrable on chest X-ray films.

Surgical removal of the thyroid gland is called **thyroidectomy.**

(*a*) **Types of Goitre**—some important types of goitre are:

(i) **Simple Goitre** (Non-toxic goitre)—this condition is unassociated with any abnormality of endocrine secretions. One form of this condition is thought to result from a deficient intake of iodine. In another type, known as **non-toxic adenomatous goitre,** single or multiple nodular overgrowths of glandular tissue, called **thyroid adenomas,** develop in the gland.

(ii) **Toxic Goitre**—a name used to describe any goitre associated with hyperthyroidism (i.e. overactivity of the thyroid gland) resulting from oversecretion of the thyroid hormone, thyroxin.

The presence of abnormally high amounts of this hormone leads to a general increase of cellular metabolic processes throughout the body. This is evidenced clinically by signs and symptoms such as rapid pulse, excessive sweating, loss of weight, restlessness, nervousness and tremor of the hands, i.e. the so-called "toxic" features of the disorder which lead to it also being referred to as **thyrotoxicosis.**

In one form of toxic goitre, known as **exophthalmic goitre,** or **Graves' disease,** in addition to evidence of hyperthyroidism there develops also **exophthalmos,** i.e. a condition of protrusion of the eyballs.

In another type of toxic goitre, thyrotoxic features may develop in a patient who has had a non-toxic adenomatous goitre for many years. This type is sometimes called a **toxic adenoma.**

Toxic goitres in middle-aged and elderly subjects may be complicated by the development of a form of heart disease known as **thyrotoxic heart disease.** Atrial fibrillation is common in this condition.

The treatment of toxic goitres may be by surgery, anti-thyroid drugs (e.g. carbimazole) or radioactive iodine.

(iii) **Malignant Goitre**—this is due to the development of carcinomatous changes in the thyroid gland and is thus also termed **carcinoma of the thyroid gland.** This neoplasm is not usually associated with overactivity of the gland but it often produces metastases at an early stage of its growth. These develop most frequently in lymph glands in the neck and in the lungs and bones.

(*b*) **Hypothyroidism.** Underactivity of the thyroid gland is, as already noted, termed **hypothyroidism.** This condition is associated with defective secretion of thyroxin and consequent diminution of metabolic activities of cells throughout the body.

In certain cases of hypothyroidism occurring in adults, there is a characteristic thickening of the subcutaneous tissues which simulates swelling of the tissues due to oedema. This type of hypothyroidism is called **myxoedema** and among its other features are an abnormally slow pulse rate, obesity, lethargy, slowing of mental processes, loss of hair, and enlargement of the heart. Treatment is by administration of thyroxin.

Cretinism (infantile hypothyroidism) is another type of hypothyroidism. It may occur as a congenital condition due to absence, or marked underdevelopment of the thyroid gland. It can also develop in early childhood, when it appears to result from iodine deficiency and may be associated with a goitre.

Among the clinical features of cretinism are lethargy and retardation of mental and skeletal development. The tongue is enlarged and protruding, and the infant is pot-bellied. Treatment is by administration of thyroxine.

(*c*) **Other Diseases**—other diseases of the thyroid gland include a number of uncommon inflammatory disorders, e.g. **acute thyroiditis, Hashimoto's thyroiditis, Riedel's thyroiditis.**

3. DISEASES OF THE PARATHYROID GLANDS

The parathyroid glands are normally situated on the posterior aspect of the thyroid gland. They are variable in number; four usually being present. Rarely, ectopic (abnormally placed) parathyroid glands may be sited in the superior mediastinum.

The parathyroids secrete a hormone, called **parathormone** which is concerned with the maintenance of a normal level of calcium in the blood plasma and a normal balance between the amounts of calcium and phosphorous in the blood.

(*a*) **Hyperparathyroidism**—in this uncommon condition there is overactivity of parathyroid tissue resulting in oversecretion of parathormone, and increased amounts of calcium are found in the blood. This latter feature is termed **hypercalcaemia.**

Primary hyperparathyroidism may result from the presence of a benign tumour called a **parathyroid adenoma** or from hyperplasia (overgrowth) of the parathyroids. **Secondary hyperparathyroidism** may develop as a secondary effect of certain kidney diseases in which there is increased loss of calcium in the urine.

In both types of hyperparathyroidism there is increased absorption of calcium from the bones. The bones become osteoporotic and may develop a condition termed **generalized osteitis fibrosa.** Renal stones are also common as a result of the increased blood calcium leading to increased excretion of calcium in the urine; the latter condition being called **hypercalciuria.**

(*b*) **Hypoparathyroidism**—is a rare condition, resulting from deficiency of parathormone, and is usually seen as a result of accidental removal of the parathyroid glands during thyroidectomy (surgical removal of the thyroid gland).

In this disorder the blood calcium is below normal, resulting in an undue excitability of nervous and muscular tissue. This excitability may lead to the development of **tetany,** a condition characterized by painful muscle spasms. (*Note:* tetany occurs in other disorders in which blood calcium levels are below normal and in diseases in which the blood has a more alkaline reaction than normal, i.e. in various forms of **alkalosis**).

4. DISEASES OF THE SUPRARENAL GLANDS

The suprarenal (adrenal) are two in number and each lies in close apposition to the upper pole of the corresponding kidney, in the posterior part of the abdomen.

Each gland consists of an outer part called the cortex and inner part called the medulla. These structures are of different developmental origin and thus differ from each other in structure and function (cf. the anterior and posterior lobes of the pituitary gland):

(*a*) **The suprarenal cortex**—produces a large number of endocrine secretions and its principal functions are concerned with the metabolism of carbohydrates, minerals and water. It also produces sex hormones of both male and female type. These latter play some part in the development of secondary sexual characteristics and the functioning of the sex glands; but the production of sex hormones by the suprarenals is small in relation to production of these substances by the gonads (i.e. the testes and ovaries). It is interesting to note that small quantities of androgens (male sex hormones) are secreted normally by the adrenals in females and small quantities of oestrogens (female sex hormones) are secreted in males both by the suprarenals and by endocrine cells in the testes.

The secretion of hormones by the adrenal cortex is stimulated by the anterior pituitary hormone called **corticotrophin** or A.C.T.H. (adrenocorticotrophic hormone).

The prefixes **adrenocortico-** and **cortico-** are both used with reference to the suprarenal cortex.

Adrenocortical hormones may thus be classified into three main groups:—(i) **glucocorticoids**—which affect carbohydrate metabolism, e.g. cortisone and hydrocortisone, (ii) **mineralocorticoids**—which affect mineral metabolism and in particular are concerned with the retention of sodium and water in the body. These are thus referred to by Strong (2) as the **sodium retaining hormones,** e.g. aldosterone, deoxycorticosterone, (iii) **sex hormones,** i.e. **androgens** (e.g. testosterone) and **oestrogens** (e.g. oestriol, progesterone). (See also "Note re. Corticosteroid Therapy").

Diseases of the suprarenal cortex are not common. Over-activity of the adrenal cortex is often referred to as **hyperfunction of the suprarenal cortex** (adrenocortical overaction) and may be associated with hyperplasia (overgrowth) of adrenocortical tissue on both sides, the presence of one or more benign tumours called **cortical adenomas,** or in rare instances, **carcinoma of the adrenal cortex.**

The principal diseases which occur as a result of **adrenocortical hyperfunction** are:

(i) **Cushing's Syndrome**—a condition associated predominantly with overproduction of carbohydrate-regulating hormones (glucocorticoids) and sometimes accompanied by changes in the basophil cells of the anterior lobe of the pituitary, or the presence of a tumour of this structure called a **basophil adenoma.**

Among the clinical features of Cushing's syndrome are obesity of the face (producing the characteristic "moonface" appearance), obesity of the trunk with accompanying wasting of the limbs, hypertension and glycosuria, osteoporosis, impotence in males and amenorrhoea and virilisation in females. (**Virilisation** means the development, in female subjects, of male secondary sexual characteristics, e.g. deepening of the voice, growth of a beard, etc.). The disorder is associated with increased excretion, in the urine, of substances called **17-ketosteroids.**

Treatment of the condition may be surgical, or by the administration of hormones or irradiation of the pituitary gland: or by various combinations of these three methods. Surgery is indicated in cases in which a cortical neoplasm is found to be present.

(ii) **Conn's Disease**—a rare condition associated with overproduction of the mineralocorticoid called aldosterone, and thus also known as **primary aldosteronism.**

It is characterized by retention of sodium and water which may result in oedema. Muscular weakness is a prominent clinical feature and hypertension develops in some cases.

(iii) **Adrenogenital syndrome**—a disorder associated with overproduction of sex hormones, usually of androgens but sometimes of oestrogens. Richardson (3) states this syndrome results in virilisation (see under Cushing's syndrome) in females and sexual precocity in boys with, very rarely, feminisation in adult males.

Hypofunction of the adrenal cortex may result from bilateral atrophy or destruction (e.g. by tuberculous infection) of the suprarenal glands and is seen clinically in the form of Addison's disease.

Addison's Disease (Adrenal insufficiency) was so-called after Thomas Addison, an English physician after whom Addisonian anaemia was also named. It most commonly develops in middle-aged subjects and is associated with a deficiency of cortical hormones concerned with carbohydrate metabolism (glucocorticoids) and with metabolism of minerals (mineralocorticoids). Among its clinical features are severe general weakness, mental apathy, low blood pressure, brownish pigmentation of the skin and gastro-intestinal disturbances. Treatment is by administration of corticosteroids.

[**Note re. Corticosteroid therapy:** the word **steroid** literally means "fat-like" and describes a class of substances to which belong the

corticosteroids, i.e. steroid hormones produced by the suprarenal cortex, e.g. cortisone, aldosterone.

The treatment of diseases by corticosteroid hormones and certain synthetic substances with similar properties is called **corticosteroid therapy,** or alternatively **steroid therapy.**

Substances such as naturally occurring cortisone and hydrocortisone, and synthetic corticosteroids are widely employed in the treatment of a variety of different conditions, e.g. rheumatoid arthritis, ulcerative colitis, sarcoidosis, following bilateral adrenalectomy, in the emergency treatment of hypersensitivity reactions and for vomiting resulting from courses of radiotherapy.

Some patients receiving corticosteroid therapy may develop undesirable side-effects as a result of treatment, e.g. signs and symptoms similar to those of Cushing's syndrome, peptic ulceration, etc.

Disorders of this nature which are the direct result of remedies prescribed in treatment of the primary condition are often referred to as **iatrogenic diseases** meaning literally "diseases caused by physicians". (Other examples of iatrogenic diseases include insulin coma, reactions to treatment with ionizing radiations, etc.).

Sudden cessation of corticosteroid therapy is dangerous as it may produce so called **"withdrawal symptoms"** among which may be generalized muscular weakness and sometimes circulatory collapse. Patients on routine treatment with steroids may be given a "steroid card" to carry on their persons giving particulars regarding such treatment.

(*b*) **The suprarenal medulla** is derived from nervous tissue and secretes two hormones, *adrenaline* and *noradrenaline*.

Adrenaline acts on the nerve endings of the sympathetic nervous system. It increases the output of blood by the heart, and the blood supply of the skeletal muscles during times of stress, whilst diminishing the circulation in the skin and gastro-intestinal tract. As stated by McNaught (4) in a concise account of the endocrine system, "adrenaline reinforces the action of the sympathetic nervous system in preparing the various systems of the body to meet emergencies".

The functions of noradrenaline are as yet incompletely understood but it has the property of raising the blood pressure.

Several rare types of tumour may develop in the suprarenal medulla, viz:

(i) **Phaeochromocytoma**—a rare tumour, of cells called phaeochromocytes, which may be benign or malignant. It secretes the suprarenal medullary hormones, adrenaline and noradrenaline, and consequently produces hypertension (high blood pressure).

The hypertension may be persistent or occur in intermittent attacks. In this latter event it is referred to as **paroxysmal hypertension.**

(ii) **Neuroblastoma**—a rare but highly malignant tumour which is composed of nerve cells of primitive type called neuroblasts. It occurs in childhood and frequently produces metastases at an early stage in sites such as the lungs, liver and bones.

(iii) **Ganglioneuroma**—a very rare benign tumour of nerve cells.

4. DISEASES OF THE GONADS

Diseases of the ovaries are referred to in Section E and diseases of the testes in Section D.

5. DISEASES OF THE PANCREAS ISLETS

The cells of the pancreas, which belong to the endocrine system, are arranged in collections known as the **pancreas islets** or **islets of Langerhans.** These cells secrete a hormone called **insulin,** which plays an important role in carbohydrate metabolism.

Overproduction in insulin is associated with a rare tumour of the pancreas called an **islet cell tumour** (insulinoma).

Deficient production of insulin or defective action of insulin gives rise to a common and important disease called diabetes mellitus.

Diabetes mellitus—is due to defective action of insulin which may result from (i) deficient secretion of this hormone by the islet cells of the pancreas, (ii) oversecretion of **insulin antagonists,** i.e. other hormones in the body which render the action of insulin less effective than normal (the adrenocortical hormone cortisone and anterior pituitary growth hormone are examples of insulin antagonists), (iii) increased requirements of the body for insulin due to the development of obesity (when such requirements are in excess of what the pancreas can meet).

Defective action of insulin interferes with the normal utilisation of glucose by tissue cells and also with the production of glycogen and its storage. (*Note:* carbohydrates are converted into glucose during digestion and absorbed into the blood in this form. The absorbed glucose is then either utilized by tissue cells, or converted into a starch called glycogen and stored in the liver and muscles). Such defective hormone action leads to **hyperglycaemia** (excessive amounts of glucose in the blood) and consequent **glycosuria** (passage of glucose in the urine).

Common symptoms of diabetes are excessive thirst **(polydipsia),** the passage of excessive amounts of dilute urine **(polyuria),** and loss of weight. A variety of other symptoms and signs may occur as a result of the disease and its many complications. The milder type of case may, however, be completely symptomless.

The passage of large amounts of sugar containing urine gives the disorder its name; **diabetes** meaning "to go through" and **mellitus** meaning "honey".

(*Note:* used without qualification the term diabetes is used to indicate diabetes mellitus and not the uncommon pituitary disorder called diabetes insipidus.)

In the severer forms of diabetes, secondary disorders may develop also in the metabolism of fats and proteins. The former may result in accumulation of substances called **ketone bodies** in the blood, i.e. **ketosis** (keto-acidosis) and the presence of such substances in the urine, i.e. **ketonuria.** Diabetic ketosis is a serious development and may lead to a state of unconsciousness termed **diabetic coma** (hyperglycaemic coma).

Important diagnostic investigations in suspected diabetic subjects including the testing of the urine for sugar and ketone bodies, **blood sugar estimations,** and tests termed **glucose tolerance tests.**

Diabetes is a disease of many complications. Among these are **diabetic cataract** (opacity of the lens of the eye), **diabetic retinopathy** (also called diabetic retinitis—see p. 286), **diabetic gangrene, diabetic neuropathy** (a disease of the nervous system) which may lead to the development of **Charcot joints** (see p. 254). Diabetics show an increased liability to the development of septic infections; certain forms of renal disease, especially pyelonephritis; pulmonary tuberculosis; and the degenerative arterial disease called atheroma.

Treatment of diabetes is by dietetic measures in mild cases and generally, in more severe cases, by dietetic measures combined with the administration of insulin by injection. In some instances drugs which lower the blood sugar may be given by mouth, instead of giving insulin. Such drugs are called **oral hypoglaemic agents** (e.g. tolbutamide).

It is to be noted that overdosage with insulin may lower the blood sugar to such an extent that a type of coma termed an **insulin coma** (hypoglycaemic coma) may develop.

REFERENCES

(1) Warwick, R. *Whillis's Elementary Anatomy and Physiology,* 1961.
(2) Strong, J. A. *The Principles and Practice of Medicine* (Ed. Sir Stanley Davidson). E. and S. Livingstone, 1966.

(3) Richardson, Sir John. *The Practice of Medicine*. J. and A. Churchill, 1960.
(4) McNaught, Anne. *Companion to Illustrated Physiology*. E. and S. Livingstone, 1965.

Section K. THE SKIN AND SUBCUTANEOUS TISSUES

1. SOME ANATOMICAL AND PHYSIOLOGICAL CONSIDERATIONS

The **skin** consists of an outer layer called the *epidermis* and an inner layer called the *dermis*.

The epidermis consists of epithelial cells among which are cells containing the pigment *melanin* and called *melanocytes*. It does not contain any blood vessels but receives its noruishment from the blood capillaries of the dermis. The deepest cells of the epidermis are known as *basal cells*. The most superficial layer of the epidermis is called the *horny layer*.

The dermis is richly supplied with blood vessels, lymphatic vessels and nerves. It also contains *hair follicles, sebaceous glands,* and *sweat glands,* and these structures together with the hair and the nails are sometimes referred as the **appendages of the skin.**

The skin provides a waterproof protective covering for the body and the pigmentation in the epidermis protects the delicate under-lying dermis from excessive ultra-violet radiation. It has functions concerned with the regulation of body temperature and is to some extent concerned with the excretion of water and salts. It is also able to absorb certain oily substances.

The prefix **derm-** and the adjective **cutaneous** mean "pertaining to the skin".

The skin is separated from the deeper tissues of the body by the **subcutaneous tissues,** composed of connective tissue and containing some of the main fat deposits of the body.

2. SOME GENERAL ASPECTS OF SKIN DISEASES

The branch of medicine concerned with diseases of the skin is known as **dermatology.**

Skin diseases produce effects which in most instances are readily discernible on visual inspection but bacteriological examination is an important procedure in infective dermatological conditions, and biopsy is frequently required in certain cutaneous disorders.

Among the signs and symptoms of skin disorders are:—**erythema** (redness of the skin); **rashes** (eruptions) composed of lesions, referred to as **macules, papules, vesicles,** or **petechiae** (see under "Infectious Fevers" p. 45); urticaria (nettle rash); purpura (see p. 207); ulceration of the skin: crust formation, fissure formation, scarring; areas of skin thickening (such areas are termed **hyperkeratoses** when the thickening is due to overgrowth of the horny layer of the skin); areas of atrophy of the skin: localised or diffuse areas of swelling in the skin and subcutaneous tissues; small localised swellings in the skin termed **nodules;** tumour formation, etc.

There are many primary disorders of the skin and a large variety of diseases of other systems of the body may produce secondary lesions within the skin. It will only be possible herein to indicate medical terms referring to a selected number of common or otherwise important skin diseases.

Among the methods of treatment employed in dermatology are the external application of ointments, creams, lotions, paints, pastes and powders, etc., to the skin; the internal administration of drugs, the giving of injections, the use of medicated baths; surgical procedures including plastic surgery and diathermy; the use of carbon dioxide snow; graduated exposures of ultra-violet rays; and superficial X-ray treatment.

3. CONGENITAL ABNORMALITIES

As a result of errors in development, in rare instances the opening of a congenital sinus or fistula may be present in the skin at birth. Such a condition results from persistence of structures which normally disappear during intra-uterine life. Examples are **branchial sinus** and **branchial fistula** in the neck; **pilonidal sinus** found usually behind the upper part of the coccyx; and **urachal fistula** leading from the urinary bladder to the umbilicus.

4. TRAUMATIC DISORDERS

These include damage to the skin and subcutaneous tissues caused by violence, mechanical irritation, external physical agents and external chemical agents.

A breach in the continuity of the skin, caused by violence is termed a **wound.**

Mechanical irritation or pressure as a result of long periods of lying in bed may produce open sores (i.e. breaches in the skin surface, skin ulcers) called **bedsores** or **pressure sores.** Pressure sores may also result from ill-fitting plaster splints and other appliances.

Intermittent pressure over the toes, or less commonly in other sites, may cause a localised thickening in the horny layer of the skin called a **corn.**

Damage to the skin from excessive heat, electric currents, certain chemical agents (e.g. strong acids and alkalies, phosphorous) produces injuries called **burns.** These may be classified as **superficial** (partial skin thickness) and **deep** (full skin thickness) **burns.** In these latter, there may also be damage to underlying structures such as muscle and bone. The more extensive type of burn is accompanied by considerable loss of blood plasma from damaged capillaries in the burnt area and resultant shock.

5. INFECTIONS

These are of considerable variety and include inflammatory disease due to infection with bacteria, viruses, and fungi. Some examples are:

(*a*) **Pyogenic Infections**—as indicated in Part III infection with pus-producing bacteria may cause the following types of infection in the skin and subcutaneous tissues:

> (i) due to staphylococci—**furuncle** (boil), **carbuncle, paronychia** (whitlow), **pulp infection of a finger, wound infection.**
>
> (ii) due to streptococci—**cellulitis, erysipelas.**

In addition to the above, either staphylococcal of streptococcal infection may cause a contagious infection of the skin called **impetigo contagiosa.** The lesions of this disorder occur most frequently in the skin of the face and scalp in the form of small blisters known as **vesicles** and larger blisters termed **bullae.** These rupture and their contents form thick yellow crusts on the skin surface.

(*b*) **Tuberculosis of the Skin**—this may occur in the form of (i) **primary tuberculosis of the skin,** which is very rare, (ii) **Lupus vulgaris** —an uncommon type of post-primary tuberculous infection which produces small reddish brown nodules in the skin. These are seen most commonly on the face and neck and tend to heal with the production of much deformity. Carcinoma may sometimes develop in an area of lupus. (iii) eruptions called **tuberculides.**

(*c*) **Syphilis**—syphilitic infection of the skin may occur in the primary, secondary, or tertiary stages of the disease, and in congenital syphilis. The initial lesion of the disease known as the **primary sore** or **chancre** develops in the skin or a mucous membrane. In the majority of cases it occurs in the external genital organs.

Syphilitic rashes are common in secondary syphilis and in early congenital syphilis. In tertiary syphilis the characteristic lesions known as **gummas** may develop within the skin and cause ulceration.

(*d*) **Gas gangrene**—a disorder caused by putrefactive bacteria and usually seen as a result of a wound infection. The infecting organisms cause putrefaction and accompanying gas formation in skin, subcutaneous and muscle tissue. The condition is treated by administration of penicillin or other antibiotics.

(*e*) **Anthrax**—an uncommon bacterial disease in which infection is derived from infected animals such as cattle and pigs, or infected animal products such as wool, hides and bristle used in the manufacture of imported shaving brushes.

The word **anthrax** means "a carbuncle" (see p. 51) Infection of the skin with the *bacillus anthracis* causes a lesion resembling a carbuncle and known as a **malignant pustule;** or less commonly a spreading type of infection affecting the skin and subcutaneous tissues and called **anthrax oedema.**

Another type of anthrax infection may affect either the lungs or gastro-intestinal tract and is termed **wool sorter's disease.**

(*f*) **Leprosy** and **Yaws,** see Part V.

(*g*) **Herpes simplex**—a virus infection which causes redness of the skin and the formation of vesicles in affected areas. It develops most commonly in the lips and surrounding skin, but may also occur on the genital organs.

(*Note:* **Herpes Zoster,** another condition characterised by a vesicular skin eruption, is primarily a disorder of the nervous system and will be referred to later.)

(*h*) **Verruca Vulgaris** (Common Wart)—**verrucae,** or **warts** of this type are common and are localized overgrowths of epithelium due to a virus infection. They are sometimes classified as benign tumours of the skin. They have a roughened surface and occur chiefly on the hands, forearms, and soles of the feet **(plantar warts).** They are often resistant to treatment but in some instances disappear spontaneously.

(*i*) **Molluscum contagiosum**—is a term used to describe another form of warts due to virus infection. In this condition the epithelial overgrowths have a smooth surface.

(*j*) **Ringworm** (tinea) is a term used to describe a group of diseases due to infection of the skin by a number of related fungi called **ringworm fungi.** The commonest members of the group are (i) **tinea capitis** (ringworm of the scalp), (ii) **tinea pedis** (ringworm of the foot)—also known as **epidermophytosis,** or **athlete's foot,** (iii) **tinea cruris** (ringworm of the leg)—also known as **dhobie's itch.** (*Note:* "dhoby" is the Hindu name for a washerman). This condition usually commences on the inner side of the upper part of the thigh and may spread from there to the skin of the groin, abdomen and genital organs

(*k*) **Skin Eruptions due to Infectious Fevers**—these have been referred to in Part III.

6. INFESTATIONS

These disorders are due to animal parasites which provoke an inflammatory reaction in the skin. They include:

(*a*) **Scabies**—due to infestation with a form of parasite called a **mite.** The mite which causes this highly contagious disease is called *sarcoptes scabiei* and its presence in the skin causes severe itching, and a rash composed of papules and small vesicles. The name of the disease is derived from a Latin word meaning "to scratch".

(*b*) **Pediculosis**—"pediculus" is the Latin word for "a louse" and this term describes three disorders resulting from infestation with lice. As denoted by their individual names, **pediculosis capititis, pediculosis corporis,** and **pediculosis pubis,** the infestation in these disorders affects respectively the head (scalp), body and pubic region.

7. NEOPLASMS

BENIGN NEOPLASMS

(*a*) **Papilloma**—a localised overgrowth of skin which consists of an outer covering of epithelium and an inner portion of connective tissue. In external appearance it may resemble a verruca.

(*b*) **Simple melanoma** (pigmented mole)—a tumour of cells which produce pigment. A simple melanoma may be present at birth, or first appear in adult life. It may, in some instances, undergo malignant change into a **malignant melanoma.**

(*c*) **Lipoma**—a tumour which develops from fat cells in the sub-cutaneous tissue.

(*d*) **Haemangioma**—a tumour of vascular tissue of which there are several different forms. The **"spider naevus"** and the **capillary angioma** are both due to new growth of capillaries. The latter is popularly called a "birth-mark" or "port-wine" stain.

Haemangiomas may also occur in muscles, bones and in the liver and brain. Certain types of haemangioma are treated by radiotherapy.

Clotting of blood may take place within the vessel walls of haemangiomas. Subsequently calcium salts may be deposited within the clots, producing opacities in radiographs.

(*e*) **Lymphangioma**—a tumour of the lymphatic system, which may rarely be found in the skin or subcutaneous tissues or elsewhere. A type which grows in the deep tissues of the neck is called a **cystic hygroma.**

MALIGNANT NEOPLASMS

(*a*) **Epithelioma** (squamous carcinoma)—this is a carcinomatous new growth arising from cells of the epidermis. It may be seen on any part of the skin, but is commonest on the face and lips. It may present as an outgrowth of skin, or as an ulcer.

It is rarely seen before middle age. Chronic irritation is a factor in its causation in many cases, e.g. through exposure to certain types of oil used in industry, and exposure to excessive doses of ionizing radiations. It may also develop in any area of extensive scarring, such as may follow old burns, or infection with lupus vulgaris.

The tumour is usually of slow growth, but has a tendency to spread, so as to involve deeper structures, such as bone. Bone involvement may be demonstrated on radiographs. Spread by lymphatics may be an early or late feature of this disease, but blood-borne metastases are usually only seen in its later stages.

Treatment may be by surgical excision or by radiotherapy.

(*b*) **Rodent ulcer** (basal-cell carcinoma)—this condition is also a carcinoma arising in cells of the epidermis. However, whereas an epithelioma originates from cells called **Malphigian cells,** a rodent ulcer is, in most instances, a growth of the **basal cells of** the epidermis.

Rodent ulcer is also rare before middle age. It is of slow growth and does not produce metastases. If not successfully treated however, in the course of time, it causes widespread destruction of the skin and deeper tissues. The face is by far the commonest site for its occurrence.

Treatment may be by surgical excision or radiotherapy.

(*c*) **Malignant melanoma**—is often a very rapidly growing and highly malignant tumour of the pigment-producing cells of the skin or their ancestral cells. It may arise as a result of malignant change in a pigmented mole, or alternatively, in an apparently normal area of skin. It may also originate within the eye.

Lymphatic and blood-borne metastases are frequently early features of a malignant melanoma. Such metastases are commonly seen in lymph glands, lungs and liver, and not infrequently in bone.

(*d*) **Metastases**—metastatic growths from primary carcinomas of other organs (e.g. breast), are sometimes found in the skin.

8. URTICARIA (NETTLERASH)

This term describes a type of inflammatory reaction which occurs in skin as a manifestation of allergy (hypersensitivity) to various agents. The reaction may be localized or generalized and is evidenced by the presence in the skin of areas of erythema, which cause itching and which often develop into wheals.

The name **urticaria** derives from the Latin word for "a nettle" and the condition may result from nettle stings, insect bites, ingestion of certain protein foods and drugs, and the injection of iodine-containing radiographic contrast media, etc.

A type of urticaria of unknown causation, called **papular urticaria** is of common occurrence in childhood and is popularly referred to as "heat spots". It is usually provoked by insect bites.

9. ECZEMA AND DERMATITIS

The term eczema is used to indicate a number of skin diseases which exhibit a special type of cutaneous inflammation called the **eczema reaction.** This reaction appears, in the majority of instances, to be a manifestation of skin allergy.

In allergic or otherwise predisposed subjects, the eczema reaction may result from agents which reach the skin (i) from the exterior, e.g. the external application of certain drugs and chemicals (e.g. penicillin, certain chemical dyes and detergents, photographic chemicals), contact with certain plants (e.g. primulas), exposure to sunlight, micro-organisms, (ii) via the bloodstream, e.g. ingested proteins.

Terms referring to different forms of eczema include the following: **contact eczema, infective eczema, infantile eczema.**

Eczema may present in acute or chronic form and among the clinical features produced by the eczema reaction are erythema, itching, the formation of vesicles and sometimes bullae, weeping (i.e. exudation of fluid from the skin lesions), crust formation and the development of areas of skin thickening.

Some authorities classify eczema as a form of dermatitis. The term

dermatitis when used in its widest sense may be employed to indicate any form of inflammation of the skin. Other authorities use the term in a more restricted sense and differentiate between eczema and conditions which may be described as forms of dermatitis.

Some individual disorders described as "dermatitis,' are **dermatitis herpetiformis, radiation dermatitis** (produced by ionizing radiations) and **neurodermatitis** (an eczematous condition in which psychological factors are thought to play a role).

The description of **industrial dermatitis** is applied to certain non-infective types of cutaneous inflammation arising as a result of the patient's occupation.

The term **generalised exfoliative dermatitis** described a condition in which there is shedding of the superficial layers of the skin over large areas of the body. (Shedding of the superficial layers of the skin is known as **exfoliation** or **desquamation**). It may develop as during the course of other skin disorders when these occur in generalized form (e.g. psoriasis, eczema, drug eruptions); as a complication of Hodgekin's disease or leukaemia: or may arise from completely unknown causes.

10. SOME OTHER SKIN DISEASES

(*a*) **Psoriasis**—the name of this inflammatory disorder means "itching". It is a common disease, of unknown origin and chronic course. The characteristic lesions consist of red papules covered by white scales. They may occur in any part of the skin, but are commonest over the knees and elbows and in the scalp. In older patients there is not infrequently an accompanying arthritis (inflammation of joints) referred to as **psoriatic arthritis.**

(*b*) **Chilblains** (Erythema pernio)—these lesions represent an abnormal response to cold in affected areas of skin. They are due to the action of cold on the capillaries in sites such as the fingers and toes, heels, lobes of the ears, and tip of the nose.

(*c*) **Cutaneous sarcoidosis**—sarcoidosis is a chronic inflammatory disease of unknown origin. It lesions bear a similarity to those seen as a result of chronic tuberculosis, They occur most frequently in sites such as the skin, lungs, hilar glands and other lymph glands, bone, the eye and the parotid gland.

In bone, sarcoid lesions occur most commonly in the phalanges producing a condition known as **osteitis multiplex cystoides.** A combination of eye lesions and lesions in the parotid glands constitutes the condition called **uveo-parotitis**. (*Note:* the uveal tract comprises the iris diaphragm, ciliary body and choroid coat of the eye.)

In the skin, sarcoidosis may produce a nodular condition called **Boeck's sarcoid** or more rarely a condition called **lupus pernio** which affects the cheeks and nose.

Erythema nodosum (see below) may also develop in patients with sarcoidosis.

(*d*) **Drug eruptions** (Drug Rashes)—this term is used to indicate skin rashes which develop as a result of the internal administration of certain drugs. It does not include eczema or dermatitis caused by the external application of drugs to the skin.

Percival (1) states that drug eruptions are examples of allergy but that "the allergic processes involved in urticaria, eczema and drug rashes, differ basically from one another."

Among the drugs which may cause eruptions are penicillin, sulphonamides, bromides and iodides.

(*e*) **Erythema nodosum**—a condition in which, as indicated by its name, tender reddish rounded areas of thickening appear in the skin, usually on the shins but sometimes on the forearms. The lesions are usually few in number.

In many instances this disease appears to be an allergic response to primary tuberculous infection or streptococcal infection elsewhere in the body. Erythema nodosum may also follow the taking of certain drugs and is seen, not infrequently, in patients with sarcoidosis.

(*f*) **Pemphigus**—this word means "a blister" and is used to denote a group of uncommon diseases, of unknown origin, which are characterized by rashes in which the essential feature is the formation of bullae (i.e. fluid-containing blisters, larger than vesicles). The condition called **pemphigus vulgaris** is the least uncommon member of this group.

(*g*) **Angioneurotic oedema**—is a condition which can affect both the skin and mucous membranes. It is of rapid onset and produces marked oedematous swelling of affected tissues, as a result of excessive leakage of fluid from the blood capillaries therein. It occurs most commonly in the region of the mouth and face. It can affect the throat and larynx and in severe cases the swelling may cause a degree of respiratory obstruction which necessitates tracheostomy.

(*h*) **Ichthyosis**—a condition of abnormal dryness of the skin. Areas of the skin surface may present an appearance resembling those of fish scales and the name of the disease derives from the Greek word meaning "a fish".

(*i*) **Dupuytren's Contracture**—a disorder in which thickened bands of fibrous tissue develop in the subcutaneous tissues of the palm and produce flexion deformities of fingers; usually the middle and ring fingers.

11. SOME DISORDERS OF THE SKIN APPENDAGES

(*a*) **Acne Vulgaris**—is a common disorder in adolescents of both sexes but occurs more frequently in males. Endocrine factors appear to play some part in its causation and it appears to be aggravated in some individuals by certain foodstuffs.

In acne, lesions called **blackheads** or **comedones** form in the openings of the hair follicles, blocking these latter structures and causing a surrounding inflammatory reaction which results in the formation of papules which are red in colour. Secondary infection of the follicles with staphylococci occurs and causes many of the papules to develop into pustules. The basic patholocigal features of the disease are enlargement of sebaceous glands, increased secretion of **sebum** (i.e. the oily material secreted by sebaceous glands) and blocking of the openings of these glands.

Increased secretion of sebaceous glands is called **seborrhoea** and is associated with other disorders besides acne (e.g. with the occurrence of dandruff of the scalp).

The lesions of acne occur mainly in the skin of the face, neck and upper part of the back. They tend to disappear spontaneously during early adult life.

(*b*) **Alopecia**—this term means "baldness", i.e. absence of hair from the scalp.

Diffuse baldness may be associated with seborrhoea (i.e. increased secretion of sebum by sebaceous glands) or following severe infections, injuries or operations.

Localized areas of baldness may develop as a result of diseases or injuries of the scalp or treatment with X-rays etc. They may also occur in a condition of unknown origin called **alopecia areata.**

(*c*) **Prickly heat,** (Miliaria)—is a disorder in which blockage of sweat glands results in the development of an irritating skin rash. It is predominantly a disease of hot climates.

REFERENCE

(1) Percival, G. H. *An Introduction to Dermatology.* (E. and S. Livingstone, 1967).

Section L. THE LOCOMOTOR SYSTEM

The *bones* and *joints* together with the *skeletal muscles* and their *tendons* and *aponeuroses* constitute the **locomotor system.** As indicated by its name this system is concerned with movement (i.e. **locomotion** means movement from one place to another).

The bones are sometimes referred to as constituting the **skeletal system** and the joints as constituting the **articulatory system.**

Also connected with the locomotor system are certain of the structures called *bursae* (see later).

1. SOME ANATOMICAL AND PHYSIOLOGICAL CONSIDERATIONS. OSTEOPOROSIS. OSTEOMALACIA

(*a*) **Bones** are structures composed of specialised connective tissue and are of four principal types:— *flat bones* (e.g. skull vault), *irregular bones* (e.g. vertebrae), *long bones* (e.g. femora,) and *short bones* (e.g. phalanges).

Individual bones when fully developed possess:

(i) An investing membrane—the *periosteum*. This surrounds the bone, except in such areas where bony surfaces entering into the formation of joints have a protective covering of *articular cartilage*.

The periosteum consists of an outer layer of fibrous tissue and an inner layer, containing cells called *osteoblasts,* which readily lay down new bone if it is injured or affected by certain disease processes (e.g. infection; neoplastic disease).

(ii) A complete outer shell of bone tissue of the type called compact or cortical bone—the *cortex*.

(iii) An inner portion composed of bone tissue of the type called cancellous or spongy bone—the *medulla*.

In long bones there is a hollow space in the middle of the medulla. This is called the *medullary cavity* and is lined by a fibrous membrane called the *endosteum*.

Compact bone consists of tightly packed layers of bony tissue within which are spaces containing blood vessels and nerves. Cancellous bone contains numerous plates of bony tissue, which are called *bone trabeculae* and are arranged in such a manner as to produce a spong-like appearance. Between the trabeculae are spaces called *marrow spaces* which contain soft tissue known as *bone marow.*

Bone marrow is of two types (i) *yellow marrow,* which consists mainly of fat, and (ii) *red marrow* which is very vascular and contains cells which form red blood corpuscles, granulocytic leucocytes and blood platelets. In childhood red marrow is found in all bones but, in the adult, it is limited chiefly to the vertebrae, sternum, ribs, skull and pelvic bones, and upper ends of the humeri and femora.

During foetal life bones are preformed in either *cartilage* (another type of specialised connective tissue, referred to in lay language as "gristle"), or a type of fibrous connective tissue called "*membrane*". The processes of bone formation are referred to collectively as **ossification** or **osteogenesis,** and according to the type of tissue in which it originates, bone formation may take the form of **ossification-in-cartilage** (e.g. as in the bones of the limbs) or **ossification-in-membrane** (e.g. as in the bones of the skull vault and clavicle).

Ossification in the great majority of bones commences in foetal life but in some (e.g. the carpal bones and some of the tarsal bones), it starts in childhood. The site, or sites, at which bone form commences within a developing bone are called *primary centres of ossification,* Some bones during their period of growth also develop *secondary centres of ossification.* These are generally all referred to as *epiphyses,* although certain of them (i.e. those which do not enter into the formation of joints) are more strictly termed *apophyses.*

During the formation of bone tissue, cells called *osteoblasts* lay down *osteoid tissue* which possesses an abundant intercellular substance called *matrix* (**osteoid** means "bone-like" and **matrix** a "mould"). This latter contains large amounts of a protein substance called *collagen,* which is an important constituent of all forms of connective tissue.

Osteoid tissue is converted into *bone tissue* proper by the deposition in the matrix of calcium salts from the bloodstream (mainly in the form of calcium phosphate) and matrix is then often referred to as *calcified matrix.* It is this process of calcification that gives bone tissue its characteristic rigidity.

The cells of fully formed bone are known as *osteocytes.* During the processes of bone formation, other cells called *osteoclasts* which have the ability to absorb bone, model the newly formed bone tissue to its required shape.

Osteogenesis does not cease when growth of the bony skeleton is complete. The activities of osteoblasts and osteoclasts continue throughout life and all bone tissue is subject to a continual process of absorption of old bone and its replacement by newly formed bone.

In early adult life and middle age the processes of bone production and bone replacement are exactly counterbalanced but with the onset of old age, the formation of new bone tissue decreases.

A generalised or localised upset in the processes of normal ossification may result in the development of:

(i) **Osteoporosis**—a condition in which the formation (but not the calcification) of osteoid tissue is defective. Osteoporotic bones contain less bone tissue and thus less calcium than normal. They are more brittle than normal bones, and accordingly fracture more easily. They also show a diminished density on X-ray films.

In accordance with the decreased formation of new bone referred to above as a normal feature of old age, a generalized osteoporosis is common in elderly subjects and is referred to as **senile osteoporosis.** The increased liability of the old to sustain fractures of their bones is well known.

Disuse is another common factor in osteoporosis. Lack of normal mobility of a part, or parts of the body, may produce a localized or generalized form of the condition termed **disuse osteoporosis.**

Endocrine disorders may also diminish bone formation and cause generalized osteoporosis, (e.g. **post-menopausal osteoporosis**), as also may the therapeutic administration of hormones, (e.g. osteoporosis due to cortisone and other forms of steroid therapy).

Vitamin C is essential for the production of collagen, the protein substance which has been noted above as an important constituent of bone matrix. Thus osteoporosis is one of the predominant features of scurvy, a disease due to deficiency of this vitamin.

Protein deficiency states may also interfere with the formation of osteoid tissue causing osteoporosis.

Localized osteoporosis may be produced as a result of certain infective process (e.g. tuberculosis) and neoplasms affecting bone.

(ii) **Osteomalacia**—a generalized condition in which osteoid tissue is formed in normal amounts but, owing to a defective supply of calcium and/or phosphorous from the blood, calcification of bone matrix is deficient. The bones as a result, are less rigid than normal and if the disorder is marked, severe bony deformities may develop, particularly in weight-bearing bones.

The name "osteomalacia" means "softening of bone".

Osteomalacia may result from a diet which contains inadequate amounts of calcium and/or phosphorous, and/or Vitamin D (a fat soluble vitamin which controls the absorption of these substances from the bowel and their utilization by the tissues of the body). It may also be due to **malabsorption syndromes** (e.g. coeliac disease, idiopathic steatorrhoea, see p. 129), which prevent absorption of these substances from the small bowel; or due to **renal causes,** i.e. certain types of congenital and acquired kidney disease which cause an undue loss of calcium and phosphates in the urine.

Some types of osteomalacia due to renal causes may also be complicated by changes which are due to **secondary hyperparathyroidism** (see p. 213) a condition which develops as a reaction to a certain type of disorder of calcium and phosphate metabolism.

Some reference to the clinical manifestations of osteomalacia will be made when discussing metabolic diseases of bone.

Concise and detailed accounts of osteoporosis and osteomalacia and the radiological appearances produced by these conditions have been given by Grainger (1).

(*b*) **Joints** (articulations) are formed wherever two or more bones come into contact. The opposing bone ends may be connected by fibrous tissue (e.g. sutural joints of skull), or cartilage (e.g. symphysis pubis). In the majority of the joints of the body however, the bone ends are covered in *articular cartilage* and separated from each other by a joint cavity containing *synovial fluid.* This fluid is formed by the *synovial membrane* that lines the *joint capsule* surrounding the joint. The joint capsule is strengthened by *supporting ligaments* composed of connective tissue. Joints of this type are called *synovial joints* (e.g. shoulder, hip, etc.).

(*c*) **The skeletal muscles** are all composed of muscle tissue of the type called *voluntary (striated) muscle.* [*Note:* the other two types of muscle tissue found in the body are known as *involuntary (smooth, non striated) muscle* and *cardiac muscle*].

These muscles are attached to bones by bands of dense white fibrous tissue called *tendons,* or sometimes by sheets of white fibrous tissue called *aponeuroses.* The fleshy part of a muscle is referred to as its *belly.*

The skeletal muscles are all surrounded by coverings of fibrous connective tissue called *deep fascia,* and lie beneath the *superficial fascia,* a layer of fibrous tissue which is found immediately below the skin.

All forms of muscle tissue possess powers of contraction, which are subject to the control of the nervous system, and are thereby able to effect movement of joints.

(*d*) **Bursae**—these are small fluid containing sacs which lie between certain structures and facilate their movements, e.g. between a tendon and a bone, a bone and overlying skin, or between two muscles. As they are related to the skeletal system, it is convenient to refer later in this section to disease conditions affecting certain of bursae.

The prefix **osteo-** means "pertaining to bone"; **chondro-**, "pertaining to joints"; **arthro-.** "pertaining to joints"; and **myo-,** "pertaining to muscle".

2. SOME GENERAL ASPECTS OF DISEASES OF THE BONES AND JOINTS

Bones may be the subject of congenital disorders, traumatic disorders, infective diseases, neoplasms, and cyst formation. They may also be affected by metabolic diseases, chemical poisons, endocrine and idiopathic diseases.

Many diseases of bone produce secondary effects on neighbouring joints. There are also a number of important primary diseases of joints, among which are certain congenital, traumatic, inflammatory and degenerative conditions.

Bone and joint diseases may give rise to clinical features such as pain, deformity, limitation of movement, bony swelling, soft tissue swelling, secondary wasting of muscles.

Radiological investigation is both of great value in the diagnosis, and in assessing the response to treatment of many types of bone and joint disease and injury, whilst in some, pathological investigation (e.g. by bacteriological examination, biopsy, etc.), is also required.

Many diseases of the bones and joints, and also of the muscles and tendons, fall within the scope of the orthopaedic surgeon, particularly traumatic diseases (i.e. injuries) and deformities. The word **orthopaedics** derives from the Greek words "straight" and "child" and thus indicates one of the main concerns of this branch of medicine, namely the correction of deformities in children.

The orthopaedic surgeon is concerned both with operative and non-operative methods of treatment. Adams (2) describing non-operative methods of treatment in orthopaedic disorders lists "rest: support, physiotherapy, local injections, drugs, manipulation and radiotherapy".

The work of physiotherapists, occupational therapists and remedial gymnasts frequently plays a very important part in the treatment and rehabilitation of patients suffering from injuries and diseases of the bones, joints and muscles. (Note: **rehabilitation** means the process of rendering a disabled person both mentally and physically fit to resume some form of occupation).

3. CONGENITAL ABNORMALITIES OF BONES AND JOINTS

Congenital abnormalities of the bones and joints are of considerable variety. They range from small isolated developmental errors, affecting a single bone, to gross changes which may be widespread throughout the skeleton. Structural abnormalities are found in some of these disorders unassociated with any upset in the normal processes of ossification, e.g. in polydactyly extra digits are found and these may be normally ossified. In other types, some of which are described as skeletal **dysplasias** and others as skeletal **dystrophies,** there are abnormalities of osteogenesis (bone formation).

Both the nomenclature and the systems of classification used in the description of these disorders are complex and reference here will only be made to some of the commoner or more interesting forms of congenital lesions of the skeletal and articulatory systems.

(*a*) **Cervical rib**—is an accessory rib and may be formed on one or both sides of the body, articulating with the seventh cervical vertebra. A cervical rib is generally symptomless but, in some instances, may cause pain and disability through pressure on the lowest trunk of the brachial nervous plexus or subclavian artery. Surgical excision of the accessory rib may then be required.

(*b*) **Spondylolisis**—is a congenital abnormality in which an affected vertebra has a gap in one, or both sides of its posterior arch. The condition is usually confined to a single vertebra: usually the fifth lumbar but sometimes the fourth lumbar vertebra. The importance of this condition is that its presence may result in a forward slipping of the affected vertebra, carrying with it all the spinal vertebrae which lie above. The condition is then referred to as **spondylolisthesis,** i.e. **spondyle**—"a vertebra", **listhesis**—"slipping".

(*c*) **Spina Bifida**—is a congenital abnormality in which the two halves of the posterior arch of one or more spinal vertebrae fail to unite. They are thus divided by a cleft, i.e. they are "bifid".

If the resultant gap in the posterior arch is large the spinal meninges may protrude through it constituting a **meningocele,** or there may be a protrusion of both meninges and spinal cord, when the condition is called a **meningo-myelocele.** The presence of a spinal meningocele or meningo-myelocele is evidenced by a soft-tissue swelling of variable size in the midline of the back. The severer degrees of these conditions may be associated with various forms of paralysis and necessitate operative treatment within the first twenty-four hours after birth.

The simplest form of spina bifida is symptomless and unassociated with any protrusion of the contents of the spinal cord and is referred to as **spina bifida occulta**; the word **occulta** meaning "hidden".

(*d*) **Congenital Dislocation of the Hip**—a **dislocation** is a displacement of bone surfaces which form a joint. In this condition, in addition to dislocation or subluxation (see p. 239) of the hip joint on one or both sides, there is usually defective development of the upper part of the acetabulum. Many authorities regard this latter feature as the basis of the disorder and the displacement of the femoral head as secondary to the malformation of the acetabulum (i.e. the cup-shaped cavity on the outer side of the hip bone, which articulates with the head of the femur).

Congenital dislocation of the hip is much commoner in female than in male children.

This condition is due to some incompletely understood abnormality of the hip joint which results in a dislocation of one or both hips which is either present at birth, or develops shortly afterwards. Undue laxity of the ligaments of the hip joint appears to be a factor of considerable importance in many cases of the disorder.

Early diagnosis is of prime importance in this condition and a simple clinical test can be employed to demonstrate the presence of dislocation, or of a predisposition to dislocation, in newborn babies.

Treatment in the majority of instances is by closed reduction and splinting. Some cases, however, may require operative treatment.

(*e*) **Achondroplasia**—the name of this disease derives from its being due to defective growth (aplasia) of bones that are pre-formed in cartilage ("chondro"—meaning "pertaining to cartilage"). Thus **achondroplasiacs,** i.e. individuals affected with achondroplasia, have abnormally short arms and legs and small skull bases; whilst the bones of their skull vaults, which are ossified in membrane, grow to a normal size. Their intelligence is normal and their muscular development is usually very strong. Many of the dwarfs seen in circuses are achondroplasiacs.

Related to achondroplasia are two other types of congenital bone dysplasia called **Morquio's disease** (chondro-osteodystrophy) and **gargoylism** (Hurler's syndrome). Both these disorders are rare. The latter is associated with disordered metabolism of fatty substances called lipoids.

(*f*) **Osteogenesis imperfecta**—this uncommon disease affects the whole skeleton. Owing to defective bone formation, the bones are abnormally fragile and fracture easily when subjected to mild trauma. The liability to fracture may develop in foetal life, or alternatively may not occur until early or late childhood. In the course of time the disorder shows a tendency towards spontaneous cure.

Many patients with osteogenesis imperfecta have an intense blue colour of the sclerotic coats of their eyes and may develop deafness in early adult life, due to a condition called otosclerosis.

(*g*) **Some other congenital abnormalities**—these include:

(i) **Arachnodactyly** (spider digits)—in this condition, the fingers, and sometimes the toes, are of abnormal length. In a disorder called **Marfan's syndrome** arachnodactyly occurs in association with congenital heart disease and dislocation of the lenses of the eyes.

(ii) **Cleido-cranial dysostosis**—a condition in which defects of ossification occur in the clavicles and skull.

(iii) **Congenital coxa vara**—**coxa** is the Latin term for the "hip joint" and in this disorder the hip joint is the subject of a **varus** deformity, i.e. a deformity in which the angle between the neck and shaft of the femur is reduced so as to approach a right angle. Varus deformity of the hip joint may be due to causes other than congenital abnormality, e.g. slipping of the femoral head epiphysis (adolescent coxa vara), fracture of the femoral neck in old age.

(iv) **Congenital pes cavus**—congenital claw foot. (**Pes** means "foot").

(v) **Congenital pes planus**—congenital flat foot. This condition may occur together with **congenital vertical talus.**

(vi) **Congenital talipes equino-varus**—congenital club foot. **Talipes** means "club foot" and the term **equino-varus** indicates that the foot is both turned inwards (**varus**) and that the anterior part of the foot is dropped with raising of the heel (**equinus**— so called by comparison with a horse's hoof).

(vii) **Congenital Torticollis**—congenital wry-neck.

(viii) **Hemivertebra**—a condition of failure of development of half of a vertebral body. It is one of the causes of **congenital scoliosis** (lateral curvature of the spine).

(ix) **Craniostenosis**—this is a rare disorder of ossification-in-membrane affecting the bones of the skull vault. It leads to premature fusion of one or more of the sutures which separate these latter bones and consequent deformity of the skull. Such deformity may take various forms according to the suture or sutures involved. The least uncommon variety is known as oxycephaly (tower skull). (Note: the sutures of the skull vault normally commence to fuse afout fifteen years of age).

(x) **Hereditary multiple exostoses** (diaphyseal aclasia, dyschondroplasia)—a condition in which multiple small outgrowths, called *exostoses,* arise from the growing ends of bones which are pre-formed in cartilage.

(xi) **Hypertelorism**—a deformity of the base of the skull resulting in a greatly widened space between the orbits.

(xii) **Osteopetrosis** (Marble bones)—an uncommon generalized disease in which affected bones show a greatly increased density on radiographs.

(xiii) **Polydactyly**—the presence of extra digits (i.e. fingers or toes).

(xiv) **Sacralisation**—a condition of partial or, less commonly, complete fusion between the lowest lumbar vertebra and the first sacral vertebra.

(xv) **Sprengel's Shoulder**—congenital elevation of the scapula.

(xvi) **Syndactyly**—web-fingers or web-toes, with which may be associated bony fusion in the affected digits.

(xvii) **Amelia** (absent limbs) and **phocomelia** (rudimentary limbs)—two severe forms of developmental error.

4. TRAUMATIC DISORDERS OF BONES AND JOINTS

These may take the form of fractures of bones, dislocations or sprains of joints, and subperiosteal haematomas.

(*a*) **Fractures**—A **fracture** is a break in the continuity of a bone, which usually results from a severe degree of direct or indirect injury, or sometimes from violent muscular contraction (e.g. as in some fractures of the patella and ribs). Rarely a fracture may occur as a result of repeated minor injuries producing a so-called **stress fracture** (fatigue fracture). The commonest site for a stress fracture is in the shaft of a metatarsal, when it is referred to as a **March fracture.**

A fracture may also occur, with or without violence through an area of bone weakened by disease, being then termed a **pathological fracture.** Carcinomatous secondary deposits in bone are a common cause of pathological fracture.

Fractures are of two main types (*a*) **simple** (closed)—where no wound connects the fracture site and the surface of the body; and (*b*) **compound** (open)—where there is an external wound which leads down to the fracture site.

Simple or compound fractures may be described as **complicated**

fractures when associated with injury to nerves, important blood vessels or internal organs, or **comminuted fractures,** when the bone is broken into several fragments.

(Note: in all fractures there is injury to small blood vessels with consequent swelling and bruising of adjacent soft tissues).

Fractures are generally named according to their site, e.g. fracture of neck of the femur. A number, however, are named after surgeons, e.g.:

Bennett's fracture—a fracture of the base of the first metacarpəl, involving its lower articular surface and showing outward displacement of the distal fragment.

Colles' fracture—a fracture of the lower end of the radius about half to one inch above the wrist joint, with outward and backward displacement of the lower fragment. There is often an accompanying fracture of the ulnar styloid process.

Smith's fracture—is often called a reversed Colles. It is a fracture of the lower end of the radius with forward displacement of the lower fragment.

Pott's fracture—this term is nowadays generally used to indicate a variety of fractures, which involve the lower ends of the tibia and fibula in the region of the ankle joint.

Guérin's fracture—a fracture of the maxilla with detachment of the tooth-bearing segment. The injury is usually bilateral.

Clinically, fractures may be evidenced by pain and tenderness over the fracture site, swelling and interference with normal function. If the fracture has caused displacement of the fractured bone ends, there may be visible or palpable deformity. Shock is also a common associated feature; its degree varying with the severity of the injury.

Radiological examination plays an essential role in both the diagnosis of suspected fractures and in the control of treatment, when the diagnosis has been established.

Fracture treatment involves considerations regarding first aid and the treatment of associated shock, wounds and complications, besides treatment of the injured bone or bones. The latter, in most types of fracture, consists basically of (i) firstly, correcting, as far as possible, any displacement of the fractured bone ends. This is called **reduction** (setting of the fracture). [**Closed reduction** comprises manipulative procedures or the exerting of gradual **traction** to reduce the fracture, i.e. by exerting a pull on the skin (**skin traction**) or on a pin inserted into bone (**skeletal traction**). **Open reduction** involves carrying out a surgical operation to set a fracture.] (ii) secondly, preventing movement between the fractured bone ends until they are firmly joined together by new bone. This is termed **immobilisation** and may be effected by the use of Plaster of Paris splints or casts, metal splints, etc., or after an open reduction by various **internal fixation** methods such as **screwing, plateing, nailing, pinning, wiring,** or **bone grafting.** (iii) thirdly, preserving the function of muscles and joints in the vicinity of the fracture. [*Note:* Reduction is not possible in every type of fracture, and it is to be noted that early movements are prescribed for some comminuted fractures.]

Fractures heal by production of new bone, and firstly a rudimentary type of new bone, called **callus** is laid down between the fragments and joins them together. Callus is at first soft but gradually becomes hardened. When it is sufficiently hard to prevent any movement between the fragments, **union** of the fracture is stated to have taken place. Callus is gradually converted into mature bone and, when this process is complete, **consolidation** of the fracture is said to have occurred.

Fractures, owing to a variety of causes (e.g. inadequate immobilisation, infection, etc.) may be the subject of **delayed union** or of **non-union** with the formation of a **false joint** between the ununited fractured bone ends.

One cause of non-union is known as **avascular necrosis,** a term indicating death of cells in a localized area, through loss of their blood supply. This condition is seen when an injury causing a fracture, is such as to deprive one of the fragments of the injured bone of an adequate blood supply. This complication occurs most commonly in fractures of the femoral neck and carpal scaphoid.

(*b*) **Dislocations**—a dislocation is a condition of displacement of the ends of bones which form a joint. If the displacement is such that the articular surfaces of these bones retain some degree of contact, the dislocation is described as being **incomplete,** or as a **subluxation.**

Most dislocations result from severe trauma but they can be due to congenital malformation (e.g. congenital dislocation of the hip) or, as in the case of **pathological dislocations,** they may result from disease of a joint or its motor muscles.

(*c*) **Sprains**—"sprain" is a term used to describe a soft tissue injury due to the tearing of the ligaments or articular capsule of a joint.

Traumatic damage to a joint capsule may result in the secretion of excess of synovial fluid into a joint, a condition referred to as **traumatic synovitis.**

(*d*) **Subperiosteal haematomas**—an injury, insufficient to cause a fracture, may sometimes result in the formation of a haematoma (i.e. a swelling due to a localized collection of blood) beneath the periosteum in the affected part of a bone. Subsequently, ossification may occur in the swelling.

An **ossifying haematoma** may produce appearances on an X-ray film very similar to those of malignant bone tumour called an osteogenic sarcoma.

(*e*) **Internal Derangement of the Knee Joint (I.D.K.)**—is a term used to describe several varieties of injury to the knee joint including sprains due to tearing of the capsule of the knee joint or its collateral ligaments, tearing of the cruciate ligaments within the joint, and tears of the external or internal semilunar cartilages (menisci). Tears of the latter structures are commonly referred as **"torn cartilage"** and are especially common in footballers and others who follow athletic pursuits.

5. INFECTIONS OF BONES AND JOINTS

Infective micro-organisms may invade the soft tissues of the bone marrow causing an inflammatory reaction in these tissues termed **osteomyelitis.** They may also cause inflammation of the periosteum producing **periostitis.** Both these conditions are forms of **osteitis,** a comprehensive term indicating the presence of inflammation in any part of a bone.

In some types of bone infection thrombosis of blood vessels in the affected area may result in fragments of bone undergoing necrosis through loss of their blood supply. Such dead fragments of bone are called **sequestra** (singular: **sequestrum**).

When an infective lesion in a bone is situated near a joint, secondary joint infection may result in **infective arthritis** (joint inflammation). Infective arthritis can also commence primarily in the synovial membrane of a joint and then develop a secondary spread into adjacent bone.

If a joint infection leads to much destruction of articular cartilage, a common sequel is **ankylosis,** i.e. union of the opposing joint surfaces by fibrous tissue **(fibrous ankylosis)** or by newly formed bone **(bony ankylosis).**

Inflammatory changes in bone may be either acute or chronic. They may result in stimulation of osteoblasts and consequent new bone formation; or stimulation of osteoclasts with bone destruction. Frequently a combination of both these types of reaction is produced.

Both processes produce changes demonstrable on X-ray films.

Infection of bones and joints may be (i) haematogenous (i.e. blood borne), the micro-organisms being carried in the blood from a focus of infection elsewhere in the body; (ii) by direct spread from a focus of infection in nearby tissues; or (iii) via the wound of a compound fracture or a penetrating missile injury.

Some important types of infections of bones and joints are:

(a) **Acute Osteomyelitis** (Acute Suppurative Osteomyelitis, Acute Pyogenic Osteomyelitis)—this is an acute suppurative infection of bone usually commencing in the marrow spaces within the medulla but frequently spreading to involve cortical bone and periosteum.

The disease is commoner in children than in adults. It can affect any bone in the body but occurs most frequently in the metaphysis of a long bone, i.e. in the end of the diaphysis just below the epiphyseal plate.

The causal micro-organism is usually a staphylococcus but some cases of osteomyelitis are due to streptococci or other pyogenic (pus-producing) micro-organisms. In the majority of cases infection is haematogenous (blood borne) from some other infective focus within the body, e.g. a boil in the skin.

The diagnosis is made on clinical grounds as, although the disease produces radiographic changes due to bone destruction and reactive periostitis, these do not appear until about seven or more days after the onset of infection.

Treatment consists initially of injection of large doses of penicillin or other antibiotics, sometimes followed by surgical measures to release pus from the affected areas of bone.

In some instances the infection leads to chronic osteomyelitis. Complications include metastatic (secondary) infections in other bones and other tissues, septicaemia, and the formation of infective sinuses which discharge on the skin surface. Sinus formation is associated with the presence of sequestra in the area of bone infection.

(b) **Chronic Osteomyelitis**—chronic infection of bone may occur in the form of a low grade infection which is of chronic nature from its onset, or as a sequel to an acute osteomyelitis which has failed to resolve. The inflammatory changes in this condition may be diffuse or localized. One form of chronic osteomyelitis occurs in the form of a localized abscess cavity, often containing a small central sequestrum, and known as a **Brodie's abscess.**

(c) **Acute Suppurative Arthritis**—this is a disease in which pus is formed within a joint either as a result of infection of its synovial membrane by blood-borne pyogenic micro-organisms, spread of infection into a joint from an adjacent area of osteomyelitis, or direct infection of a joint by a penetrating wound.

As with acute osteomyelitis, the commonest causal organism of the condition is the staphylococcus.

Acute suppurative arthritis may lead to bony ankylosis and to the formation of infective sinuses, leading from the infected joint to the skin surface.

(*d*) **Tuberculous infections of Bones and Joints**—these are metastatic forms of tuberculosis (see p. 53) and produce a chronic inflammatory reaction in affected structures. They are not nowadays very common.

Tuberculous infection of bone is generally referred to as **tuberculous osteitis.** It occurs more frequently in children and adolescents than in adults. It can, however, affect any bone and develop at any age.

When *tubercle bacilli* infect an area of bone near a joint, spread to this joint with resultant tuberculous arthritis is a usual sequel. Conversely, when tuberculous infection occurs in the synovial membrane of a joint, secondary spread to the adjacent bone ends usually follows. Thus tuberculous osteitis in the spine, ends of long bones, and in small bones such as those of the tarsus and carpus, is usually seen with accompanying joint involvement.

The formation of chronic abscesses of a type referred to as **"cold abscesses"** and sinus formation are common features of skeletal tuberculosis. Pathological calcification is common in old abscess cavities.

Tuberculosis of the spine is an important form of tuberculous osteitis and is frequently referred to as **Pott's disease.** It may cause collapse of vertebral bodies, and changes in adjacent intervertebral discs. It may also lead to formation of abscesses which press on the spinal cord and cause neurological signs and symptoms, and also, according to the site of infection, **retropharyngeal** (cervical spine), **paravertebral** (dorsal spine), **lumbar** or **psoas abscess** (lumbar spine).

Rarely, tuberculous osteitis may occur in the fingers or toes producing **tuberculous dactylitis;** the word **dactyl** meaning "a digit".

Tuberculous lesions in bones and joints characteristically produce a persistent aching type of pain. When there is joint infection, limitation of movement of the affected joint and muscle wasting are usual features. Radiological investigation is an essential procedure in all suspected cases.

Treatment involves the administration of anti-tuberculosis drugs and immobilisation of the diseased area. Surgical measures are employed to drain abscesses when these have formed.

(e) **Syphilitic Infection of the Bones and Joints**—syphilitic infection of bone, referred to as **syphilitic osteitis,** occurs in congenital syphilis and in the secondary and tertiary stages of acquired syphilis.

Syphilitic arthritis is very uncommon but may occur in both the congenital and acquired forms of the disease. Syphilitic infection of the nervous system may lead to the development of one or more **Charcot joints** as a result of **neuropathic arthritis,** a condition in which the joint changes are due to involvement of the nerves supplying joints and not to joint infection.

(f) **Uncommon Infections of Bone**—among these, Rohan Williams (3) listed the following: typhoid fever, undulant fever (brucellosis), leprosy, ecchinococcus disease (hydatid disease), actinomycosis and yaws.

6. NEOPLASMS OF BONE

Bone, as already noted, is composed of cells called osteocytes and calcified intercellular substance called bone matrix. It also contains cells called osteoblasts and osteoclasts. In addition to bone tissue proper, bones contain in their inner spaces fibrous, vascular, nervous and reticulo-endothelial tissue. They are moreover ensheathed by a fibrous membrane, the periosteum, and their articular ends are covered by articular cartilage. During early development bone is preformed in either cartilage or membrane.

It is thus not surprising that in view of the many different types of tissue which it contains, a large variety of primary tumours may arise in bone. Bone is also a common site for metastases from carcinomatous neoplasms arising elsewhere in the body.

Plain X-ray films are extensively employed in the diagnosis of bone tumours and frequently specialized radiological investigations such as tomography, angiography, and methods using radioactive isotopes are also employed. Biopsy is often an essential procedure when a primary malignant neoplasm of bone is suspected.

Neoplasms of bone may be classified as benign or malignant. Malignant neoplasms may be of primary or secondary type. Some of the more important varieties are as follows:

BENIGN NEOPLASMS

(a) **Osteoma**—a benign tumour of bone tissue proper. It may consist of cancellous bone (**cancellous osteoma**) or compact bone (**ivory osteoma**). The former type generally arises from a long bone and the latter from a skull or facial bone.

(*b*) **Chondroma**—a benign tumour of cartilage. It may be single or multiple. A chondroma which projects from the outer surface of a bone is called an **ecchondroma**, whilst one growing within the interior of a bone is known as an **enchondroma**.

(*c*) **Osteochondroma**—a benign tumour composed of both bone and cartilage. It may sometimes undergo malignant change with the formation of a chondrosarcoma.

(*d*) **Osteoclastoma** (Giant-cell tumour of bone)—a tumour which is composed of cells resembling osteoclasts. This condition holds an intermediate position between the benign and malignant tumours in that, whilst possessing a number of benign characteristics, it may infiltrate widely into surrounding tissues, in a similar fashion to a malignant tumour.

Note: An osteoma or osteochondroma may be described as an **exostosis**; a term used to describe any form of localized bony outgrowth, and which thus includes certain conditions which are not of a neoplastic nature (e.g. the condition called **traumatic exostosis** wherein, as a result of injury, bone is formed in the insertion of a tendon).

(*e*) **Haemangioma** (Benign angioma)—a benign tumour of blood vessels which may occur in many different tissues, including bone.

(*f*) **Other Benign Neoplasms**—these include **osteoid osteoma, benign chondroblastoma, osteogenic fibroma** (benign osteoblastoma) and **non-osteogenic fibroma**.

PRIMARY MALIGNANT NEOPLASMS

(*a*) **Osteogenic Sarcoma** (Osteosarcoma)—a sarcoma is a malignant tumour arising from connective tissue, and, as stated by Campbell Golding (4) "The term **osteogenic** indicates an origin from tissue capable of forming bone".

This neoplasm is usually highly malignant, local extension being rapid and metastases in the lungs and other organs frequently being early features. Its highest incidence occurs in late childhood and adolescence. A certain number of cases are seen in elderly subjects as a result of osteogenic sarcoma developing as a complication of Paget's disease of bone.

The commonest site for the tumour to originate is at the end of a long bone, particularly in the region of the knee joint.

Severe pain in the affected region is usually the first symptom of the disease.

Radiological investigation and biopsy are important complementary diagnostic procedures.

Treatment is primarily by radiotherapy, followed subsequently, in some instances, by amputation when the site of tumour renders this operation practicable.

There are a number of different types of osteogenic sarcoma and, according to their pathological features, these may be described by names such as **chondrosarcoma, fibrosarcoma of bone, simple sarcoma of bone,** etc.

(*b*) **Ewing's Tumour of Bone** (Ewing's Sarcoma)—a rare malignant neoplasm of bone, named after J. Ewing, who was an American pathologist. Its exact nature is in dispute but many authorities regard it as a sarcomatous growth of the reticulo-endothelial cells of the bone marrow. Like osteogenic sarcoma it occurs principally in late childhood and adolescence. Unlike this latter condition, however, it usually arises in the middle of a long bone and it may produce metastases in other bones and lymph glands.

(*c*) **Myelomatosis**—the word **myeloma** means "a tumour of bone marrow". This disease is uncommon and whilst it can occur in the form of a single tumour referred to as a **solitary myeloma,** it usually has a multicentric origin presenting in the form of multiple tumours of the bone marrow when it is referred to as a **multiple myeloma**.

Common sites for the lesions are the bones of the spine, ribs, skull and pelvis (i.e. sites of red marrow in adult life) where they produce areas of bone destruction which may be demonstrated on X-ray films.

The diagnosis may be confirmed by microscopic examination of a fragment of bone marrow tissue obtained by marrow puncture, and by demonstration of abnormal protein substances in blood plasma, using an electrical method called **electrophoresis**.

Patients with multiple myeloma often excrete in their urine an abnormal substance called **Bence-Jones protein.**

Treatment is by radiotherapy and chemotherapy.

(*d*) **Other Malignant Bone Tumours**—among these may be listed **reticulosarcoma, angiosarcoma** and **liposarcoma.**

SECONDARY MALIGNANT NEOPLASMS

Metastases are the commonest neoplasms occurring in bone and develop most frequently from primary carcinomas of the breast, prostate and bronchus. They occur principally in those sites where red bone marrow persists in adult life (see p. 230).

Less common primary tumours with a predilection for producing bony metastases are carcinomas of the thyroid, kidney and body of the uterus, and also neuroblastomas of the suprarenal gland.

Metastatic growths in bone may be single, but are more frequently multiple. They may cause bone destruction or may lead to reactive new bone formation or frequently a combination of both these processes.

Metastases are occasionally painless and evidence of their presence first revealed as a result of an X-ray examination or by the patient sustaining a pathological fracture. In most instances, however, they cause severe pain and this may be present for a long time before typical X-ray changes can be demonstrated.

Scanning methods after administration of a radio-active isotope are sometimes employed to investigate the presence and distribution of these lesions.

Radiotherapy is extensively used as a form of pallative treatment for bony metastases. Hormone treatment is much employed when such metastases arise from carcinomas of the breast or prostate.

7. CYSTS OF BONE

Cysts may occur in bone as a result of various causes e.g. (i) developmental abnormalities—**simple cysts,** (ii) trauma—**post traumatic cysts,** (iii) endocrine disease, e.g. **generalized osteitis fibrosa** (due to hyperparathyroidism), (iv) idiopathic disease, e.g. **aneurysmal bone cyst, polyostotic fibrous dysplasia, osteitis multiplex cystoides** (a manifestation of sarcoidosis).

8. METABOLIC DISEASES OF BONE

These may be:

(i) due to lack of Vitamin C or deficiency of certain types of protein. This form of metabolic bone disease is characterized by generalized **osteoporosis** (see p. 231), the bones containing less calcified bone matrix than normal (see p. 230).

(ii) due to lack of adequate supply, to the bones, of calcium and phosphorous or due to Vitamin D deficiency, causing **osteomalacia** (see p. 231).

(iii) associated with raised amounts of calcium in the blood (i.e. hypercalcaemia) in a rare but interesting disease of infancy called

infantile hypercalcaemia. This condition is generally believed to be due to hypersensitivity to Vitamin D and, in the more severe cases, areas of increased bone deposition (referred to as areas of **osteosclerosis)** can be demonstrated in radiographs of the bones.

The following are some important clinical types of metabolic bone disease:

(*a*) **Scurvy**—a nowadays uncommon disease due to deficiency of Vitamin C. This vitamin is found chiefly in fresh fruit and vegetables and is essential for the formation of the protein substance collagen, an important constituent of bone matrix and other types of connective tissue. The disease may occur in adults who are deprived of these foodstuffs, or in bottle-fed infants who are not given fruit juice to supplement their bottle feeds.

Scurvy is a generalized disease affecting other connective tissues as well as bone. Its principal features are capillary haemorrhages, which are especially common from the gums, in the skin and below the periosteum of long bones; anaemia, osteoporosis (see p. 231) and delay in the healing of wounds.

Treatment is by administration of Vitamin C.

(*b*) **Simple Rickets**—a disease of infancy due usually both to a lack of calcium and phosphorous, and also Vitamin D in the diet. Lack of exposure to sunlight may also be a factor as Vitamin D is synthesized, in small amounts, in the fat cells of the skin when these are exposed to the sun's rays.

This condition is a type of osteomalacia (see p. 231) and accordingly the bones are softer than normal. As a result, in severe cases, marked deformities may develop especially in the lower limbs and pelvis. Deformities of the chest may also occur.

In some cases of rickets the blood calcium is low and these may show various manifestations of **tetany** (spasmophilia), a condition of hyperexcitability of the nervous system evidenced by various types of intermittent muscular spasms.

Treatment of rickets is by administration of Vitamin D and a diet with adequate content of calcium and phosphorus.

(*c*) **Dietetic Osteomalacia**—this disease occurs when adults are subjected to the dietetic deficiencies which cause simple rickets in infants; and treatment is along similar lines.

The disease is more frequent in females than in males, and nowadays is rare, except in some under-developed countries.

As in simple rickets the basic pathological feature is defective calcification of bone matrix. This defect in normal maintenance of bony tissue leads to softening of bones and may lead to marked skeletal deformities. These and general rarefaction of bone may be readily demonstrated on radiographs.

In severe cases, localized areas of marked rarefaction may simulate fractured bones. Such areas are termed **pseudo-fractures** or **Looser's zones.** (*Note:* The presence of pseudo-fractures is the main feature of an unusual type of osteomalacia called **Milkman's syndrome).**

(*d*) **Other types of Rickets and Osteomalacia**—("Vitamin D-resistant" Rickets and Osteomalacia).

(i) Due to **malabsorption syndromes.**

Although the diet may contain adequate amounts of calcium, phosphorous and Vitamin D, disorders of the digestive system may prevent their adequate absorption. This occurs in a group of disorders, known collectively as malabsorption syndromes, which may thus be associated with the development of rickets in childhood or osteomalacia in adult life, e.g. coeliac disease and idiopathic steatorrhoea (see p. 129).

(ii) Due to **renal causes.**

In certain types of congenital and acquired kidney disease, undue loss of calcium and phosphorous in the urine may result in rickets or osteomalacia. In some of these diseases the radiological appearances of rickets or osteomalacia in the bones may be complicated by changes which are due to **secondary hyperparathyroidism** (see p. 213). This latter occurs as a reaction to a certain type of upset of calcium and phosphate metabolism.

The term **renal osteodystrophy** may be used to refer to any metabolic disorder of bone due to renal causes, but is commonly applied to one such disorder, known also as **renal rickets.**

Among a number of uncommon kidney disorders associated with metabolic bone disease may be mentioned **renal tubular acidosis,** also known as **Lightwood-Albright syndrome** (see p. 159) and **Fanconi's syndrome,** a congenital disorder of the renal tubules.

9. IDIOPATHIC DISEASES

(*a*) **Paget's Disease of Bone** (Osteitis Deformans)—this disease was so-called after Sir James Paget, a nineteenth century English surgeon. It is a fairly common condition in elderly male subjects and its cause is quite unknown. It is not an inflammatory condition as might be suggested by its alternative name of **osteitis deformans.**

The pathological changes comprise a mixture of diffuse absorption of existing bone and the excessive deposition of new bone of spongy type. Affected bones are thickened but are weaker than normal. The changes may be limited to a single bone but usually involve a number of bones; common sites for the disease being the pelvis, femora, tibiae, lumbar spine and skull.

Pain is often a prominent feature. Deformity of affected bones is common. Pathological fractures are of frequent occurrence and the development of an osteogenic sarcoma may complicate the disease.

Characteristic changes are seen on radiographs but these are sometimes simulated by carcinomatous metastases especially from carcinoma of the prostate.

There is no specific treatment. Pain may sometimes be considerably relieved by X-ray therapy.

(*b*) **Juvenile Osteochondritis** (Osteochondrosis)—this term describes a condition in which a localized death of bone and cartilage cells (i.e. a necrosis) occurs in the primary or secondary centres of ossification of one or more growing bones.

The necrosis occurring in osteochondritis is thought to result from a defective blood supply to the affected area and this condition is thus described as being a type of **avascular necrosis.** It is not an inflammatory condition as its name would suggest and the cause of the deficient blood supply is unknown. It is, however, thought that this latter may, in many cases, be the result of injury, especially of a minor nature.

Pain and, in some sites, deformity are common clinical features of juvenile osteochondritis.

Radiologically, increased density of the bone in the affected area, and later an appearance of fragmentation are usually the principal signs.

Juvenile osteochondritis is found in a variety of ossific centres. The different types are named either by the name of the person who first described them, or better, according to their site of occurrence.

Site of osteochondritis	*Alternative name*
Vertebral epiphyseal plates	Scheuermann's disease
Semilunar bone of carpus	Kienbock's disease
Epiphysis of femoral head	Perthes' disease (Pseudo-coxalgia)
Epiphysis of the tibial tubercle	Osgood-Schlatter's disease
Navicular bone of tarsus	Köhler's disease
Epiphysis Apophysis of os calcis	Sever's disease
Second and third metatarsal head epiphysis	Freiberg's disease

Juvenile osteochondritis bears a resemblance to a number of conditions, seen in adults, and known collectively as **adult osteochondritis.** It is thought probable, however, that many of these latter are the late results of minor undiagnosed, and consequently untreated, fractures.

(*Note:* The majority of secondary centres of ossification are at the growing ends of bones where they take part in the formation of joints and known as **epiphyses.** Secondary centres of ossification which take no part in the formation of joints are called **apophyses** (singular: apophysis).

(*c*) **Osteochondritis Dissecans**—this is a disorder in which a small localized area of necrosis of articular cartilage, and bone lying immediately beneath it, develops at a joint surface. Like juvenile osteochondritis (see above) the condition is thought to be a type of avascular necrosis, probably resulting from injury.

The dead area of bone and cartilage gradually separates from the surrounding live tissue and may ultimately become completely detached so as to form a **loose body** within the joint.

Osteochondritis dissecans is seen most frequently in adolescents and young adults and usually occurs in the larger joints, especially the knee joint. It gives rise to pain, effusion of synovial fluid and when a loose body has formed it may produce a condition of sudden fixation of an affected joint called "**locking**".

(*d*) **Slipped Upper Femoral Epiphysis** (Adolescent Coxa Vara)—in this condition, which may affect one or both hips, the capital epiphysis (epiphysis of the head of the femur) slips downwards and backwards on the neck of the femur. The disorder develops in adolescence and causes pain and a limp. It occurs more frequently in males than in females. It cause is unknown. Some authorities consider that it is of traumatic origin and others that endocrine factors play a part in its causation.

(*e*) **Idiopathic Scoliosis**—the term **scoliosis** denotes a lateral curvature of the spine. (*Note:* a backward curvature is called a **kyphosis** and a forward curvature, a **lordosis**). Scoliosis may be due to a large variety of causes (e.g. congenital abnormality, disease of the vertebral bodies, muscular paralysis following anterior poliomyelitis, etc.) but the majority of cases develop in childhood, or adolescence, and form a group of unknown origin, called **idiopathic scoliosis.**

(*f*) **Hypertrophic Pulmonary Osteopathy**—an uncommon condition in which periosteal new bone formation occurs around short and long bones in the upper and lower limbs. Its cause is unknown but it develops in association with certain lung diseases and bronchial carcinoma, usually in association with finger clubbing (see p. 88).

10. CHRONIC ARTHRITIS

It is to be noted that whilst the term **arthritis** strictly speaking means joint inflammation, it is also employed to indicate certain joint conditions which are of a degenerative nature. The latter are sometimes described as **arthroses** (singular—arthrosis).

Chronic suppurative arthritis may develop as a sequel to acute suppurative arthritis (see p. 241) and **tuberculous arthritis** is another important type of chronic arthritic disorder (see p. 242). Other important types of chronic arthritis include **osteoarthritis,** which is a degenerative disorder, **rheumatoid arthritis** and **ankylosing spondylitis,** which are inflammatory diseases, and the **gouty arthritis** due to a metabolic disease called gout.

Chronic arthritis and also some forms of acute arthritis commonly produce symptoms referred to as being due to **rheumatism.** Duthie (5) states "the term 'rheumatism' has been loosely applied to all conditions causing pain and stiffness of the muscles and joints".

(*a*) **Osteoarthritis** (Osteoarthrosis, Hypertrophic Arthritis, Degenerative Arthritis) is a very common type of degenerative arthritis, occurring predominantly in middle and old age and commoner in males than in females.

It may develop in a single joint but often affects a number of joints. Malalignment of joint surfaces, as a result of injury or disease, and the pursuit of occupations causing strain on joints appear to be important contributory factors in the causation of many cases. Obesity appears to predispose to osteoarthritis in weight-bearing joints.

The chief pathological features of the condition are degenerative changes and destruction of articular cartilage of affected joint surfaces: reactive new bone formation in areas of bone underlying destroyed articular cartilage; and the formation of projecting spurs of new bone around joint margins. These spurs are referred to as **osteophytes** and are readily demonstrable on radiographs. Radiographs will also show loss of joint space (due to the destruction of articular cartilage) and increased density of bone ends (due to the reactive new bone formation).

The chief clinical features are pain, stiffness, deformity and decreased movement in affected joints.

There is no curative treatment as the joint changes are permanent. Pain relieving drugs, physiotherapy, and manipulation together with the injection of hydrocortisone are employed to produce some relief of symptoms. Surgical measures (e.g. arthrodesis or arthroplasty) may be required in cases with severe pain and disability.

(*b*) **Rheumatoid arthritis**—this term describes an inflammatory disorder of connective tissue, the principal clinical manifestations of which result from an arthritis, which affects multiple joints and is thus referred to as a **polyarthritis.** Anaemia is also a common feature in the established disease and other factors which may develop include subcutaneous nodules called **rheumatoid nodules;** and lung changes, the different varieties of which are sometimes referred to as **rheumatoid lung.**

The disorder belongs to a group of conditions described as **connective tissue diseases** (see p. 300).

The chronic inflammatory changes in the joints are reversible in their early stages, but later often lead to much destruction of articular cartilage and underlying bone. Muscle wasting is frequently severe around affected joints and pathological dislocations of not uncommon occurrence.

When damage to articular cartilage is severe, opposing joint surfaces may become united by fibrous tissue, formed as a result of the inflammation. This is termed **fibrous ankylosis.** Subsequently, osteoblasts may deposit bone in the fibrous tissue converting the condition into one of **bony ankylosis.**

The cause of rheumatoid arthritis is unknown. Whilst it shows certain features resembling those of an infection, no infective micro-organism has ever been established as its cause.

The disease usually commences in early adult life and shows a much higher incidence in femal subjects than in males. Common sites for its onset are the small joints of the hands and feet which become painful, stiff and swollen. Later it may spread so as to involve the larger joints of the limbs and the joints of the trunk.

Periodic attacks of active inflammation and remissions are common in the course of the disease. During the former, some degree of fever and increase in pulse rate may occur. Psychological stress possibly plays some ill-understood role in many patients.

X-ray investigation is of value in the demonstration of joint changes, the earliest sign of which is osteoporosis around affected joints.

Examination of the blood will demonstrate the anaemia resulting from the disease and tests such as the **Rose-Waaler agglutination test** and the **latex flocculation test** may show a factor, called the rheumatoid factor, to be present in the blood serum during the active stages of rheumatoid arthritis.

As in many other inflammatory disorders, a test called the **erythrocyte sedimentation rate (E.S.R.)** shows increased values in phases of activity of the disease.

Treatment comprises (i) measures to improve general health, (ii) physiotherapy with measures designed to try and prevent deformities from developing, (iii) the giving of drugs such as aspirin, butazolidine, gold salts, or corticosteroids, (iv) occupational therapy.

An operation called **synovectomy** (excision of the synovial membrane of a joint) is sometimes employed in the treatment of acutely inflamed joints in the early stages of rheumatoid arthritis.

When the active phase of the disease has subsided surgical treatment may be employed to correct or improve residual deformities.

A type of rheumatoid arthritis which occurs in children is called **Still's disease,** after Sir George Frederick Still, an English paediatrician, and is associated in many instances with enlargement of lymph glands and the spleen.

(c) **Ankylosing Spondylitis**—**ankylosis** is a term indictaing "fusion of joints" and **spondylitis** means "inflammation of a vertebra or vertebrae".

Ankylosing spondylitis commences in the sacro-iliac joints, which join the spine to the pelvic girdle, with inflammatory changes which lead to destruction of articular cartilage and subsequent bony ankylosis. As the disease progresses, arthritic changes develop in other joints of the spine and the costo-vertebral joints between the spine and ribs. These changes are also of inflammatory nature and involve the ligaments of affected joints, leading to varying degrees of **ligamentous ossification** (i.e. the formation of bone within ligaments). In advanced cases resultant immobility and rigidity of the spine produces a condition known as "poker-back". The lesions in the sacro-iliac joints and spine may sometimes be accompanied by arthritic changes in limb joints. In some cases, spontaneous arrest of the disease may occur in its earlier stages.

The cause of ankylosing spondylitis is unknown. Its onset is usually in early adult life and its incidence is much higher in males than in females.

Radiology is of great value in the early diagnosis of the condition and in assessing its progress. In the advanced stages, ossification of ligaments may give rise to an X-ray appearance referred to as "bamboo-spine".

Treatment with deep X-rays is frequently effective in arresting the progress of the disease.

(*d*) **Gouty Arthritis**—the development of inflammatory changes in joints, first of acute type but later becoming chronic, is one of the outstanding features of a disorder of purine metabolism called **gout.**

(*Note:* **purines** are derivatives of a class of proteins which are constituents of cell nuclei and are called **nucleoproteins.** One of the end products of purine metabolism is an acid called **uric acid**).

Gout is an uncommon condition which rarely develops before middle age, although hereditary factors are important in its causation. It occurs much more frequently in males than in females. It is characterized during its active phases by increased amounts of uric acid in the blood, as can be shown by **estimation of the serum uric acid,** and by the deposition of salts of uric acid, called **urates,** in soft tissues around joints, in cartilage and bone in the vicinity of joints, in the cartilage of the external ear, and in bursae, especially the olecranon bursa.

Deposits of urate crystals produce nodules called **tophi.** These produce palpable swellings in the subcutaneous tissues and may lead to ulceration of overlying skin. In the bones they produce localized areas of bone absorption demonstrable on radiographs.

Hypertension and renal disease are frequent accompaniments of gout.

(*e*) **Neuropathic Arthritis**—this term describes the occurrence in joints of chronic arthritic changes which are secondary to some form of **neuropathy,** i.e. disease of the nervous system. Joints affected by neuropathic arthritis are frequently referred to as **Charcot joints** after Jean Martin Charcot, a nineteenth century French physician. They develop most frequently as a complication of tabes dorsalis or syringomyelia, but are sometimes due to diabetic neuropathy.

Owing to pathological changes in the nerves supplying it, a neuropathic joint is characteristically painless although severe joint disorganization frequently develops. Either single or multiple joints may be the subject of this condition in the same individual. Large joints are more often affected than small joints.

11. DISORDERS OF THE INTERVERTEBRAL DISCS AND SPONDYLOSIS

The intervertebral discs act as shock absorbers in the spinal column. They may be the subject of congenital abnormality or involvement by infective lesions in adjacent vertebral bodies (e.g. as in spinal tuberculosis), or they may be damaged as a result of degenerative changes or trauma Disc damage, from the two latter causes may result in a portion of a disc slipping out of the space between the vertebral bodies. A condition of **prolapsed disc,** or **slipped disc,** is then said to be present.

Prolapsed disc is commonest in the lower lumbar and lower cervical regions of the spine, but may occur elsewhere in these regions and also in the dorsal region.

(*a*) **Lumbar disc prolapse**—In this condition the protruding portion of the disc may press on nerves, or nerve roots, causing a type of pain in the lumbar region of the back, called **lumbago,** and pain in the distribution of the sciatic nerve referred to as **sciatica.**

The commonest site for lumbar disc prolapse is the lumbo-sacral disc space.

The diagnosis is made principally on the clinical features. Plain radiography is limited in value to excluding some other cause of the symptoms, such as spinal tuberculosis, metastases in the spine, etc. Evidence that a disc is damaged is revealed in plain films by narrowing of the disc space. It cannot, however, be stated from such examination if the damage has resulted in actual proplapse of the damaged disc or not. It is also well recognized that demonstration of a normal disc space, on conventional films, does not exclude there being prolapse of the disc which lies within it. A certain proportion of prolapsed discs can, however, be demonstrated by myelography, and this examination may be employed when the clinical features are equivocal.

Various forms of treatment are employed in this condition, e.g. manipulation, traction, immobilisation by a spinal corset, etc. Operative treatment to remove the protruding portion of the affected disc is occasionally necessary. Access to the affected disc is obtained by removing one or both of the laminae of the overlying vertebral arch. This operation is called **laminectomy.**

(*b*) **Cervical disc prolapse**—This condition occurs most frequently in the lower cervical region and may affect either a single disc or several discs. The disc protrusion may press on cervical nerves, causing among other features pain in the arm or shoulder. Less commonly pressure may be exerted on the spinal cord itself, causing nervous signs and symptoms in the lower limbs. As in the lumbar region, plain radiography is of value in indicating disc damage and excluding other vertebral conditions. Among these latter is the presence of a cervical rib. Disc protrusions in this region may be shown by myelography.

Initial treatment may be by manipulation, traction or immobilisation by some form of support. Laminectomy is occasionally necessary in cases which fail to respond to non-operative measures.

SPONDYLOSIS

Is a degenerative condition of the spine, in which bony spurs form outgrowth in relation to the margins of the vertebral bodies. These spurs are similar to the spurs which form around osteoarthritic joints and are referred by a similar name, i.e. as **osteophytes.** Spondylosis is thought to develop as a secondary result of degenerative changes in the intervertebral discs. It is extremely common in older subjects of both sexes. It is usually symptomless unless, as may happen particularly in the cervical region, the bony outgrowths develop so as to press on nerve roots, or as described by Lodge (6), on the spinal cord itself.

Pressure on the roots of the brachial plexus may cause a condition known as **brachial radiculitis,** in which there is pain and other evidence of nerve root irritation.

As stated by Brain (7), **cervical spondylosis** is an important cause of headache and can intensify the symptoms of **vertebro-basilar ischaemia.** In this latter condition atheroma in the vertebral and basilar arteries causes interference with the blood supply to the brain stem, with resultant symptoms such as dizziness, disturbances of vision and gait, etc.

12. SOME OTHER BONE AND JOINT DISEASES AND DEFORMITIES

(*a*) **Loose Bodies in Joints**—loose bodies, composed of bone and cartilage, may be found in bones and joints as a result of injury; osteochondritis dissecans (see p. 250); in association with osteoarthritis: or in a condition of unknown origin called **synovial osteochondromatosis.**

Locking of an affected joint (see p. 250) is a common indication of the presence of a loose body.

(*b*) **Chondromalacia patellae**—an uncommon disorder in which degenerative changes occur in the articular cartilage covering the posterior surface of the patella. It is sometimes secondary to recurrent dislocation of the patella.

(*c*) **Metatarsalgia**—a term used to describe pain in the forefoot arising from a variety of causes including pes planus and March fracture.

(*d*) **Hallux Valgus**—a very common deformity, especially in females, in which the great toe deviates outwards. It is often associated with varus deformity (inward deviation) of the first metatarsal. This latter condition is known as **metatarsus primus varus.**

(*e*) **Hallux rigidus**—a condition due, in its chronic form to osteoarthritis of the first metatarsophalangeal joint and causing pain and stiffness of this joint.

(*f*) **Subungual exostosis**—an **exostosis** is an outgrowth of bone and **subungual** means beneath the nail. This condition principally occurs in the great toe.

(*g*) **Genu valgum** (knock knee) and **genu varum** (bow legs)—in both these disorders the great majority of cases are, in the U.K., due to unknown causes which operate during childhood and, usually, the deformity rights itself during growth. A small proportion of cases, however, result from disease (e.g. rickets) or bony injury in the region of the knee joint.

(*h*) **Hammer Toe**—a name used to describe a toe with flexion deformity at either its proximal or distal interphalangeal joint. This condition occurs most commonly in the second toe. Its cause is unknown.

(*i*) **Mallet finger**—a condition of flexion deformity of the distal interphalangeal joint of a finger, due to an injury causing detachment of the extensor tensor tendon from its insertion into the base of the terminal phalanx.

(*j*) **Coccydynia**—a condition of chronic pain in the region of the coccyx which usually develops as a sequel to an injury in this region.

13. DISEASES OF SKELETAL MUSCLES

Pathological conditions of the skeletal muscles may be due to primary diseases of muscle, or occur secondary to (i) diseases and injuries to bones and joints, (ii) diseases and injuries primarily affecting the nervous system, or (iii) disease of other structures.

Atrophy (wasting) and weakness or paralysis (loss of function) of muscles are common features of many muscle disorders. In some types of disorder, an investigation called **electromyography** (E.M.G.) may be employed to differentiate between primary muscle disease and disease of muscle occurring secondary to lesions in the nervous system.

Muscle biopsy is another type of investigation sometimes employed in the investigation of lesions in skeletal muscles.

Diseases of the skeletal muscles include:

(*a*) **Traumatic conditions**—injuries of a certain type may produce marked tearing of fibres resulting in a condition of partial or complete loss of continuity of tissue in a tendon, or less commonly in muscle fibres. This is referred to as a partial or complete **rupture** of tendon or muscle, e.g. rupture of the Achilles tendon.

Following injury to a muscle or tendon, occasionally bone may be laid down in the area of tissue damage producing a condition known as **traumatic myositis ossificans.** This occurs most frequently in the brachialis muscle, following a fracture in the region of the elbow joint or dislocation of this joint.

(*b*) **Inflammations**—these may result from infection of muscular tissue with pathogenic micro-organisms; parasitic infestations such as **cysticercosis** (see p. 306) and **trichiniasis,** a disease due to a worm called the muscle worm; or as a manifestation of **collagen diseases** (see p. 300).

Inflammation of muscular tissue is called **myositis.** Pain of muscular origin is called **myalgia.** The disease called **epidemic myalgia** or **Bornholm disease** is an inflammatory disease characterized by causing severe pain in the chest as a result of inflammatory changes in intercostal muscles. It is believed to be due to a virus infection.

Inflammation of a tendon is termed **tendinitis.** Tendon sheaths possess an inner synovial lining and outer fibrous sheath. As indicated by Adams (8) inflammatory changes in the former are referred to as **tenosynovitis,** and in the latter as **tenovaginitis.** Tenosynovitis may be of traumatic causation or due to infection. Tenovaginitis is a condition of unknown origin.

Inflammation of fascia is known as **fasciitis.** Inflammatory changes occurring in the plantar fascia, in the sole of the foot, in the region of its attachment to the os calcis produce a painful disorder called **plantar fasciitis.**

(*Note:* The use of the term "rheumatism" to describe conditions causing pain and stiffness in muscles and joints has already been referred to (see p. 251).)

It was formerly widely held that besides being due to various forms of acute and chronic arthritis, symptoms of rheumatism also frequently resulted from non-specific inflammatory changes in muscles and surrounding soft-tissues. Thus rheumatic symptoms were often ascribed as being due to **muscular rheumatism** or **fibrositis** (inflammation of fibrous connective tissue). Such diagnoses are made much less frequently nowadays and Duthie (9) writing of the pathology of **non-articular rheumatism** states that "the opinion is now widely held that muscular pain and spasm arise most commonly as a result of strain or injury to related ligamentous or articular structures".

(*c*) **Neoplasms**—of rare occurrence is a malignant tumour of striated muscle tissue called a **rhabdomyosarcoma.**

(*d*) **Muscular Dystrophies**—(Myopathies)—this term describes a group of primary diseases of muscular tissue in which degenerative changes develop in skeletal muscles, causing atrophy of muscle fibres and muscular weakness. They result from hereditary factors and develop in childhood or early adult life.

Among the different types of muscular dystrophy are the conditions called **pseudo-hypertrophic muscular dystrophy** and **facio-scapulo-humeral-dystrophy.**

(*e*) **Myotonia**—is a term used to describe a form of sustained contraction and gradual relaxation of muscles. It occurs in a hereditary disorder called **myotonia congenita** (Thomsen's disease) and in another hereditary condition called **dystrophia myotonica.** In the latter the myotonia is accompanied by degenerative changes in affected muscular tissue.

(*f*) **Myasthenia Gravis**—the name of this disease means "severe muscular weakness" and it is characterized by a rapid onset of fatigue in voluntary muscles. The muscles involved vary, but those responsible for movement of the eyes and limbs and those concerned with speech are often affected.

The cause of myasthenia has not been established but in many cases there is some associated disorder of the thymus gland. In some this latter takes the form of a tumour called a **thymoma** and in others there is hypertrophy of the thymus gland.

The drug called neostigmine is extensively used in treatment. Selected patients may derive considerable benefit from thymectomy or irradiation of thymus, or from a combination of both these procedures.

(*g*) **Volkmann's Ischaemic Contracture**—this is an uncommon disorder in which as a result of ischaemia (localized deficiency in blood supply) there occurs a replacement of muscular tissue by fibrous tissue, in the flexor muscles of the forearm. Contraction of the fibrous tissue leads to deformity of the wrist and fingers.

The condition usually occurs as a complication of injuries around the elbow joint which interfere with the blood supply to the flexor muscles of the forearm.

14. BURSITIS

Bursitis, i.e. inflammation of a bursa (see p. 232) may be acute or chronic in type and may occur as a result of mechanical irritation, e.g. as in **prepatellar bursitis** (housemaid's knee); or as a result of infection, e.g. pyogenic infection or tuberculous infection.

Olecranon bursitis is sometimes seen as a complication of gout.

SOME ORTHOPAEDIC OPERATIONS

(*a*) **Arthrodesis**—operative fusion of a joint.

(*b*) **Arthroplasty**—operative reconstruction of a joint, e.g. Austin-Moore arthroplasty in which the head and neck of the femur are replaced by a metallic prosthesis—used in the operative treatment of osteo-arthritis of the hip and sometimes for fractures of the femoral neck in old people.

(*c*) **Arthrotomy**—making an opening into a joint.

(*d*) **Bone Grafting**—a procedure in which a portion of bone (i.e. a graft) is transferred from another bone in the patient's body (or sometimes from a bone of another human subject) and inserted into, or fixed to a bone which is the site of some defect, e.g. an ununited fracture, or a cavity produced by removal of a tumour or cyst.

(*e*) **Internal fixation operations employed in fracture treatment**—e.g. fixation of a fracture of the femoral neck by a metallic pin and plate (see also p. 239).

(*f*) **Laminectomy**—removal of the lamina from one or both sides of the posterior arch of a spinal vertebra to gain access to the spinal canal.

(*g*) **Osteotomy**—cutting through a bone.

(*h*) **Synovectomy**—excision of the synovial membrane of a joint.

(*i*) **Tenotomy**—cutting through a tendon.

(*j*) **Tendon Transplant** (Tendon transfer)—the operative detachment of a tendon from its normal site of insertion and its transfer to another site of insertion.

REFERENCES

(1) Grainger, R. E. *Recent Advances in Radiology* (Ed. T. Lodge). J. and A. Churchill, 1964.

(2), (8) Adams, J. C. *Outline of Orthopaedics,* E. and S. Livingstone, 1967.

(3) Rohan Williams, E. *A Textbook of X-ray Diagnosis* (British Authors). H. K. Lewis, 1959.

(4) Campbell Golding, F. *A Textbook of X-ray Diagnosis* (British Authors). H. K. Lewis, 1959.

(5) and (9) Duthie, J. J. R. *The Principles and Practice of Medicine* (Ed. Sir Stanley Davidson). E. and S. Livingstone, 1966.

(6) Lodge, T. *Recent Advances in Radiology* (3rd Edn.). J. and A. Churchill, 1955.
(7) Brain, W. R. *Brit. Med. J.,* 1.771. 1963.

Section M.—THE TEETH

Whilst the diagnosis and treatment of diseases of the teeth is principally the concern of those engaged in the dental profession, understanding of some of the terms referring to such diseases is of importance to medical workers. Some important dental disorders are as follows:

(*a*) **Developmental Abnormalities of the Teeth**—these include the presence of:—(i) extra teeth called **supernumerary teeth,** (ii) a deficiency in the number of teeth, (iii) delay or failure in the eruption of teeth, (iv) misplaced teeth, (v) abnormally formed teeth.

Misplaced teeth frequently develop so as to become wedged against adjacent teeth in such a manner that they are unable to erupt normally through the gums. This condition is termed **impaction** and occurs most commonly in the lower third molar teeth (wisdom teeth).

The treatment of many forms of developmental abnormality is the concern of a branch of dentistry called **orthodontics,** the name of which derives from the Greek words meaning "straight" and "tooth'.

(*b*) **Fractures of the Teeth**—these may occur in either the crown, neck or roots of an affected tooth.

(*c*) **Inflammatory disorders.**

(i) **Dental caries**—an infective disorder, also referred to as "dental decay".

(ii) **Periapical infection**—a condition resulting in spread of infection from a tooth whose pulp has been killed by caries, into the bony tissues of the tooth socket. It results in the formation of either an **acute** or **chronic apical abscess** (dental abscess) in the part of the socket around the apex of the root, or roots of the dead tooth; or less commonly in certain other types of infective process (e.g. root absorption).

(iii) **Pyorrhoea** (paradontal disease, periodontal disease)—a disease of unknown origin in which inflammatory changes first appear in the gums (*gingivitis*) and later spread to the underlying bony margins of the mandible and maxilla.

(*d*) **Odontomes**—these comprise certain neoplasms and malformations which arise in connection with dental tissues. There are a variety of types, e.g. **adamantinoma** (ameloblastoma), **dentigerous cyst** (associated with an unerupted tooth), etc.

(*e*) **Dental Cyst**—a cyst which usually arises in connection with an infected tooth root and develops in the mandible or maxilla.

(*f*) **Buried Tooth Roots** (Retained Roots)—these may result from breaking of a tooth during extraction or destruction of the distal part of a tooth by severe caries.

Section N.—THE NERVOUS SYSTEM

1. SOME ANATOMICAL AND PHYSIOLOGICAL CONSIDERATIONS

The nervous system consists of (i) the *central nervous system* (the *brain* and *spinal cord*), often referred to as the C.N.S., (ii) the *peripheral nervous system* (the *cranial* and *spinal nerves*), (iii) the *autonomic nervous system* (the *sympathetic* and *parasympathetic nervous systems*).

Nervous tissue is composed of units called *neurones* which consist of nerve cells together with processes called *dendrites* and other elongated processes which are called *nerve fibres (axons)*.

In the brain and spinal cord nervous tissue is arranged in the form of *grey matter* which mainly comprises collections of nerve cells, and *white matter* which consists of nerve fibres. Also found within the nervous system is a specialized type of supporting tissue called *neuroglia*.

Outside the central nervous system are found collections of nerve fibres arranged in cord-like structures referred to as *nerve trunks,* or *nerves*. In certain sites, composite arrangements of nerve-trunks, resembling a network, constitute what are termed *nervous plexuses* (e.g. the brachial plexus).

All nerve fibres are surrounded by *nerve sheaths* and according to whether this sheath contains a fatty substance called *myelin*, or not, they are referred to as *medullated* or *non-medullated nerve fibres*.

In addition to the nerve cells in the grey matter, small collections of nerve cells are found, in certain sites outside the central nervous system, in structures called *ganglia* (singular: ganglion). These latter occur in association with certain cranial nerves and the dorsal roots of spinal nerves, and also in the sympathetic and parasympathetic nervous systems.

The brain and spinal cord are completely surrounded by membranous structures called *meninges*. These comprise three membranes known as the *dura mater, arachnoid mater* and *pia mater*; the dura mater providing the outer covering and the pia mater the inner covering of the central nervous system. The *cerebrospinal fluid* (C.S.F.) which is formed in the *ventricles of the brain,* circulates in the *subarachnoid space* (i.e. between the arachnoid and pia mater). The portion of the meninges covering the spinal cord is referred to as the *spinal theca,* the word "theca" meaning a sheath.

Functionally, the nervous system comprises:—

(i) *Sensory (afferent) neurones*—concerned with the reception and appreciation of sensory impulses from both the external environment and the interior of the body.

(ii) *Motor (efferent) neurones*—which control the movements of both voluntary and involuntary muscle tissue.

(iii) *Connector neurones*—linking the sensory and motor components of the system.

By this arrangement of neurones, the nervous system is enabled to regulate and co-ordinate the activities of all the other systems of the body and to control the processes by which the individual adapts to his external environment.

The prefix **neuro-** means pertaining to the nervous system and the branch of medicine which is concerned with diseases of the nervous system is termed **neurology.**

The adjective **cerebral** means "pertaining to the brain" and the prefix **encephalo-** has the same meaning. **Myelo-** means "pertaining to the spinal cord" but it is to be noted that this prefix is also used in other contexts with reference to the bone marrow (e.g. a myeloma is a tumour of the bone marrow).

2. SOME GENERAL ASPECTS OF DISEASES OF THE NERVOUS SYSTEM

Diseases of the nervous system may be congenital, traumatic, infective, neoplastic, or degenerative. They may also occur as a result of vascular disorders or be due to a number of other causes.

They are evidenced by a wide variety of signs and symptoms arising from disturbances in the functions of the sensory and motor neurones of the system, and the resultant effects of these disturbances in other tissues.

Thus among the many clinical features of nervous diseases are found disorders of smell, vision, hearing, balance and speech; abnormalities of sensibility to touch, temperature and pain; defects of positional sense; pain in the course of nerve trunks; weakness or paralysis and subsequent wasting of muscle groups, supplied by nerves which are the subject of injury or disease; abnormal muscular contractions and incoordination of muscular actions; disorders of bladder and bowel control; abnormalities of reflexes; associated mental changes, etc.

(*Note:* **reflexes** are involuntary reactions produced automatically by certain stimuli, e.g. the tendon reflex, called the **knee jerk,** which comprises involuntary contraction of the quadriceps muscle in response to a sharp tap over the lower part of its tendon just below the patella).

The following are some of the terms used to indicate clinical signs and symptoms which may arise from different types of diseases of the nervous system:—

amnesia—loss of memory.

anaesthesia—loss of sensation, particularly loss of sensibility to pain; but the term can be used to indicate loss of sensibility to temperature (**thermal anaesthesia**) and touch (**tactile anaesthesia**). (See also p. 27).

aphasia—this term is used to refer to a number of disorders in which the power of speech is partially or completely lost. Such loss may be due to inability to understand spoken and/or written words (**sensory aphasia**), or from inability to express thought in the form of articulated speech and/or in writing (**motor aphasia**).

ataxia—an absence of proper co-ordination of muscular action.

Babinski sign—also referred to as an **extensor plantar response**—consists of an upward movement of the great toe (the normal movement is downwards) when the outer side of the sole of the foot is stroked with a blunt object. It is a sign of great value in indicating disease affecting certain motor neurones in the central nervous system.

coma—a state of unconsciousness from which the sufferer cannot be aroused.

convulsions—attacks of involuntary contractions of muscles which may be of localized or widespread distribution.

diplegia—motor paralysis of the same members of both sides of the body (e.g. both legs).

dysarthria—a defect of articulated speech resulting from incoordination or paralysis of the muscles which produce the spoken voice. It thus differs from the disorders of speech described above as being due to aphasia.

fit—a term used widely to indicate various types of organic and functional disorders which are of sudden onset and often of periodic occurrence.

In neurology this term is commonly used as a synonym for convulsions (see above).

hemianaesthesia—loss of sensation involving one side of the body.

hemiplegia—motor paralysis of one side of the body.

neuralgia—pain of severe type in the distribution of a sensory nerve.

nystagmus—a variety of abnormal involuntary movements of the eyes.

palsy—a synonym of paralysis (see below).

photophobia—dislike of light.

papilloedema—swelling of the optic disc as a result of oedema of this structure; a condition demonstrable on examination of the interior of the eye by an ophthalmoscope. It is also referred to as "**choked disc**".

paraesthesiae—abnormal sensations such as feelings of numbness, tingling sensations and the sensations described as "pins and needles".

paralysis—loss of function. Used without qualification this term indicates **motor paralysis** i.e. a loss of the power of movement. Loss of sensation is sometimes, however, described as **sensory paralysis.**

Loss of function in motor nerves results in paralysis and wasting of the muscles which they supply. According to the site of the nerve lesions the muscular paralysis may occur in the form of **spastic muscular paralysis** or **flaccid muscular paralysis.**

paresis—a condition of partial paralysis.

quadriplegia—motor paralysis of all four limbs.

seizure—a synonym of fit (see above).

stupor—a condition of partial unconsciousness.

tinnitus—a sensation of ringing or noises in the ears.

tremor—abnormal coarse or fine movements, of a vibratory nature, in voluntary muscles.

vertigo—a sensation of giddiness.

3. SPECIAL EXAMINATIONS

These include:

(*a*) The taking of pressure readings from the cerebrospinal fluid and the examination of specimens of this fluid by microscopy and various other pathological procedures; chemical, bacteriological, etc. Such specimens are most commonly obtained by **lumbar puncture;** a procedure which involves insertion of the tip of a needle into the subarachnoid space within the spinal theca. The puncture is made in the lower lumbar region, well below the termination of the spinal cord, the lower limit of which lies at the lower border of the first lumbar or upper border of the second lumbar vertebra.

In special instances **cisternal puncture** is employed as an alternative method to **lumbar puncture,** the needle being inserted, between the occipital bone and first cervical vertebra, into the cisterna magna which is a part of the subarachnoid space lying just below the brain, and just above the posterior part of the foramen magnum.

(*b*) **Radiological procedures:**

(i) *Plain radiography*—to show changes in the skull, spine and other structures secondary to, or associated with diseases of the nervous system. In suspected space-occupying lesions within the cranium, one important procedure is the taking of films to demonstrate any displacement of the pineal gland (pineal body), which lies in the midline behind the upper part of the third ventricle of the brain. This gland, particularly in older individuals, often shows calcium deposits in its substance thus rendering it visible on skull radiographs.

(ii) *Specialised radiological investigations*—such as demonstration of the ventricles of the brain by **ventriculography** or **encephalography;** demonstration of the cerebral blood vessels by **carotid** or **vertebral angiography;** and investigation of the spinal cord and theca by **myelography.**

(iii) *Investigations employing radioactive isotopes.*

(*c*) **Electro-encephalography (E.E.G.)**—a procedure whereby tracings of electrical discharges from the brain are recorded in wave-form.

(*d*) **Ultrasonography**—this procedure is of particular value in showing displacement of midline structures by intracranial space-occupying lesions. It involves the use of vibrations of high frequency, called **ultrasonics,** which travel through matter in the form of a beam and are beyond the range of audible sound. Such vibrations have both diagnostic and therapeutic applications in neurology.

(*e*) Investigation of the electrical responses in muscle groups supplied by damaged motor nerves, e.g. **electromyography** (see p. 257).

4. CONGENITAL ABNORMALITIES

These include:

(*a*) **Spastic diplegia** (Little's Disease)—this is one type of a group of disorders known collectively as **cerebral palsy.** Thomson and Cotton (1) state "it may possibly be due to birth trauma but more probably is a developmental abnormality of brain tissue". Its principal clinical feature is spasticity of muscle groups in the legs (spastic paraplegia), or in both legs and both arms (spastic quadriplegia), resulting in various degrees of paralysis of the affected limbs.

Sufferers from this condition and other forms of cerebral palsy are commonly known as **"spastics"**. They frequently show some degree of associated mental defect.

(*b*) **Anencephaly** (see p. 185).

(*c*) **Microcephaly**—a condition in which there is defective development of the brain and the cranium is abnormally small.

(*d*) **Abnormalities associated with spina bifida**—meningocele, meningo-myelocele, etc. (see p. 234).

(*e*) **Mongolism**—a congenital disorder resulting in a severe degree of defective development of mental processes.

Sufferers from mongols are called **mongols** and possess flat faces and obliquely-set eyes, thus bearing a facial resemblance to members of the Mongolian race. A proportion of mongols suffer from congenital heart disease.

(*f*) **Congenital Hydrocephalus**—hydrocephalus is a condition of excessive accumulation of cerebrospinal fluid within the cranium. The congenital variety is due to factors present during intra-uterine existence and may develop in foetal life (**foetal hydrocephalus**—see p. 185) or shortly after birth. It results from some form of obstruction to the normal circulation of cerebrospinal fluid and may be produced by developmental defects, or certain infective conditions which affect the foetus. Hydrocephalus can also occur as an acquired condition in post-natal life.

(*g*) **Arnold-Chiari Malformation**—a developmental abnormality in which there is protrusion of parts of the cerbellum and medulla oblongata, through the foramen magnum, into the upper part of the spinal canal.

5. TRAUMATIC DISORDERS

(*a*) **Injuries to the Brain.** Traumatic injury to the brain may occur with, or without, associated **fracture of the cranium** (i.e. the part of the skull which contains the brain). Compound fractures with brain damage may lead to infection in the meninges and underlying brain tissue.

In its simplest form, brain injury may be evidenced by an instantaneous but temporary loss of consciousness, termed **simple concussion.** This condition is frequently accompanied by a loss of memory **(amnesia)** for incidents immediately prior to the causal trauma, and for subsequent happenings over a variable period of time.

A more serious injury may lead to haemorrhage from blood vessels supplying the meninges or brain tissue (**intracranial haemorrhage**) and the formation of an **intracranial haematoma** (i.e. a swelling composed of blood) which constitutes what is termed an **intracranial space-occupying lesion.** Such a lesion causes a rise in intracranial pressure and thus causes compression of brain tissue, evidenced by a clinical condition known as **cerebral compression.**

Severe injuries may also lead to **contusion** (bruising) or **laceration** (tearing) **of the brain** and these conditions may occur together with, or in the absence of, haematoma formation within the cranium.

Simple concussion usually recovers without giving rise to any long-lasting after-effects. In cases in which there is contusion or laceration of the brain, concussion may be followed by signs and symptoms of brain damage termed **cerebral irritation,** which may last several weeks before recovery ensues. This latter condition is evidenced by features such as stupor, restlessness, mental irritability, etc.

More serious degrees of contusion or laceration may be evidenced, immediately after the causal trauma, by signs and symptoms of more severe neurological disorders and may produce after-effects such as permanent paralyses, **traumatic epilepsy** (Jacksonian epilepsy), etc.

In cases with intracranial haemorrhage, concussion may be followed by evidence of compression but commonly these two states are separated by an interval during which consciousness is regained. This interval is called the **"lucid interval"** and during its duration, which is of variable length, there is frequently little or no clinical evidence of brain injury.

With the development of compression, however, there appear signs such as abnormalities of pulse rate, respiration and body temperature; abnormalities of the pupils of the eyes, drowsiness and unconsciousness, disordered reflexes; muscular paralyses, etc. (*Note:* cerebral compression may also be caused by conditions other than trauma, see "Space-occupying Lesions in the Cranium".)

According to the site of the haemorrhage, intra-cranial haematomas which produce cerebral compression, are described as **extradural haematomas** (between the dura and overlying skull); **subdural haematomas** (between the dura and arachnoid mater) and **intracerebral haematomas** (within the brain).

Extradural haematomas are frequently the result of injury to the middle meningeal artery and associated with a fracture of the temporo-parietal region of the skull. Subdural haematomas occur in both acute the chronic form; the latter sometimes being the result of a relatively minor injury which results in a slow leakage of blood into the subdural space.

Intracranial haematomas are treated surgically, the skull being opened and the haematoma evacuated. Radiological investigations and ultrasonic methods frequently play an important role in the diagnosis of these disorders.

(*b*) **Injuries to the spinal cord**—these usually, but not invariably, occur in association with fracture-dislocations or dislocations of the vertebrae. They may take the form of **contusions** or **lacerations of the spinal cord substance**; or of **compression of the spinal cord** as a result of haemorrhage (c.f. cerebral compression) or pressure of displaced bony parts on the cord (see p. 278).

Injury to the cord, according to its extent and severity, may cause varying degrees of temporary, or permanent, motor paralysis; sensory loss below the level of the damage to the cord tissue; and accompanying disorders of bowel and bladder function. Injuries which tear through the substance of cord, or cause irreversible damage involving part or the whole thickness of the cord at the site of injury, are referred to as causing **partial** or **complete transection of the spinal cord.**

(*c*) **Peripheral Nerve Injuries**—these comprise **contusion** (bruising), **compression, partial division** and **complete division of nerves** and result in a loss of nervous function in affected nerves. This loss may affect motor or sensory functions, or both, according to whether an injured nerve is of motor, sensory or mixed type. The resultant effects may be temporary or permanent according to the nature of the injury. Damage to motor nerve fibres results in paralysis of muscles supplied by such fibres and subsequent muscle wasting.

Damaged nerve fibres possess certain powers of regeneration and eventual complete recovery is common in injuries in which there is no actual division of nerve fibres, (i.e. in contusion and compression nerve injuries). In these, treatment is directed to the care of paralysed muscles with various forms of physiotherapy, while recovery of nervous function is proceeding.

In order to obtain restoration of function in cases of partial or complete division, when practicable, the cut nerve ends must be stitched together; the operation being called **nerve suture.** In some instances it is necessary to fill in a gap between the nerve ends by a short segment obtained from another nerve in the patient's body. This procedure is called **nerve-grafting.**

Various investigations are employed in cases of nerve injury in order to estimate the degree of nerve damage, and also the progress of regeneration when this occurs. Included among these are the testing of the responses, to galvanic and faradic currents, of muscles supplied by the affected nerve and the investigation called electromyography (see p. 257).

6. INFECTIVE DISEASES

Inflammatory changes in the various structures of the nervous system are denoted by the following terms—brain tissue—**encephalitis;** meninges—**meningitis;** brain and meninges—**meningo-encephalitis;** spinal cord tissue—**myelitis;** brain and spinal cord—**encephalo-myelitis;** grey matter of spinal cord—**poliomyelitis;** nerves—**neuritis.**

(*a*) **Meningitis**—inflammation of the meninges may be due to a variety of causes including bacterial infections and infections with viruses (viral meningitis).

Infective bacteria may reach the meninges (i) by the blood stream as in meningococcal meningitis (see p. 50), tuberculous meningitis, and meningitis occurring as a complication of streptococcal infections elsewhere in the body, (ii) by direct spread from infective processes in sites such as the frontal sinuses and mastoid air cells, and (iii) as a result of penetrating wounds of the skull.

Viral meningitis may occur rarely as a complication of virus infections such as mumps and measles, or sometimes as a primary infective condition of the meninges.

In addition to general signs and symptoms of infection, e.g. headache, pyrexia, increase of pulse rate, etc., patients with meningitis show signs due to **meningeal irritation** such as limitation of the movements of the neck due to muscle spasm (neck rigidity), and a sign called **Kernig's sign** which consists of inability to extend the knee when the thigh is flexed to a right angle on the trunk. In severe cases there may also be a condition of marked extension of the neck called **head retraction. Photophobia** (dislike of light) is also common in meningitis.

Signs of meningeal irritation due to meningitis have to be differentiated from similar signs occurring in a condition called **meningism,** which may occur during the course of pneumonia and other acute febrile infections in childhood.

Examination of the cerebrospinal fluid is an important diagnostic procedure in meningitis. Antibiotics are widely used in the treatment of meningeal infections.

(*b*) **Encephalitis**—inflammation of brain tissue may result from infection with pyogenic (pus-producing) bacteria (see "Brain Abscess"), spirochaetes (see "Neurosyphilis"), and viruses. Encephalitis also occurs in the form of malaria called **cerebral malaria** and in another infection called **toxoplasmosis,** which is also due to a protozoan parasite.

In rare instances blood-borne infection of brain tissue with tubercle bacilli may occur and lead to the formation of a solitary lesion called a **cerebral tuberculoma.**

Among the types of encephalitis due to viruses are a disease called **encephalitis lethargica** which may give rise to a condition called **Parkinsonism** (see p. 279); **rabies** (hydrophobia) a virus infection transmitted to human subjects by dogs or less commonly other animals; and encephalitis occurring as a rare complication of acute infectious fevers such as chicken pox and smallpox, or consequent on vaccination against smallpox.

(*c*) **Brain Abscess**—infection of brain tissue with pyogenic micro-organisms may result in the formation of a brain abscess (i.e. a cavity containing pus), which constitutes a space-occupying lesion within the cranium and results in raised intracranial pressure. The infection may be blood-borne, derived from a neighbouring focus such as an infected frontal sinus or infected mastoid air cells; or due to a penetrating wound of the skull.

A brain abscess occurs most commonly in one of the cerebral hemispheres or in the cerebellum. Treatment is by aspiration or surgical operation.

(*d*) **Infective Sinus Thrombosis**—this condition is a serious complication which occurs when a nearby infective process spreads to involve venous sinuses lying in the dura mater. With the increased use of antibiotics in the treatment of infections it is nowadays uncommon. The principal types of sinus thrombosis are **cavernous sinus thrombosis,** which may occur secondary to a carbuncle of the face, and **lateral sinus thrombosis** which may complicate mastoid infection.

(*e*) **Neurosyphilis,** i.e. syphilis of the nervous system is not nowadays common but can develop in the tertiary and quaternary stages of acquired syphilitic infection.

In the tertiary stage it presents in the form of **meningo-vascular syphilis,** so called because in this disorder the infective lesions chiefly affect the meninges and blood vessels of the brain and spinal cord. A variety of clinical pictures may result from this condition and these may not infrequently mimic those of other diseases of the central nervous system.

The manifestations of quaternary syphilis may take the form of a condition called **general paralysis of the insane,** when the lesions affect the brain, and **tabes dorsalis** when they chiefly involve the spinal cord and the posterior roots of the spinal nerves.

General Paralysis of the insane (dementia paralytica) as indicated by its name, is associated with severe mental changes and the development of weakness and paralysis in various groups of muscles.

Tabes dorsalis is also called **locomotor ataxia** and one of its features is a staggering gait as a result of incoordination of muscular action (ataxia) in the muscles of the lower limbs. Other features include pains around the chest referred to as "girdle pains"; bladder and bowel disturbances; areas of sensory loss which may lead to painless ulcers developing in the feet and legs; and Charcot joints.

The term "tabes" means "wasting" and the name "tabes dorsalis" refers to degenerative changes which occur in structures, composed of white matter, called the posterior (dorsal) columns of the spinal cord.

In tabes and other forms of neurosyphilis the lesions may also affect the nerve supply of the pupils of the eyes producing a condition referred to as **Argyll-Robertson pupils,** i.e. pupils which possess normal powers of accommodation but show a loss of normal reflex reaction to light (**accommodation** is the mechanism by which adjustments are effected in the lens of the eye to permit clear visualization of objects at different distances).

(*f*) **Acute Anterior Poliomyelitis**—this is an infection due to a virus called the *poliovirus.* It is thought to be carried by droplet infection and also in contaminated food and water, and thus to gain access to the blood stream, and thence to the central nervous system, via the nasopharynx and alimentary tract.

The disease commences with a febrile illness known as the **pre-paralytic stage** of the disease. In so-called **non-paralytic cases,** the infection does not progress beyond this stage. In others, however, it proceeds to a **paralytic stage** as a result of involvement and resultant inflammatory changes in structures, within the grey matter (polio) of the spinal cord, called the **anterior horns.** These changes give the disease the name of anterior poliomyelitis.

Whilst poliomyelitis not infrequently occurs in adults below middle age, its chief incidence is in childhood and it thus is sometimes referred to as **infantile paralysis.**

The inflammatory changes affect motor nerve cells in the anterior horns of the spinal cord and, sometimes motor nerve cells in the brain also, causing muscular paralysis of variable distribution.

Poliomyelitis occurs both in the form of isolated cases and epidemics.

The extent of the muscular paralysis varies greatly from case to case as does the degree of permanent damage caused. Thus during the **convalescent stage** of the disorder, which can last about two years, the paralysis may recover completely, improve to a varying extent, or alternatively show no evidence of recovery at all.

There is no specific treatment for poliomyelitis. Therapy comprises rest and measures to prevent deformity in the acute phase of the disease, and intensive physiotherapy to assist recovery of muscle function during convalescence. Special methods of feeding are required in patients with paralysis of the muscles used in swallowing, and those with paralysis of the respiratory muscles need some form of artificial ventilation of the lungs. This latter may be effected by some form of mechanical respirator (e.g. an "iron lung") or by performing a tracheostomy and using some form of positive pressure ventilation apparatus.

Protection against poliomyelitis may be given by vaccination with either injection of the Salk-type or oral administration of the Sabin-type of anti-poliomyelitis vaccine.

(*g*) **Herpes Zoster** (Shingles)—is a virus infection of the nervous system in which inflammatory lesions develop in sensory ganglia of cranial nerves, or the posterior root ganglia of spinal nerves. The causal virus is closely related to the virus of varicella (chicken pox).

Severe pain is experienced in sensory nerve fibres connected with affected ganglia and a vesicular rash (i.e. a rash consisting of small blisters) appears in areas of skin supplied by such fibres. The pain may persist long after the rash has disappeared, the condition then being referred to as **post-herpetic neuralgia.**

7. NEOPLASMS

INTRACRANIAL NEOPLASMS

These commonly produce the signs and symptoms of a space-occupying lesion within the cranium (see p. 277). They are of the following main types:

(*a*) **Gliomas**—these tumours arise from the neuroglia (i.e. the specialized supporting connective tissue of the central nervous system). They tend to be locally malignant but never produce metastases outside the central nervous system. There are various types of glioma distinguished by names such as **astrocytoma, glioblastoma multiforme, medulloblastoma, spongioblastoma, oligodendroglioma, ependymoma** etc.

Medulloblastomas are the commonest type of glioma in childhood.

273

They may spread via the subarachnoid space producing secondary deposits which involve the spinal cord.

Few gliomas are amenable to surgical removal and radiotherapy is extensively used in their treatment.

(*b*) **Meningioma**—a benign tumour arising from the meninges. Surgical removal of this tumour is frequently possible. Inoperable cases are treated by radiotherapy.

(*c*) **Pituitary Tumours**—these have already been referred to in connection with diseases of the endocrine system (see p. 209).

(*d*) **Acoustic neurofibroma** (auditory nerve tumour, acoustic neuroma) —a benign tumour arising from the fibrous sheath of the eighth cranial nerve (acoustic or auditory nerve). It causes deafness on the affected side and vertigo (giddiness). This neoplasm sometimes occurs in association with general neurofibromatosis (see p. 275).

(*e*) **Angioma**—the term "angioma" means "a tumour of blood vessels" but many authorities regard angiomas of the brain as congenital malformations rather than true neoplasms. Rupture of abnormal blood vessels within an angioma may give rise to intracranial haemorrhage.

(*f*) **Cerebral Metastases**—carcinomatous metastases in the brain develop most frequently from primary carcinomas of the breast and bronchus, but may be secondary to carcinomas in other sites and rarely to sarcomas.

TUMOURS ARISING WITHIN THE SPINAL CANAL

These comprise tumours of the spinal cord; the spinal meninges; the spinal nerve roots and their sheaths; and blood vessels and soft tissues within the spinal canal.

The spinal cord is sometimes referred to as the **spinal medulla** and tumours arising within the cord are known as **intramedullary tumours,** whilst the other tumours arising within the spinal canal are termed **extramedullary tumours** (comprising **intradural** and **extradural** tumours).

These tumours are not common but the most frequently seen of the intramedullary variety are gliomas, arising from the neuroglia and of the same nature as those which occur in the brain. Among the different types of extramedullary tumours encountered are meningiomas, neurofibromas, cauda equina tumours, and neoplasms arising in the spinal vertebrae (e.g. metastases).

A meningioma arises from the meninges and a neurofibroma from a nerve sheath. A **cauda equina tumour** arises in the collection of nerve

274

roots which lie in the lower part of the spinal canal below the termination of the spinal cord.

GENERALIZED NEUROFIBROMATOSIS

A neurofibroma is a benign tumour which arises in a nerve sheath from cells called Schwann cells and is thus sometimes referred to as a **Schwannoma.** This type of neoplasm, as has already been noted, may develop from the sheath of the acoustic nerve (acoustic neurofibroma), or arise from a nerve sheath within the spinal canal. In either of these sites it may be solitary or occur as part of a disorder wherein multiple neurofibromata arise in the same patient. In this latter instance the disorder is known as **generalized neurofibromatosis** or **von Recklinghausen's disease.**

The tumours produce rounded nodules in the course of both superficial nerves and deep nerves and are associated with areas of brown pigmentation in the skin, referred to as "café au lait" patches. The tumours may cause a mixture of bone destruction and reactive new bone formation as a result of pressure on neighbouring bony structures.

OTHER TUMOURS ARISING IN NERVOUS TISSUE

These include **ganglioneuromas** and **neuroblastomas** which arise from the tissues of the sympathetic nervous system, or from the suprarenal medulla, which is derived from nervous tissue of similar origin to that of the sympathetic nervous system.

8. CEREBRAL VASCULAR DISEASE

The term cerebral vascular disease is generally taken as referring to disorders of the blood vessels of the brain and its covering meninges, other than those occasioned by traumatic injury (e.g. extradural and acute and chronic subdural haematomas—see p. 268).

The commonest cause of the condition is cerebral atheroma (see p. 78). Other causes include congenital and acquired aneurysms in the cerebral circulation (see p. 79), malformations of the type known as angiomas (see p. 274) and syphilitic infection of the cerebral and meningeal arteries (see p. 271).

Important complications of cerebral vascular disease are the types of intracranial haemorrhage known as cerebral haemorrhage and subarachnoid haemorrhage, and also the disorder called cerebral ischaemia.

Investigation of the circulation in the cerebral, carotid and vertebral vessels, by radiology, is an important diagnostic procedure, which is nowadays frequently employed in demonstrating lesions causing intra-cranial haemorrhage and cerebral ischaemia.

(*a*) **Cerebral haemorrhage** (intracerebral haemorrhage)—this is a condition of spontaneous bleeding into the brain substance which is usually due to rupture of an arterial vessel and, according to Dimsdale (2), is due most commonly to rupture of an atheromatous artery in a subject with hypertension (high blood pressure).

In its more severe forms, the onset of cerebral haemorrhage, and also subarachnoid haemorrhage and cerebral thrombosis, is frequently marked by what is termed a **cerebral vascular accident** (C.V.A.) causing **apoplexy.** Brinton (3) states "by apoplexy is meant the abrupt cessation of the function of the brain as a consequence of interference with blood supply, an event commonly known as a stroke".

A variety of different forms of motor paralysis and sensory loss may follow on the occurrence of a non-fatal stroke. Disturbances of speech and hemiplegia (paralysis of one half of the body), of either a transient or permanent nature, are not uncommon sequels.

It has already been noted that, occasionally, a large haemorrhage into the brain tissue may cause an intracerebral haematoma, and this latter condition gives rise to the signs and symptoms of an intra-cranial space-occupying lesion.

(*b*) **Subarachnoid Haemorrhage**—is a condition in which bleeding occurs into the subarachnoid space between the arachnoid mater and pia mater. It is most commonly due to rupture of a congenital aneurysm of one of the arteries forming the Circle of Willis, which lies in the subarachnoid space at the base of the brain. It may, however, develop as a complication of cerebral atheroma or other vascular disease.

As with intracerebral haemorrhage, subarachnoid haemorrhage is often first evidenced as a cerebral vascular accident (see above) but, when the bleeding is subarachnoid, the diagnosis may be confirmed by performing a lumbar puncture and demonstrating the presence of blood in the cerebro-spinal fluid. Cerebral angiography is an important procedure when a diagnosis of subarachnoid haemorrhage is made, in order to determine whether an aneurysm of a cerebral artery can be demonstrated.

(*c*) **Cerebral Ischaemia**—this is a condition in which, as a result of diseases which cause narrowing or blockage of the cerebral, carotid or vertebral arteries, there is a localized deficiency of blood supply to a part or parts of the brain. It is also referred to as **cerebral vascular insufficiency.**

Blockage of a cerebral artery may lead to death of an area of brain tissue, such an area then being referred to as a **cerebral infarct.** This may occur as a result of **cerebral thrombosis,** i.e. thrombus (clot) formation in cerebral arteries (developing most frequently secondary to atheroma); and **cerebral embolism**—resulting in occlusion of cerebral vessels by emboli derived from the heart or elsewhere in the circulation.

As with cerebral haemorrhage, cerebral thrombosis and cerebral embolism, diseases affecting the carotid and vertebral arteries may produce various serious disturbances of the sensory and motor functions of the nervous. system. These disturbances when due to cerebral thrombosis are usually of gradual development but, when produced by embolism may first present in the form of a cerebral vascular accident (see p. 276) causing sudden loss of consciousness.

In addition to cerebral thrombosis and embolism, Houston, Joiner and Trounce (4) describe as important causes of cerebral ischaemia the arterial disorders called **internal carotid artery disease, vertebro-basilar disease** (see also p. 256), and **diffuse cerebral atherosclerosis.**

9. INTRACRANIAL SPACE-OCCUPYING LESIONS

Reference has been made in the foregoing account of diseases of the nervous system that certain pathological conditions constitute what are termed space-occupying lesions within the cranium. Such lesions, by causing an increase in the amounts of fluid or tissue, or both, within the restricted space contained by the walls of the cranium cause a rise of intracranial pressure. They thus commonly produce general signs and symptoms due to this increase of pressure within the cranium such as headache; vomiting; **papilloedema** (i.e. swelling of the optic discs which may be detected with an instrument called an ophthalmoscope) and convulsions. In addition, they frequently also produce localizing signs and symptoms resulting from pressure on, or involvement of structures in the vicinity of the lesion, e.g. paralysis of muscles supplied by cranial nerves, paralysis of limbs, loss of sensation in various parts of the body, mental changes, disturbances of speech, vision and hearing, vertigo, abnormalities of posture and gait, etc.

The following are some of the principal types of intracranial space-occupying lesions: intracranial tumours and cysts, brain abscesses, intracranial haematomas (e.g. chronic subdural haematomas) large blood clots within the brain due to haemorrhage from a cerebral artery, large intracranial aneurysms, cerebral tuberculomas.

Special investigations employed in the diagnosis of space-occupying lesions include plain radiography, cerebral angiography, contrast radiography of the cerebral ventricles, electro-encephalography, and scanning with radioactive isotopes.

[*Note:* Lumbar puncture is seldom carried out in these disorders as it may be dangerous when there is raised intracranial pressure.]

10. SPINAL CORD COMPRESSION

It was noted when discussing traumatic injuries that these could cause compression of the spinal cord as a result of haemorrhage within the spinal canal, or pressure from displaced bony parts of the spinal column due to dislocations or fracture-dislocations.

More commonly, however, the clinical signs and symptoms of compression are of gradual development and non-traumatic origin. Among the conditions responsible for this condition may be mentioned: central protrusion of an intervertebral disc; pressure from a bony outgrowth in cervical spondylosis; metastases in the spine, primary neoplasms arising within the spinal canal, and tuberculosis of the spine.

The effect of spinal compression is to cause muscular weakness, or paralysis, and sensory disorders below the level of the lesion, the extent of these varying considerably according to the site and severity of the lesion responsible for the cord compression. There is often pain at the level of the lesion. Disorders of bowel and bladder function are common with compression at certain sites.

11. SOME OTHER DISORDERS OF THE CENTRAL NERVOUS SYSTEM

(*a*) **Idiopathic Epilepsy**. The name epilepsy is derived from a Greek verb meaning "to seize hold of" and derives from the fact that in ancient times the disease was attributed to possession of the sufferer's body by evil spirits.

Epilepsy is a functional disorder of the brain which may be of unknown causation (**idiopathic epilepsy**) or develop secondary to some other disease which affects the brain (**symptomatic epilepsy,** e.g. due to brain injury, cerebral tumour, etc.). It may present as a generalized disturbance of cerebral function (**general epilepsy**) or as a localized disturbance of such function (**focal epilepsy**).

In general epilepsy, and some forms of focal epilepsy, patients are subject to attacks in which consciousness is partially or completely lost.

The severe forms of general epilepsy are known as **major epilepsy** ("grand mal") and in them loss of consciousness is accompanied by muscular convulsions producing what are termed **epileptic fits** or **epileptic seizures.** Such fits do not occur in the milder forms of the disease which are termed **minor epilepsy** ("petit mal").

Radiological investigations and electro-encephalography are valuable aids in differentiating between idiopathic and symptomatic epilepsy.

Idiopathic epilepsy is treated by the daily administration of anti-convulsant drugs (e.g. phenobarbitone) with the object of preventing the attacks or diminishing their severity and frequency.

(*b*) **Migraine.** This is a condition characterized by the occurrence of severe periodic headaches which are preceded by some form of temporary disturbance of vision or other sensation, known as an **aura,** and are frequently accompanied by nausea and vomiting. The headache is frequently experienced in only one side of the head.

Sufferers from migraine are generally highly conscientious individuals and given to worrying excessively about their affairs. They themselves may describe their symptoms as being due to **"bilious attacks".**

(*c*) **Parkinsonism**—a condition in which tremors and rigidity develop in the muscles of face, trunk and limbs as a result of degenerative or inflammatory lesions in structures called the basal ganglia which lie in the lower parts of the cerebral hemispheres.

It may occur as a primary disease of degenerative type when it is known as **paralysis agitans,** or as a secondary manifestation of various other diseases which affect the central nervous system. Among these latter is the virus infection called **encephalitis lethargica.**

Treatment is principally by drugs but surgical procedures may be employed in selected cases to destroy certain parts of the basal ganglia.

(*d*) **Chorea**—as already noted (see p. 68) this disease is a manifestation of acute rheumatism produced by inflammatory changes in the central nervous system. Its chief feature is the occurrence of abnormal jerky involuntary movements which led in earlier times to the disease being called **St Vitus Dance.** Chorea is frequently associated with rheumatic heart disease.

(*e*) **Disseminated Sclerosis (Multiple Sclerosis)**—this is a common disease in which widespread lesions develop in the brain and spinal cord causing destruction of nerve sheaths, nerve fibres and reactive proliferation of the surrounding neuroglia.

The name of the disease derives from the disseminate (widespread) nature of the lesions and the areas of sclerosis (i.e. hardening) which develop in the central nervous system as a result of the overgrowth of neuroglia.

The cause of disseminated sclerosis is unknown. Its maximum incidence is in early adult life. It pursues an intermittent course in its early stages, the first symptoms often disappearing completely and then reappearing, sometimes after the lapse of a number of years. In accordance with the disseminate nature of the lesions, the clinical features are very variable and may mimic those of many other disorders of the nervous system. Thus, although the disease produces no radiological signs, patients with disseminated sclerosis are frequently referred for X-ray examination, to exclude some other lesion (e.g. spinal tumour, cervical disc lesion) as being the cause of the signs and symptoms.

Among the many clinical features which may result from disseminated sclerosis are disturbances of vision, speech and hearing; disturbances of gait; disturbances of bladder function; various forms of muscular paralysis and sensory disturbance; and mental changes. Mental changes often lead to an unwarranted felling of well-being, termed **euphoria.**

There is no specific treatment.

(*f*) **Syringomyelia**—an uncommon disease of unknown origin which develops in adult life. Its basic feature is over growth of neuroglia in certain regions of the spinal cord and sometimes in the medulla oblongata (syringobulbia). Proliferation of neurolgial tissue results in degeneration and destruction of nerve cells in affected areas resulting in clinical features such as wasting and weakness in the muscles of the hands and arms, spastic weakness of the lower limbs and characteristic sensory disturbances in the upper limbs (i.e. loss of sensibility to heat, cold and pain without loss of sensibility to touch).

The name of the disease derives from the occurrence of cavitation in areas of proliferation of the neuroglia, as in such areas the spinal cord bears some resemblance to a hollow tube (c.f. "syringe" a type of hollow tube).

Complications of syringomyelia include the development of Charcot joints in the upper limbs, pes cavus (claw foot) and painless ulceration of the soles of the feet.

(*g*) **Subacute Combined Degeneration of the Cord**—this disorder develops as a complication in about 10% of patients with pernicious anaemia and is due to deficiency of Vitamin B.12. Sensory and motor changes develop in this condition as a result of degenerative changes in structures called dorsal (posterior) and lateral columns of the spinal cord (hence the name "combined degeneration"), and also in peripheral nerves.

Treatment is by the administration of vitamin B.12.

(*h*) **Hereditary Ataxias**—these are a group of uncommon hereditary disorders in which ataxia (incoordination of muscular movements) is the most prominent feature. In the type called **Friedreich's ataxia** there is usually associated bilateral pes cavus (claw foot) and a scoliosis. The ataxia results in an unsteady gait, incoordination of the movements of the upper limbs, and disordered speech.

(*i*) **Motor Neurone Disease**—this term describes a rare group of diseases of unknown causation, in which muscle wasting develops as a result of degenerative changes in motor neurones in the spinal cord and brain. The individual diseases of the group are named **progressive muscular atrophy, amyotrophic lateral sclerosis** and **progressive bulbar palsy.**

12. SOME OTHER DISORDERS OF THE PERIPHERAL NERVOUS SYSTEM

The peripheral nervous system comprises the cranial and spinal nerves. Some reference has already been made to certain **traumatic peripheral nerve injuries** and to the benign tumours called **neurofibromas** which arise from the sheaths of cranial and spinal nerves. Some of the other disorders which may affect such nerves include the following:

(*a*) **Optic neuritis**—a disorder due to inflammatory or degenerative changes in the second cranial (optic) nerve. It may lead to atrophy of this nerve, a condition referred to as **optic atrophy.**

(*b*) **Trigeminal neuralgia** (*Tic Douloureux*)—a disorder of unknown origin in which periodic attacks of severe pain occur within the distribution of the fifth cranial (trigeminal) nerve, i.e. in the face, forehead, teeth, jaws and anterior part of the tongue.

(*c*) **Facial Palsy** (Bell's Palsy)—a condition of unknown origin and sudden onset which affects the seventh cranial (facial nerve) causing a unilateral paralysis of the facial muscles.

(*d*) **Radiculitis**—a term used to indicate inflammatory conditions and other disorders of the roots of the spinal roots. Pressure on nerve roots from prolapsed intervertebral discs; bony spurs occurring in spondylosis; and carcinomatous metastases in the spine are common causes of radiculitis.

Pressure on certain of the roots of the brachial plexus by a cervical rib or other abnormalities in the region of the thoracic inlet (e.g. prolapsed intervertebral disc) may cause disturbances of motor and sensory function in the head and forearm, which, sometimes together with associated disturbances of the blood supply resulting from pressure on the subclavian artery, produce clinical signs and symptoms described as being due to **thoracic inlet syndrome.** (*Note:* some authorities refer to this condition as **thoracic outlet syndrome).**

(*e*) **Mononeuritis**—a term used to indicate inflammatory conditions or other disorders affecting a single spinal or cranial nerve. Examples of these conditions are **optic neuritis; neuritis of the median nerve** due to compression of this nerve at the wrist in the disorder called **carpal-tunnel syndrome;** and **ulnar neuritis,** due to compression of the ulnar nerve in the region of the medial epicondyle of the humerus (e.g. as a result of a fracture in this region).

(*Note:* Where a condition similar to mononeuritis affects several nerves it may be referred to as **multiple neuritus.**

The term **neuritis** is also applied to certain disorders of nerve plexuses, e.g. **brachial neuritis**—a condition of acute onset causing pain in distribution of nerves arising from the brachial plexus and paralysis of muscles around the shoulder girdle.

The term **polyneuritis** (see below) is applied to another type of disorder which affects many of the peripheral nerves and which usually produces lesions with a symmetrical distribution.)

(*f*) **Peripheral Neuropathy**—a large variety of diseases may be complicated by degenerative changes (in most instances of non-inflammatory causation) in peripheral nerves producing a disorder described as peripheral neuropathy, or alternatively as **polyneuropathy, peripheral neuritis,** or **polyneuritis.**

The term **neuropathy** means a disease of nervous tissue. The prefix **poly-** indicates that a number of nerves are affected simultaneously.

The degenerative changes occur most commonly in the nerves of the limbs, especially the lower limbs, and tend to have a symmetrical distribution. Common features resulting from the disorder are muscular weakness, various forms of sensory disturbance and loss of normal reflexes in the areas supplied by the affected nerves.

Among the many causes of peripheral neuropathy may be mentioned: diabetes, various form of chemical posioning (e.g. lead poisoning, arsenical poisoning); nutritional deficiency diseases (e.g. **beriberi** due to lack of Vitamin B.1, chronic alcoholism, malabsorption syndromes); **malignant neuropathy** (due most commonly to bronchial carcinoma); and the uncommon disorder called **acute infective polyneuritis.**

Peripheral neuropathy may also occur as a manifestation of **hereditary porphyria,** a rare disorder the other features of which include mental disturbances, the development of skin lesions as a result of exposure to sunlight, and the passage of urine which is dark red owing to the presence of pigments called porphyrins.

(*g*) **Ménières Disease**—see p. 296.

SOME NEUROSURGICAL OPERATIONS

(*a*) Surgical Methods of Opening the Cranium

These comprise:

(i) The drilling of one or more **burr holes,** e.g. for the purpose of tapping the cerebral ventricles in order to inject air or myodil for ventriculography, or draw off cerebrospinal fluid in order to decompress the brain.

(ii) **Trephining**—the cutting out of one or more circular discs of bone, which can subsequently be replaced, by means of an instrument called a **trephine,** e.g. for biopsy of a tumour, elevation of a depressed fracture, etc.

(iii) **Craniotomy**—an operation which is performed when it is thought that an intracranial lesion (e.g. an operable type of neoplasm) can be dealt with by surgical treatment. A large flap of scalp, bone and dura mater is cut and turned back in such a manner that it can be replaced at the end of the operation. This flap is known as an **osteoplastic flap.**

(iv) **Leucotomy**—the cutting of certain nerve fibres in the frontal lobes of the brain. This operation is occasionally used as a form of treatment in certain types of severe mental disorder, e.g. schizophrenia.

(v) **Laminectomy**—removal of one or more vertebral laminae in order to gain access to the interior of the vertebral canal, e.g. to remove a spinal tumour, or protrusion of an intervertebral disc.

(*d*) **Nerve Suture and Nerve Grafting**—see p. 269.

REFERENCES

(1) Thomson, A. D. and Cotton, R. E. *Lecture Notes on Pathology.* Blackwell Scientific Publicaions, 1968.
(2) Dimsdale, Helen *The Practice of Medicine* (Ed. Sir John Richardson). J. & A. Churchill, 1960.
(3) Brinton D. *Conybeare's Textbook of Medicine* (Ed. W. N. Mann). E. and S. Livingston, 1964.

(4) Houston, J. C., Joiner, C. L. and Trounce, J. R., *A Short Textbook of Medicine.* English Universities Press, 1966.

Section O. THE EYE

1. SOME GENERAL CONSIDERATIONS

The *eye* is the organ of vision. Each *eyeball* is contained within a bony cavity called the *orbit,* which also contains the *orbital muscles* and *orbital fat.* Three coats of tissue surround the eyeball: (i) an outer fibrous coat consisting in its posterior two thirds of the *sclera* and anteriorly of a transparent layer called the *cornea,* (ii) a middle pigmented vascular coat called the *uveal tract,* consisting of the *choroid, ciliary body* and *iris,* (iii) an inner coat of nervous tissue called the *retina.*

The *optic nerve,* which is the nerve of vision, transmits visual stimuli from the retina to the brain. Its fibres leave the retina at the *optic disc.*

In the interior of the eye are situated the *anterior* and *posterior chambers,* partially separated by the iris and containing a liquid substance called *aqueous humour;* the *crystalline lens* and its *suspensory ligament;* and posteriorly a jelly-like substance called the *vitreous humour.*

The amount of light entering the eyball is controlled by the action of muscle fibres within the iris which can contract or dilate the *pupil,* i.e. the central aperture in the iris.

Within the eyeball light rays are bent so as to be focussed on the retina and form clear images of objects from which they are reflected. This process of bending of light rays is called **refraction.** In order that the focus of the eye may be adjusted to view objects at different distances the eye possesses a property called **accommodation,** whereby alterations in focussing are made by altering the convexity of the anterior surface of the lens. Such alterations are effected by the action of muscle fibres in the ciliary body which can tighten or relax the suspensory ligament of the lens.

Under normal conditions, impulses are received by both eyes and slightly differing images are formed on each retina and then fused into a single image by the brain. This is termed **binocular single vision.** (*Note:* vision with one eye is called **monocular vision**).

Associated with the eyeball are a number of accessory structures such as the *orbital muscles and fascia,* the *orbital fat,* the *eyebrows,* the *eyelids* and *eyelashes,* the *conjunctiva* and the *lacrimal apparatus.*

The *conjunctiva* is a mucous membrane which covers the exposed anterior portion of the white of the eye and lines the inner surfaces of the eyelids.

The *lacrimal apparatus* of each eye comprises the *lacrimal gland* and its *ducts,* which secrete and carry tears into the conjunctival sac; and the *lacrimal passages,* i.e. the *lacrimal canaliculi, lacrimal sac* and *naso-lacrimal duct,* through which the tears are conveyed from the conjunctival sac into the nasal cavity.

The prefixes **"ophthalmo-"** and **"oculo-"** both refer to the eye whilst **"opto-"** may refer to the eye or to vision. **Optics** is a branch of science relating to light and to vision. **Ophthalmology** is the branch of medicine concerned with disorders of the eye and its accessory structures.

Methods of investigation employed in ophthalmology include ordinary visual inspection; inspection of the interior of the eye with an **ophthalmoscope;** visual inspection with magnifying devices and special illumination, e.g. **slit lamp microscopy;** investigation of visual acuity by **Snellen's test types; perimetry,** i.e. measurement of the extent of the field of vision; **refraction** (see p. 284).

In the succeeding account it will only be possible to indicate a limited number of the many medical terms that refer to various disorders encountered in ophthalmic practice.

2. DISEASES OF THE EYEBALL

These may be congenital, traumatic, infective, neoplastic, or of other types. Among the most important are:

(*a*) **Intra-ocular Foreign Body**—this may be metallic or less commonly non-metallic. It is a serious condition as it may result in permanent visual damage, particularly if the lens is injured, and in other serious complications. Among these latter is the development of chronic **iridocyclitis** (inflammation of the iris and ciliary body) in the injured eye which may later be followed by a condition called **sympathetic ophthalmia** (sympathetic iridocyclitis) in which iridocyclitis also develops in the uninjured eye.

Ophthalmia is a term used to indicate certain forms of inflammation affecting the eyeball or conjunctiva.

(*b*) **Inflammatory Disorders**—terms used to indicate inflammatory disorders occurring in various parts of the eyeball include the following: **keratitis** (cornea), **scleritis** (sclera), **iritis** (iris), **iridocyclitis** (iris and ciliary body), **uveitis** (uveal tract, i.e. iris, ciliary body and choroid), **choroiditis** (choroid), **retinitis** (retina), **papillitis** (optic disc), **panoph-**

thalmitis (inflammation affecting all the tissues of the eyeball).

Corneal ulceration is a common result of inflammatory processes, due to trauma or other causes, which affect the cornea. **Hypopyon** is a condition in which an inflammatory exudate is found in the anterior chamber of the eye and may develop as a complication of corneal ulceration.

Chronic inflammation of the cornea occurs in the condition called **interstitial keratitis** which is a manifestation of congenital syphilis.

Iritis, usually accompanied by inflammatory changes in the ciliary body and thus generally more correctly referred to as **iridocyclitis**, is a not uncommon condition. It may occur in association with dental abscesses, infected paranasal sinuses or infective lesions elsewhere in the body; as a manifestation of sarcoidosis, tuberculosis, gonorrhoea or syphilis; or be due to other causes. In patients with sarcoidosis lesions in iris and ciliary body are frequently associated with lesions in the parotid gland (**uveo-parotid sarcoidosis**).

The term **retinitis** is used to include not only true inflammatory disorders of the retina, but also a number of degenerative and other disorders.

As stressed by Martin–Doyle (1) it is less misleading to use the term **retinopathy** to describe various retinal manifestations of general disease in which the retinal changes are essentially of a degenerative nature. As described by the same author, retinopathy may occur as a complication of hypertension (**arteriosclerotic retinopathy**), certain forms of severe renal disease (**renal retinopathy**), and diabetes (**diabetic retinopathy**).

(*c*) **Neoplasms**—these are all rare. They include **melanomas** (see p. 224) which arise most frequently from the choroid; **retinoblastomas** malignant tumours of retinal cells which usually develop in childhood and are often bilateral; **gliomas of the optic nerve;** and **carcinomatous metastases** from primary tumours elsewhere in the body, e.g. the breast.

    (*d*) **Vascular Disorders of the Retina**—these include:
  (i) **Retinal Haemorrhages**—these may be due to a variety of causes including trauma, retinopathies (see above), etc.
  (ii) **Occlusion of the Central Artery of the Retina**—due to thrombosis or embolism.
  (iii) **Thrombosis of the Central Vein of the Retina.**

(*e*) **Glaucoma**—a condition in which accumulation of fluid and a consequent rise of pressure occurs in the fluid within the anterior chamber of the eyeball. The causation of glaucoma is a complex subject for an understanding of which reference should be made to a textbook of ophthalmology. Primary and secondary varieties of the disorder are described. The latter may develop as a result of iridocyclitis, haemorrhage into the eyeball, etc.

The treatment of glaucoma may be medical or surgical.

(*f*) **Papilloedema**—see p. 277.

(*g*) **Detached Retina**—a disorder in which, due to a number of different causes, an area of dissolution is formed within the retina and leads to detachment of a part of the retina, of varying extent, from the underlying choroid. Retinal detachment may occur as a result of trauma or complicate certain diseases of the retina, choroid, or iris and ciliary body. The condition is diagnosed by examination with the ophthalmoscope and treatment is surgical.

(*h*) **Toxic Amblyopias**—these are conditions in which a type of defective vision called **amblyopia** develops as a result of the action of certain toxic substances on the optic nerve or retina. The drinking of methylated spirits or other drinks containing methyl alcohol is a well known cause of toxic amblyopia. Other forms of this disorder may occur as a result of excessive consumption of ordinary alcoholic drinks (ethyl alcohol) and excessive smoking of pipe tobacco.

(*i*) **Cataract**—a fairly common disorder in which the crystalline lens of the eye, or its capsule, becomes partially or completely opaque. It may be of congenital or acquired type. Maternal rubella (German measles), developing in early pregnancy, is one cause of the congenital variety. The variety of the acquired disorder, called **senile cataract,** is a common disorder of old age. Among the other types of acquired cataract may be mentioned cataract occurring as a complication of diabetes (**diabetic cataract**) and cataract due to excessive exposure to ionizing radiations.

Operative removal of a cataract is called **cataract extraction.**

(*j*) **Optic Atrophy**—this is a degenerative disorder of the optic nerve leading to impairment of vision and sometimes to complete blindness. It may be due to certain diseases which affect the retina or optic disc (e.g. toxic amblyopias, papilloedema); neuritis of the optic nerve (see p. 281), or to involvement of the optic nerve in certain diseases of the central nervous system (e.g. tabes dorsalis, pressure from an intracranial neoplasm, etc.).

3. ERRORS OF REFRACTION

The process of refraction of light rays within the eye has been referred to on p. 284. The term **ametropia** indicates a condition in which the refractive power of the eyeball is defective. The most commonly encountered types of ametropia are:

  (i) **Hypermetropia**—(long sight)—a condition in which the eyeball is too short and entering light rays are brought to a focus behind the retina. It is correctable by spectacles with convex lenses.

  (ii) **Myopia** (short sight)—a condition in which the eyeball is too short and entering light rays are brought to a focus in front of the retina. It may be corrected by spectacles with concave lenses.

  (iii) **Presbyopia** (old sight)—a defect affecting near vision which develops with increasing years. It is due to defective accommodation (see p. 284) resulting from loss of the normal elasticity of the crystalline lens of the eye.

  (iv) **Astigmatism**—a condition in which rays of light coming from a point are imperfectly refracted and do not form a point image on the retina. It is most commonly due to an abnormality of the curvature of the cornea.

4. STRABISMUS (Squint)

An abnormality resulting from incoordination of the orbital muscles which are responsible for the movements of the eyeballs. In this condition the visual axes of the two eyeballs, which are normally parallel, either converge or diverge. In some types of strabismus, there is **diplopia,** i.e. double vision, a condition in which single objects form two visual images. This, however, does not obtain in all types of strabismus as the brain may be able to suppress one of the two images.

Martin-Doyle (2) describes two main forms of strabismus: **paralytic strabismus,** due to paralysis or weakness of one or more of the muscles which move the eyeballs, and **concomitant strabismus** which is due to a functional disorder affecting one or more of these muscles.

Strabismus may occur in association with refractive error.

The main types of treatment employed singly, or in combination, in cases of squint are the correction of refractive errors, orthoptic treatment (see p. 25) and operative treatment.

5. CONJUNCTIVITIS

Inflammation of the conjunctiva may present in acute or chronic form and may result from a variety of causes, among which are bacterial and viral infection, exposure to irritant gases and dusts, eyestrain; foreign body in the eye, allergy (e.g. hay fever).

Clinical features include **lacrimation** (excessive secretion of tears), discomfort in the eye, a mucopurulent or purulent discharge from the eye, and redness of the conjunctiva due to vascular congestion.

A special form of conjunctivitis, which affects the newly-born, is called **ophthalmia neonatorum** and is due to infection of the eyes derived from the tissues of the maternal birth canal. A proportion of cases are due to gonococcal infection. The disease may be prevented by instillation of antibiotic eye drops into the eyes of a new-born infant shortly after delivery.

Trachoma is a specific type of conjunctivitis which is very common in the tropics and subtropics and is due to infection with a virus.

6. DISEASES OF THE ORBIT

These include:—
  (i) **fractures of the bony walls of the orbit;**
  (ii) **orbital cellulitis**—an inflammation of the soft tissues of the orbital cavity, due to infection with pyogenic bacteria and most commonly secondary to infection in the paranasal sinuses;
  (iii) **benign** and **malignant neoplasms growing within the orbit.**

The eyeball may be pushed forward as a result of inflammatory or neoplastic processes within the orbit, a displacement referred to as **exophthalmos** or **proptosis.** Exophthalmos is also an associated feature of the disorder of the thyroid gland called exophthalmic goitre (see p. 212).

Fractures of the orbit may occasionally result in displacement of the eyeball backwards into the cavity of the orbit. This condition is known as **enophthalmos.**

7. DISEASES OF THE EYELIDS

(*a*) **Traumatic conditions**—these may take the form of bruising and haematoma formation (black eye), wounds or burns.

Wounds and burns may result in the formation of scar tissue within the eyelids and various resultant deformities of these structures (see later).

(*b*) **Blepharitis**—inflammation of the eyelids. This condition is usually of infective origin and may occur as an acute or chronic disorder.

289

10

(*c*) **Stye** (Hordeolum)—a condition due to pyogenic infection of sebaceous glands associated with the roots of the eyelashes.

(*d*) **Meibomian Cyst** (Tarsal cyst)—a swelling in the eyelid arising from one of the tarsal glands. These latter are sebaceous glands lying between the conjunctival lining of the eyelids and the tarsal plates, which are plates of dense connective tissue within the eyelids.

(*e*) **Neoplasms**—both benign and malignant neoplasms occur within the eyelids, the most common of the former being **papillomas,** and of the latter type, **rodent ulcers.**

(*f*) **Deformities of the Eyelids**—these may be congenital or due to traumatic inflammatory or neoplastic disease, or spasm or paralysis of the muscles which move the eyelids. Some terms used in the description of these deformities are:—(i) **Coloboma**—a congenital defect in the margin of an eyelid, (ii) **Entropion**—a turning inwards of an eyelid, (iii) **Ectropion**—a turning out of an eyelid, (iv) **Ptosis**—drooping of the upper eyelid, (v) **Symblepharon**—adhesion of an eyelid to the eyeball.

8. DISEASES OF THE LACRIMAL APPARATUS

These may affect the lacrimal glands or the lacrimal passages. The former group are rare. Inflammation of the lacrimal glands is termed **dacryoadenitis** and acute dacryoadenitis may occasionally occur as a complication of mumps.

Diminished secretion of the lacrimal glands, together with diminished secretion of the salivary glands is found in a disorder called **Sjogren's syndrome,** which occurs predominantly in middle-aged women and is frequently accompanied by chronic arthritis.

Rarely the lacrimal glands may be enlarged as a result of tumour formation, and enlargement of the lacrimal and parotid glands occurs in **Mikulicz's syndrome,** a rare condition which may develop as a result of sarcoidosis and certain other generalized diseases.

The lacrimal passages may be obstructed as a result of congenital malformations or traumatic or inflammatory disorders, resulting in **epiphora,** a condition in which the tears are unable to drain away normally and thus flow out of the conjunctival sac and down the cheek. One cause of this condition is **dacryocystitis,** i.e. inflammation of the lacrimal sac. Acute inflammatory changes in this latter structure may progress to the formation of an abscess in the sac termed a **lacrimal abscess.**

Obstruction of the lacrimal passages which is not relieved by simpler measures, may necessitate **dacryorhinostomy,** an operation in which a permanent communication is made between the lacrimal sac and the nasal cavity.

9. SOME OPHTHALMIC OPERATIONS

Brief reference has already been made to the operations of **cataract extraction** and **dacryorhinostomy** and it has been indicated that operative measures may be employed in the treatment of glaucoma and strabismus.

Three terms referring to surgical procedures not included in the foregoing account are:—(i) **iridectomy**—removal of a portion of the iris, (ii) **corneal grafting** (corneal transplantation—keratoplasty), an operation in which a portion of the cornea is excised from a patient's eye and replaced by a portion of cornea of similar size taken from a donor eye, (iii) **enucleation of the eyeball**—removal of the eyeball from its socket.

REFERENCES

(1) and (2) Martin-Doyle, J. L. C. *A Synopsis of Ophthalmology* (John Wright & Sons Ltd.). 1967.

Section P.—THE EAR

1. SOME GENERAL CONSIDERATIONS

The ear is the organ of hearing and of balance. It consists of three parts:
  (i) **the external ear,** comprising the *pinna* (auricle) and *external auditory meatus.*
  (ii) **the middle ear** (tympanic cavity, tympanum), is separated from the external ear by the *tympanic membrane* (*eardrum*) and contains the three *auditory ossicles,* the *malleus, incus* and *stapes.*

  The middle ear contains air at atmospheric pressure as its cavity communicates with the nasopharynx via the *Eustachian tube.* This cavity also communicates with the *mastoid air cells.*

  During part of its course the *seventh cranial nerve (facial* nerve) lies in bony canal called the *facial canal,* which runs through the medial and posterior walls of the middle ear. The *chorda tympani* (nerve of taste) joins the motor portion of the facial nerve in the facial canal.

(iii) **the inner ear** (labyrinth) comprises a number of cavities in the petrous portion of the temporal bone, i.e. the *cochlea, vestibule* and *semicircular canals,* which constitute the bony labyrinth, and a number of membranous structures contained within these cavities, i.e. the *duct of the cochlea* (containing the *organ of Corti*), the *utricle* and *saccule,* and the *membranous ducts* of the *semicircular canals.*

A fluid called *endolymph* circulates within the membranous labyrinth and another fluid called *perilymph* circulates in the space between this structure and the surrounding walls of the bony labyrinth.

The inner ear is separated from the middle ear by a bony partition in which lie two openings, the *oval window* (*fenestra vestibuli*) into which fits the foot-plate of the stapes, and the *round window* (*fenestra cochleae*) which is closed by a fibrous membrane.

The *cochlear division* of the *eighth cranial nerve* (*acoustic nerve, auditory nerve*) transmits impulses concerned with hearing to the brain from the hair cells in the organ of Corti. Impulses concerned with balance also pass to the brain, from end-organs in the membranous ducts of the semicircular canals, and in the utricle and saccule, being transmitted by the *vestibular division* of this nerve.

The inner part of the external auditory canal, the middle ear, the inner ear, and the mastoid air cells are all contained within the temporal bone.

The eighth cranial nerve leaves the petrous portion of the temporal bone through a bony canal called the *internal auditory meatus.* Before entering the facial canal, the seventh cranial (facial nerve) also traverses the internal auditory meatus.

The branch of medicine concerned with diseases of the ear is called **otology,** a name of Greek derivation. The adjectives **otic** and **aural** are both used with reference to the ear, the latter word being of Latin derivation. The surgery of the ear is sometimes called **aural surgery.** The adjective **auditory** may be used to refer to the ear or to the sense of hearing, and the adjective **acoustic** to indicate the sense of hearing.

Pathological conditions which affect the organs of hearing may be congenital, traumatic, infective, neoplastic or due to high intensity noises. Among their clinical features may be mentioned the following: **deafness** (impairment or loss of the sense of hearing), **otorrhoea** (discharge from the ear), **otalgia** (pain in the ear), **tinnitus** ("ringing" in the ears), **vertigo** (giddiness).

Methods of investigation employed in the investigation of disorders encountered in otology include: (i) visual examination of the external ear and tympanic membrane with an instrument, equipped with a magnifying lens and an illuminating device, called an **auriscope** or **otoscope,** (ii) examination by means of an operating microscope, (iii) bacteriological examination of discharges from the ear, (iv) radiological investigation of the ear by plain films and tomography, (v) **hearing tests.** These comprise testing the patient's ability to hear whispered and normal speech at different distances, ability to hear the sound produced by a tuning fork, and investigation of hearing by a method termed **audiometry.** This is carried out with an instrument called an **audiometer** which enables a record, called an **audiogram,** to be made.

Some of the disorders of the organs of hearing will now be discussed.

2. DISEASES OF THE EXTERNAL EAR

(*a*) **Congenital disorders**—these include various malformations of the pinna and complete or partial failure of development of the external auditory meatus.

(*b*) **Cauliflower Ear**—a condition of enlargement and deformity of the pinna due to trauma which causes the formation of a haematoma within this structure.

(*c*) **Otitis externa**—a term used to indicate inflammatory changes in the external auditory meatus, arising usually as a result of infection of the skin of this structure. The infection may be primary or occur secondary to otitis media complicated by perforation of the eardrum. One form of external otitis is the so-called **meatal furuncle** (boil) which is due to staphylococcal infection of a hair follicle in the meatus.

Otitis externa is often a painful disorder and causes a discharge from the ear.

(*d*) **Neoplasms**—these include **osteoma** arising from the bony wall of the external auditory meatus; **epithelioma** (squamous cell carcinoma) arising from the skin of the pinna or external meatus, or from the mucous membrane lining the middle ear; and **rodent ulcer** (basal cell carcinoma) of the skin of the pinna.

(*e*) **Impacted wax in the Meatus**—this condition results from excessive accumulation of wax produced by the ceruminous (waxproducing) glands in the outer cartilaginous part of the meatus. It may cause conduction deafness (see later) which can be relieved by softening of the wax by ear drops and subsequent syringing.

3. DISEASES OF THE TYMPANIC MEMBRANE

(*a*) **Myringitis,** i.e. inflammation of the tympanic membrane (eardrum) occurs most commonly in association with otitis media (inflammation of the middle ear) and may result in spontaneous perforation of the membrane. Spontaneous perforation may be avoided by **myringotomy,** an operation involving the making of a small incision through the tympanic membrane to permit escape of infective discharges from the middle ear.

Myringitis may also develop as a complication of otitis externa.

(*b*) **Traumatic Rupture of the Tympanic Membrane**—Robinson (1) gives the following examples of the causes of this condition: direct trauma, blast and fractured skull.

4. DISEASES OF THE MIDDLE EAR

(*a*) **Otitis media**—this term means "inflammation of the middle ear". Such inflammation is in most instances due to pathogens (e.g. streptococci, staphylococci) which reach the middle ear via the Eustachian tube and derive from some infective process in the upper respiratory tract. Otitis media may thus develop as a complication of conditions such as coryza, tonsillitis, sinusitis, enlarged adenoids, and from secondary bacterial infections of the upper respiratory tract developing in virus diseases such as measles and influenza, etc. A much less common route of infection is from the external auditory meatus via a traumatic perforation in the tympanic membrane.

Otitis media may be of acute, subacute or chronic type. It is a common disease especially in children and is often bilateral.

Acute suppurative otitis media is a serious condition in which pus forms within the middle ear and, if not controlled by treatment, or if untreated, may result in complications such as the following:

  (i) **perforation of the tympanic membrane** and resultant otorrhoea.
  (ii) spread of infection to the mastoid antrum and mastoid air cells causing **mastoiditis.**
  (iii) rarely, spread of infection to the inner ear causing **labyrinthitis.**
  (iv) spread of infection to air cells which are sometimes present in the petrous bone, causing **petrositis.**
  (v) thrombosis in neighbouring veins which may spread so as to

reach the lateral (sigmoid) sinus of the dura mater causing **lateral sinus thrombosis.**

(vi) spread of infection through the temporal bone causing **extra dural abscess, meningitis,** or **cerebral abscess.**

(vii) formation of adhesions between the auditory ossicles and resultant permanent **defect of hearing.**

(viii) **chronic otitis media** (see below).

Severe pain in the ear together with general signs of infection and deafness are common features of acute otitis media. If the tympanic membrane ruptures or myringotomy is performed there is also a purulent discharge from the external meatus. When mastoiditis complicates the disease there is also pain in the mastoid process and tenderness of this structure. Swelling of soft tissues over the mastoid process, or in front of the pinna, may also develop.

Treatment is by administration of systemic penicillin and analgesic drugs. Myringotomy may also be indicated. When acute mastoiditis complicates the disease it may be necessary to drain the pus from the mastoid process by an operation termed **cortical mastoidectomy** (conservative mastoidectomy).

Chronic suppurative otitis media may develop as a sequel to acute suppurative otitis media, or may be the result of an infective process which is of chronic nature from the outset. It is frequently associated with chronic mastoid infection and also with chronic sinusitis and enlarged adenoids. In this type of infection there is a permanent perforation of the eardrum and destructive changes occur which affect the bony walls of the middle ear, and often involve the mastoid process also. In addition there may be considerable destruction of the auditory ossicles resulting in permanent impairment of hearing.

The chief clinical features are otorrhea and deafness.

The complications of chronic otitis media include (i) overgrowth of granulation tissue (see p. 38) within the middle ear leading to the formation of a polypoid swelling, called an **aural polyp,** which may protrude through the perforation in the eardrum; (ii) formation of a **cholesteatoma,** a tumour-like mass of dead epithelial cells, bacteria and cholesterol crystals which develops in the middle ear as a result of the inflammatory process, and may extend into the mastoid process; (iii) involvement of the facial nerve and resultant **facial paralysis** as a result of involvement of the walls of the facial canal (see p. 292) in the infective process; (iv) **labyrinthitis;** (v) **intracranial spread.**

Surgical treatment, designed to eradicate the infection in the middle ear and mastoid, by the operations of **modified radical mastoidectomy** or **radical mastoidectomy** may be necessary in chronic otitis media. In suitable cases, the perforation in the tympanic membrane associated with the disease, may subsequently be repaired by a plastic operation called **tympanoplasty** (myringoplasty).

(*b*) **Neoplasms**—these are uncommon. They include **carcinoma of** the **middle ear** and a very rare neoplasm called a **glomus tumour** (*Note:* glomus tumours may arise at a number of sites in the body in minute structures which are called **chemoreceptors** and are sensitive to certain types of chemical change in the circulating blood).

(*c*) **Otosclerosis**—a disease of unknown causation in which the formation of new bone occurs within the bony labyrinth and involves the oval window, first limiting and then preventing movement of the stapes (the innermost of the auditory ossicles). Loss of mobility of the stapes interferes with the normal conduction of sound waves through the middle ear and thus causes progressive deafness of a type called conduction deafness (see later).

Otosclerosis tends to run in families. If affects both ears, is commoner in females than in males, and its onset is usually in adolescence or early adult life.

Surgical treatment, in the form of an operation called **stapedectomy**, may be employed for relief of the deafness. This operation involves removal of the stapes bone and implantation of a Teflon piston in its place.

5. DISEASES OF THE INNER EAR

(*a*) **Labyrinthitis**—as has been noted the inner ear is also known as the labyrinth and the term "labyrinhitis" thus indicates inflammation of the inner ear. This condition occurs most commonly as a result of spread of an acute or chronic infection from the middle ear but may be due to other causes (e.g. sensitivity to the drug streptomycin; virus infection limited to the labyrinth alone). Labyrinthitis causes impairment of hearing, vertigo and other disorders of balance. Another feature of this condition may be the presence of abnormal eye movements termed **nystagmus.**

(*b*) **Ménières Disease**—a disease affecting the labyrinth of one or sometimes both sides and characterised by violent attacks of sudden vertigo (giddiness), tinnitus (ringing in the ears) and also progressive loss of hearing. It is caused by an increase of tension of the fluid circulating in the semicircular canal, resulting from spasm or other changes in the blood vessels of the labyrinth. Treatment is in the first instance medical, but if this fails surgical or ultrasonic methods may be employed to destroy the labyrinth.

6. DISEASES OF THE AUDITORY NERVE

(*a*) **Traumatic**—the eighth cranial (auditory, acoustic) nerve may be damaged by fractures of the skull involving the petrous portion of the temporal bone. There may be concomitant injury to the facial nerve.

(*b*) **Infective**—various forms of meningeal infection and certain virus infections may involve the auditory nerve.

(*c*) **Neoplastic**—acoustic neurofibroma—see p. 274.

7. TYPES OF DEAFNESS

Reading (2) describes conduction deafness, perceptive deafness and central deafness.

Deafness is a condition of impairment or loss of the sense of hearing.

The normal mechanism of hearing comprises the passage of atmospheric vibrations, called sound waves, along the external auditory meatus and their transmission through the tympanic membrane and the auditory ossicles of the middle ear to the oval window. Here they set up pressure waves in the perilymph (see p. 292). These latter are transmitted to the endolymph through the membranous walls of the duct of the cochlea, where they produce stimuli which are received by the nervous end organs in the organ of Corti. These stimuli are then transmitted to the brain, by nerve fibres in the cochlear division of the acoustic (auditory) nerve, where they produce sensations of hearing.

Interference with the transmission of sound waves by the tympanic membrane or the ossicles causes **conduction deafness,** also termed **middle ear deafness.** Interference with reception of stimuli by the organ of Corti, as a result of diseases of the labyrinth which affect the cochlea, or as a result of lesions of nerve fibres which transmit hearing impulses along the acoustic nerve, cause **perceptive deafness,** also referred to as **nerve deafness** or **inner ear deafness.**

Examples of conditions which cause conduction deafness are impacted wax in the ear, otitis media, traumatic rupture of the ear drum, and otosclerosis. Among the diseases causing perceptive deafness are various forms of labyrinthitis; fractures of the petrous portion of the temporal bone causing damage to the labyrinth or acoustic nerve; acoustic neurofibroma.

Central deafness is caused by damage to the tissues of the auditory higher centres, within the temporal lobes of the brain.

The treatment of deafness is directed, where possible, to the treatment of its cause by conservative or surgical measures. The disability resulting from deafness that cannot be adequately relieved by such measures, may be alleviated by the learning of **lip reading** or the use of **hearing aids.**

REFERENCES

(1) Robinson, J. O. *Surgery* (Longmans). 1965.
(2) Reading, P. *Common Diseases of the Ear, Nose and Throat* (J. and A. Churchill). 1966.

Section Q.—THE MIND

The Greek word "psyche" means the "soul" or "mind" and the science concerned with the study of the mind and mental processes is called **psychology.**

The branch of medicine concerned with disorders of mental process is termed **psychiatry,** or **psychological medicine.**

A detailed description of terms used in psychiatry is beyond the scope of this book but it may be noted that among the important types of mental disorder encountered in psychiatric practice are:

(*a*) **Subnormality**—a condition in which development of the mind is incomplete and intelligence is below normal. In accordance with definitions given in the Mental Health Act 1959, patients with this condition are graded as being either "subnormal" or "severely subnormal".

Subnormality may result from hereditary factors, or disease or injury affecting the developing brain during foetal life or childhood.

(*b*) **Psychoneuroses** (neuroses)—these are disorders of mental function which affect large numbers of the population. Whilst they do not produce any complete breakdown of mental processes and affected patients often possess considerable insight into their own psychological problems, they may produce serious effects, both mental and physical, and adverse effects on work efficiency.

Some examples of disorders classified as psychoneuroses are: **anxiety states, obsessive-compulsive neuroses, hysteria** and **behaviour disorders of childhood.**

(*c*) **Psychoses**—severe disorders of mental function in which the patient's insight into his own psychological problems may be impaired or lost. They produce a marked breakdown of mental processes, which in some of these conditions is of a temporary nature but in others is permanent.

Psychoses are often accompanied by hallucinations, delusions and impulsive behaviour.

Important types of psychoses are:

(i) **Schizophrenia**—a major problem in psychiatric practice.

(ii) **Affective disorders**—**mania** and **depression.**

(iii) **Melancholia of Involutional Type.**

(iv) **Organic Psychoses**—i.e. wherein the mental disorder develops secondarily to some organic disorder of the brain (e.g. traumatic, infective, neoplastic, toxic effects arising from chronic alcoholism).

(v) **Psychoses of the elderly,** e.g. **senile dementia, senile confusional states, senile mania, senile melancholia.**

(*d*) **Aberrations of Sexual Behaviour,** e.g. **homosexuality** and **sexual perversion.**

(*e*) **Disorders resulting from defective development of personality,** e.g. **psychopathic personality,** a disorder in which immaturity of personality prevents the patient from adapting himself to normal social relationships. Common features of this condition include irresponsible and often aggressive behaviour, a lack of moral principles and an inability to form lasting friendships.

(*f*) **Addiction to alcohol or drugs** e.g. morphine, cocaine, heroin, amphetamines, barbiturates, cannabis (marihuana), lysergic acid diethylamide (L.S.D.25).

(*g*) **Psychosomatic disorders,** i.e. disorders in which there is thought to be a significant association between mental factors and structural changes in organs and tissues, other than those of the nervous system. Authorities who accept the concept of psychosomatic disorders differ as to the diseases which should be so regarded. Among the conditions described by many writers as being of this nature are eczema, neurodermatitis, bronchial asthma, primary thyrotoxicosis, peptic ulceration, and ulcerative colitis.

A brief reference to some forms of treatment employed in psychiatric illnesses was made on p. 24.

PART V

Medical Terms Referring to Certain Other Types of Disease

Section A.—CONNECTIVE TISSUE DISEASES

THIS term is used to describe a group of diseases, known formerly as **collagen diseases,** which are characterised by widespread lesions in connective tissues.

They are described by Thomson and Cotton (1) as "predominantly, but not exclusively, showing changes in collagen."

Under the heading of **connective tissue diseases,** these authors include **rheumatoid arthritis** and **rheumatic fever** and the following uncommon disorders: **disseminated lupus erythematosus** (D.L.E.), **polyarteritis nodosa, dermatomyositis** and **scleroderma** (progressive systemic sclerosis.)

(*Note:* **Collagen** is a protein substance which is an important constituent of all types of connective tissue.)

REFERENCE
(1) Thomson, A. D. and Cotton, R. E. *Lecture Notes on Pathology* (Blackwell Scientific Publications). 1968.

Section B.—TROPICAL DISEASES

Certain diseases, which normally occur only in the tropics or sub-tropics, or whilst occurring also in temperate and cold climates, show their greatest incidence in regions with warm climates, are classified as **tropical diseases.**

The majority of tropical diseases are of the nature of infections or infestations. Nutritional disorders, although frequently showing a high incidence among the inhabitants of many of the developing countries in the tropics and subtropics, are not generally classified under the heading of tropical diseases.

The condition of **tropical sprue,** has already been referred to when discussing terms describing various forms of malabsorption syndromes.

Some reference has been made when describing various diseases of the blood, to **sickle-cell anaemia** and **thalassaemia** (Cooley's anaemia or Mediterranean anaemia) two forms of haemolytic anaemia whose maximum incidence occurs amongst the natives of certain countries with warm climates.

Discussion in this section will be limited to terms indicating certain important infections and infestations which occur predominantly in the tropics and subtropics.

INFECTIONS

These may be due to bacteria, viruses, fungi, or protozoa.

(*a*) **Dysentery**—this term indicates a condition of disordered bowel action. The predominant feature of conditions described as dysentery is an infective colitis (inflammation of the large bowel) resulting in diarrhoea, often accompanied by the passage of blood and mucus in the stools. The causal organisms of dysentery are excreted in the faeces of infected individuals and transmitted to other individuals by contaminated food and water.

Bacillary dysentery as indicated by its name, is due to infection with bacteria of the type called *bacilli.* According to the nature of the causal bacilli it may take the form of **Shiga, Flexner** or **Sonne-dysentery.** The disease commences as an acute colitis and may occasionally result in chronic infection of the colon. Complications are rare but include a form of arthritis termed **colitic arthritis.** Bacillary dysentery is of world-wide distribution but has a considerably higher incidence in warm climates than in temperate climates.

Amoebic dysentery (Intestinal amoebiasis)—can be contracted outside the tropics but is predominantly a tropical disease. It is due to infection with a protozoon called *entamoeba histolytica.* It can cause an acute colitis which subsequently becomes chronic in nature but, more commonly, causes colonic inflammation which is chronic in nature from its onset. Chronic amoebic colitis may be complicated by spread of infection to the liver, causing **amoebic hepatitis** (hepatic amoebiasis) or **amoebic liver abscess,** and less commonly to the lungs resulting in **pulmonary amoebiasis.**

(*b*) **Malaria**—this is the commonest of all tropical infections. It is caused by a protozoon called the *malaria parasite,* which undergoes part of its life cycle in a species of mosquito called an *anopheles.* A human subject becomes infected with malaria as a result of malaria parasites gaining access to his bloodstream through the bite of an infected female anopheline mosquito. Within the human body the life cycle of the parasites is continued, firstly within the liver and then within red blood cells in the circulating blood. The red blood cells, which contain the parasites, rupture at a certain stage of development of the parasites and these latter are then set free within the bloodstream. The characteristic attacks of malarial fever develop at the times of such release of malaria parasites into the bloodstream. The coincident destruction of red cells may result in the development of anaemia of the haemolytic type.

There are four different types of malaria parasite, the two most commonly encountered being *Plasmodium vivax* and *Plasmodium falciparum*. The former causes a clinical form of disease called **benign tertian malaria,** in which bouts of fever occur every third day.

Plasmodium falciparum also tends to produce attacks of fever with a three-day periodicity but the infection is more severe and is known as **malignant tertian malaria.** This latter condition may be complicated by brain involvement causing **cerebral malaria**; or by extensive destruction of red cells within the circulation causing a disorder termed **blackwater fever,** in which haemoglobin is set free in the blood plasma (haemoglobinaemia) and is consequently passed in the urine (haemoglobinuria).

Splenomegaly (enlargement of the spleen) is of frequent development in patients with chronic or recurrent malarial infections.

Benign tertian malaria is subject to recurrences of infection which may persist for up to about two years after the infected individual has left a malarious area.

The clinical diagnosis of malaria is confirmed by demonstration of the causal parasites in a blood smear.

Quinine has been used for many centuries in the treatment of malaria but, in recent times, modern synthetic drugs such as chloroquine and primaquine have been extensively used in its therapy. Chloroquine, and other drugs, may also be used by those living in malarious areas in order to suppress the clinical features of malarial infection in the so-called **suppressant therapy of malaria.**

The incidence of infection in malarious areas may be greatly controlled by precautions taken by individuals to avoid mosquito bites and measures designed to destroy anopheline mosquitoes and prevent their breeding.

(*c*) **Cholera**—is a bacterial infection of the intestine, due to a pathogen called the *vibrio cholerae* or *comma bacillus,* which causes inflammatory changes in the small intestine, together with less severe inflammatory changes in the large bowel. These result in severe diarrhoea with typical "rice-water" stools, vomiting and dehydration.

This disease occurs most commonly in the Far East, where it appears from time to time in epidemic form, sometimes with a high mortality rate. It is spread by food and water contaminated by the excreta of sufferers from the disease. There is no specific treatment but protection against the disease may be given by prophylactic vaccination.

(*d*) **Plague**—is a bacterial infection which is endemic in some tropical and subtropical countries and sometimes appears in epidemic form. The causal pathogen is called *Pasteurella pestis*; the name *"Pasteurella"* deriving from that of the nineteenth century French bacteriologist, Louis Pasteur.

There are three clinical types of plague called **bubonic, pneumonic** and **septicaemic plague,** the first named being the most common. Infection is derived from infected rats and other rodents and transmitted to man by the bite of rat fleas.

Bubonic plague is so-called from the fact that the regional lymph glands draining the area of the flea bite form enlarged tender swellings called **buboes.**

Plague in former times was not confined in its occurrence to countries with warm climates, and in mediaeval times was referred to as the **"Black Death".**

The incidence of plague may be diminished by measures to destroy rats and fleas and by protective vaccination of subjects living in infected localities.

(*e*) **Brucellosis**—this term describes certain febrile illnesses caused by bacteria which are called *Brucella,* after Sir David Bruce, who was an English surgeon. The two main types of brucellosis are:

- (i) **Undulant Fever** (Abortus Fever)—an infective condition of world-wide distribution, which may be contracted by contact with infected cattle or drinking infected cow's milk.
- (ii) **Malta Fever** (Mediterranean Fever)—an infection caused by drinking infected goat's milk.

(*f*) **Leprosy**—this chronic bacterial infection only develops as a result of prolonged contact with other individuals who are suffering from the disease. The lesions of leprosy develop in the nerves, skin, subcutaneous tissues and mucous membranes and sometimes also affect the skeleton.

There are two principal clinical types of the disorder known as **nodular (lepromatous) leprosy** and **maculo-anaesthetic leprosy.**

(*g*) **Yaws**—this is a condition which develops in stages and shows certain clinical similarities to syphilis. It also gives rise to positive Wasserman and Kahn reactions in the blood but is not of venereal origin. The causal organism is a spirochaete called *Treponema pertenue.*

(*h*) **Tropical Ulcer**—a type of sloughing ulceration of the skin, which occurs in hot countries and appears to be associated with malnutrition and general ill-health. Middlemiss (1) states such ulceration occurs almost exclusively below the knee and describes various radiological changes seen in cases in which bone involvement complicates the ulceration.

(*i*) **Some Other Tropical Infections**—some of these and their mode of transmission are as follows:

(i) **Bacterial**—**Typhoid Fever** (see p. 49), **Relapsing Fever** (Man to man by ticks or lice).

(ii) **Rickettsiae**—**Typhus Fever** (see p. 57).

(iii) **Viral**—**Dengue** (Man to man by *Aedes* mosquitoes), **Sandfly Fever** (Man to man by sandflies), **Yellow Fever** (man to man by *Aedes* mosquitoes).

(iv) **Protozoal**—**Cutaneous Leishmaniasis** or **Oriental Sore** (man to man by sandflies); **Visceral Leishmaniasis** or **Kala Azar** (man to man by sandflies); **African Trypanosomiasis** or **Sleeping Sickness** (from man to man, or from cattle or antelopes to man, by *tsetse* flies); **South American Trypanosomiasis** or **Chagas' Disease** (from man to man, or certain animals to man, by winged bugs).

INFESTATIONS

These disorders are due to the presence in the body of organisms called *helminths* or *worms* which are *parasitic* in nature, i.e. they live in or on the tissues of another organism, referred to as a **host,** from which they draw their nutriment. Some worms require only one host for the completion of their life cycle; others undergo the earlier stages of their development in a so-called **intermediate host,** and the adult stages in a second host known as a **definitive host.**

There are three main types of helminths:—*nematodes,* e.g. *round-worms, cestodes* or *tapeworms*; and *trematodes* or *flukes.* Some nematodes have only a single host but tapeworms and flukes require both an intermediate and a definitive host.

Infestations with parasitic helminths occur with much greater frequency in the tropics and sub-tropics than in temperate regions. A minority of them, however, are confined to countries with warm climates.

Some important disorders due to such infestations are as follows:

(*a*) **Ascariasis**—a common infestation, of wide distribution and due to a round worm called *ascaris lumbricoides*. This worm, which may be as much as ten inches long, goes through its life cycle within a human host and its ova are excreted in the faeces. The infestation is spread to other humans by food or water contaminated with ascaris ova.

During their development within the body, the parasites pass through the lungs where they may cause inflammatory changes. The adult worms live in the small bowel of the host where they may be demonstrated by a barium meal follow-through examination.

(*b*) **Oxyuriasis**—(Threadworm infestation)—a condition due to nematodes called *threadworms* which live in the intestine of the human host. Threadworm infestation is of world-wide distribution and particularly common in children. It frequently leads to pruritus (itching) and inflammatory changes in the region of the anus and vulva. The ova are excreted in the faeces.

(*c*) **Ankylostomiasis** (Hookworm infestation)—an infestation due to a nematode called the *hookworm* or *ankylostoma duodenale,* which has a very high incidence in many tropical countries. The adult worms live in the intestine causing inflammatory changes and bleeding from the intestinal wall. This bleeding frequently results in severe anaemia. The ova of the parasites are excreted in the faeces and, when they are deposited in warm soil, develop into embryos which can invade the body of another human host by penetrating his skin. They then reach his intestine via the venous circulation, lungs, oesophagus and stomach.

(*d*) **Other Nematode Infestations**—these include **trichiniasis** (Muscle worm infestation) in which the pig is the intermediate host and man, the definitive host; **dracontiasis** (Guinea-worm infestation) in which a small fresh water organism of the crustacean variety is the intermediate host and man the definitive host; and **filariasis** in which the parasites are transmitted from man to man by mosquito bites. The commonest form of filariasis is due to a parasitic worm called *Wuchereria bancrofti,* and is associated with blockage of lymphatic channels in affected tissues, leading to **elephantiasis,** a condition of marked thickening of the skin and subcutaneous tissues.

The diseases called **loa-loa** and **onchocerciasis** are other varieties of filariasis.

(*e*) **Tape worm infestations**—the principal of these in man are infestations with the pork tape worm, *Taenia solium,* and the beef tape worm, *Taenia saginata*; and the disorder called hydatid disease.

Cattle are the intermediate hosts in beef tapeworm infestation.

In human infestation with the pork tapeworm the pig is usually the intermediate host and man the definitive host. Occasionally, however, a human subject may become the intermediate host of this parasite by ingesting its ova and develop a disorder called **cysticercosis;** characterized by the development of epilepsy and the presence of calcification within the bodies of parasitic embryos which, have settled and subsequently died in the tissues of the skeletal muscles.

Hydatid disease (Echinococcus disease) is due to the *Taenia echinococcus.* This tapeworm is a parasite of dogs. If its ova are ingested by a human being, embryos which develop from them may enter the circulation, and reaching sites such as the liver, lungs and bones, may then produce **hydatid cysts.** Sufferers from hydatid disease, in the majority of instances give positive reactions to a blood test called a **complement fixation test** and a skin test called the **Casoni test.**

(*f*) **Schistosomiasis** (Bilharziasis)—this is the name given to a group of diseases caused by members of a species of fluke called *schistosoma.* The intermediate host is a fresh-water snail and man, the definitive host, contracts the disorder from contact with water contaminated with immature forms of the parasite called **cercariae.** These enter the human body by penetrating the skin or the mucous membrane of the mouth. The adult worms live in the portal venous system but, according to the type of infestation, the females deposit their eggs in the walls of the host's urinary bladder, causing inflammation and haematuria; or in the wall of the bowel, causing inflammation and bleeding from the rectum. Chronic infestations may lead eventually to the development of carcinoma of the bladder or rectum.

(*g*) **Other Infestations with Flukes**—these include infestations with *liver flukes (fasciola hepatica* and *clonorchis sinensis,* the Chinese liver fluke), and **paragonimiasis** due to *lung flukes.*

REFERENCE

(1) Middlemiss, H. *Tropical Radiology* (William Heinemann Medical Books Ltd.). 1961.

Section C.—NUTRITIONAL DISORDERS

Nutritional disorders may be due to (i) Inadequate food consumption resulting in various degrees of **starvation,** (ii) Excessive food consumption resulting in pathological degrees of **obesity,** a condition in which there is excessive deposition of fat within the body, (iii) deficiency of essential food constituents, or defective absorption or utilization of these essential food constituents by the body. This latter group of disorders are often referred to as **deficiency diseases** and include conditions resulting from deficiencies of protein, minerals, and vitamins.

The condition called **Kwashiorkor,** is an important disorder due primarily to protein deficiency, and Davidson (1) states that "with the possible exception of iron deficiency anaemia and deficiency of calories it is the most important dietary deficiency disease in the world". The chief incidence of the disease is seen in young children and it is principally encountered in under-developed communities living in the tropics and sub-tropics. Common clinical features include wasting, oedema, diarrhoea and skin changes.

An important group of clinical disorders result from deficiency of certain essential accessory food factors known as **vitamins.** Examples of these are as follows:

Type of Vitamin Deficiency	*Principal Clinical Disorders*
(a) Vitamin A (fat soluble).	Night blindness. Xerophalmia (an eye disease).
(b) Vitamin B Complex (water soluble). (i) Vitamin B.1. (Thiamine, Aneurine).	Dry beri-beri. (Chief feature— polyneuritis). Wet beri-beri. (Chief features— heart disease with oedema).
(ii) Vitamin B.2. (Riboflavine).	Vascularisation of the cornea. Angular stomatitis.
(iii) Nicotinic Acid.	Pellagra.
(iv) Vitamin B.12 (Cyanacobalmin).	Pernicious Anaemia (see p. 202). Sub-acute combined degeneration of the Cord (see p. 280).
(vi) Folic Acid.	Tropical Sprue (see p. 130).
(c) Vitamin C (water soluble).	Scurvy (see p. 217).

(*d*) Vitamin D (fat soluble).   Rickets (see p. 247).
Dietetic Osteomalacia (see p. 247).

(*e*) Vitamin K (fat soluble).   Hypoprothrombinaemia (resulting in diminished coaguability of the blood).

(*Note:* It is important to note several types of vitamin deficiency may occur together in the same patient.)

REFERENCE

(1) Davidson, Sir Stanley. *The Principles and Practice of Medicine.* (E. and S. Livingstone). 1966.

Section D.—POISONINGS

The term **poisoning** describes a condition in which tissue damage, sometimes resulting in a fatal outcome, is caused by the entry into the body of a variety of harmful solid, liquid or gaseous substances termed **poisons.** Poisoning may be accidental or the result of attempted suicide or homicide.

The commonest type of poisoning is **food poisoning** which is due to the ingestion of food contaminated by certain types of infective bacteria and is evidenced by symptoms of gastritis or gastro-enteritis.

Some other well known forms of poisoning include those due to **carbon monoxide** (coal gas); drugs such as **barbiturates, aspirin** and **opium; arsenical** and **lead poisoning; corrosive poisoning** (e.g. due to lysol and phenol); **snake-bite poisoning, alcoholic poisoning; strychnine poisoning; hydrocyanic acid (prussic acid) poisoning.**

The branch of science concerned with the study of poisons is called **toxicology.**

Section E.—DISORDERS DUE TO PHYSICAL AGENTS

These disorders include:

(*a*) **Disorders due to Heat,** e.g. **heat stroke**—a condition in which hyperpyrexia develops as a result of failure of the normal mechanisms of body temperature control; and **heat exhaustion**—a condition of severe weakness, leading sometimes to circulatory collapse, and in many instances associated with salt (sodium chloride) deficiency in the blood plasma.

(*b*) **Disorders due to Cold,** e.g. **frostbite**—a condition due to exposure of the extremities to severe cold with resultant diminution of blood supply and development of gangrene in severe cases; and **hypothermia** a condition of general lowering of body temperature which may occur when heat loss by the body exceeds heat production. (*Note:* the use of artificial hypothermia with general anaesthesia was noted when discussing surgical operations on the heart in Part IV.)

(*c*) **Disorders due to Abnormal Atmospheric Pressures,** e.g. **altitude sickness** experienced at high altitudes as a result of oxygen deficiency; and **caisson disease,** a disorder which occurs in those who work under high atmospheric pressure (e.g. divers) when subjected to too rapid decompression, during the return to normal atmospheric conditions.

Section F.—RADIATION HAZARDS AND RADIATION INJURY

As is widely known, radiations of the type known as ionizing radiations (see p. 311) can, in high doses, cause damage to the tissues of the body. Such radiations in lower doses can cause changes in transmissible hereditary material contained in **genes** (units of hereditary material).

Two different types of hazard are thus associated with the use of "man-made" ionizing radiations in medicine, industry or warfare:—the risk of causing **somatic damage,** i.e. damage to the tissues of an irradiated individual; and the rish of causing **genetic damage,** i.e. damage to hereditary material contained within the genes of an irradiated individual.

(*a*) **Somatic damage**—*serious somatic damage is only produced by high amounts of radiation* but may develop as a result of the tissues receiving such amounts in a short period of time, or the cumulative effect of numerous small doses of radiation, producing a high total dosage over a lengthy period (e.g. after many years).

When tissue damage occurs it varies greatly in severity according to the amount and penetrating power of the causal radiation, and the extent and site of the irradiated area. Thus radiation injuries vary from slight reactions, which affect only a localized area of skin, to the extensive tissue damage that results from high doses of whole-body radiation.

Whilst any tissue in the body may be injured by excessive exposure, ionizing radiations tend to produce their effects mainly in certain "radiosensitive" tissues where cell multiplication is most active, i.e. in the lymphatic system and bone marrow; gastro-intestinal tract; skin; gonads (testes and ovaries); and in early foetal life, the central nervous system. Thus, radiation injury may be evidenced by effects such as depression of white and red blood cell platelets count and resultant clinical features of agranulocytosis or anaemia; inflammatory changes in the skin referred to as **radiation dermatitis;** severe skin damage, manifested by **radiation burns;** inflammatory changes in the gastro-intestinal tract, producing nausea, vomiting and diarrhoea; and impaired fertility.

Late effects of radiation injury include the development of leukaemia and also sometimes the growth of malignant tumours (e.g. skin carcinomas) in areas of tissue damage.

Illness due to the more immediate effects of somatic damage is frequently referred to as **radiation sickness,** particularly when manifested by signs and symptoms of gastro-intestinal disorder.

In view of the high doses of radiation which must often be employed in the radiotherapy of malignant neoplasms, and the small differences that may exist between an adequate treatment dose and the amount of radiation that will damage normal tissue cells in the vicinity of the treatment area, some minor damage to normal tissues may be inevitable in patients undergoing radiotherapy. A proper application of modern methods of protection against ionizing radiations will however obviate somatic hazards to patients undergoing diagnostic radiological investigations and to staff working in diagnostic X-ray and radiotherapy departments.

(*b*) **Genetic damage**—as noted above, this type of radiation injury can be produced by doses of radiation lower than those required to produce somatic damage.

Genetic damage results in alterations in genes known as **mutations.** Mutations occurring in genes within reproductive cells of an individual will be transmitted to his or her offspring. It is thought that the production of mutations within the reproductive cells of large numbers of individuals *may carry a possible risk* of causing the appearance of inherited defects after a number of generations. This potential hazard makes it important that when any person of, or below, child-bearing age is exposed to ionizing radiations, in the course of medical investigation or treatment, or as a result of his or her occupation, irradiation of the gonads should be avoided or limited to such an extent as is practicable.

Measures for protection of patients and staff against hazards arising from the use of ionizing radiations in medical and dental practice are set out in the "Code of Practice for the Protection against Ionizing Radiations arising from Medical and Dental Use". (H.M. Stationery Office, 1964).

[*Note:* **Ionizing radiations**—are so called because, when they pass through matter, they cause a process called **ionization** whereby neutral atoms acquire a temporary electric charge.)

These radiations comprise **electromagnetic radiations**—X-rays and gamma rays (γ-rays) and **corpuscular radiations**—alpha particles (α-particles), beta particles (β-particles), neutrons and protons.

X-rays are electro-magnetic waves of short-wave length produced in X-ray tubes, by bombarding a heavy metal target with fast-moving electrons.

Atoms are composed of a central nucleus, around which revolve negatively-charged particles called electrons. The central nucleus contains particles called **protons,** which are positively charged, and **neutrons** which have no charge. Atomic nuclei which contain high numbers of neutrons relative to protons are unstable and disintegrate forming stable nuclei of simpler elements.

Beta-particles (β-particles) which are fast moving electrons; **alpha-particles** (α-particles) which are the nuclei of helium atoms; and **gamma-rays** (γ-rays) which are electro-magnetic waves of very short wave-length, are all forms of radiation which may be emitted when the nuclei of atoms undergo disintegration.

The spontaneous emission of ionizing radiations which accompanies nuclear disintegration, is termed **radioactivity.** This property is possessed by a few naturally occurring elements which have unstable nuclei (e.g. radium) and by a number of man-made "isotopes". **Isotopes** are differing forms of the same element, all of which have identical chemical properties and the same atomic number, but possess different atomic weights. Some isotopes have unstable nuclei which disintegrate with the emission of ionizing radiations, and these are thus known as **radioactive isotopes.**]

Appendix

Standard Works and Journals consulted by the Author

ANATOMY AND PHYSIOLOGY

Davies, D. V. (edit. by). *Grays Anatomy*. (Longmans, Green & Co. Ltd., 1967.)

McNaught, Anne B. *Companion to Illustrated Physiology*. (E. and S. Livingstone Ltd., 1965.)

Pearce, Evelyn. *Anatomy and Physiology for Nurses*. (Faber and Faber, 1962.)

Warwick, R. (edit. by). *Whillis's Elementary Anatomy and Physiology*. (J. and A. Churchill Ltd., 1961.)

MEDICINE, DERMATOLOGY, GASTRO-ENTEROLOGY, HAEMATOLOGY, NEUROLOGY AND PSYCHIATRY

Altschul, A. *Aids to Psychiatric Nursing*. (Baillière, Tindall & Cox, 1964.)

Davidson, Sir Stanley (edit. by). *The Practice and Principles of Medicine*. (E. and S. Livingstone, 1966.)

Forster, Francis M. *Synopsis of Neurology*. (The C. V. Morby Company, 1966.)

Houston, J. C., Joiner, C. L. and Trounce, J. R. *A Short Textbook of Medicine*. (English Universities Press Ltd., 1966.)

Hutton, J. H. *Practical Endocrinology*. (Charles C. Thomas, 1966.)

Lightwood, R. and Brimblecombe, F. S. W. *Paterson's Sick Children*. (Cassell, 1963.)

Mann, W. N. (edit. by). *Conybeare's Textbook of Medicine*. (E. and S. Livingstone, 1964.)

Naish, J. M. and Read, A. E. A. *Basic Gastroenterology*. (John Wright & Sons Ltd., 1965.)

Oswald, N. C. and Fry, J. *Diseases of the Respiratory System*. (Blackwell Scientific Publications, 1962.)

Percival, G. H. *An Introduction to Dermatology*. (E. and S. Livingstone, 1967.)

Richardson, Sir John (edit. by). *The Practice of Medicine.* (J. and A. Churchill, 1960.)

Rodger, T. Ferguson, Ingram, I. M., Timbury, G. C., Mowbray, R. M. *Lecture Notes on Psychological Medicine.* (E. and S. Livingstone Ltd., 1967.)

Thompson, R. B. *A Short Textbook of Haematology.* (Pitman Medical Publishing Co., 1965.)

OBSTETRICS AND GYNAECOLOGY

Barnes, Josephine. *Lecture Notes on Gynaecology.* (Blackwell Scientific Publications, 1966.)

Baynes, Trevor L. S. *Handbook of Gynaecology.* (Sylviro Publications, 1951.)

Gibberd, G. F. *A Short Textbook of Midwifery.* (J. and A. Churchill Ltd., 1965.)

Ten Teachers. Diseases of Women (edit. by F. W. Roques, S. G. Clayton and T. L. T. Lewis.) (Edward Arnold Ltd., 1964.)

Ten Teachers. Midwifery, 10th Edition. (Edward Arnold, Ltd., 1961.)

PATHOLOGY

Boyd, William A. *A Textbook of Pathology.* (Henry Kimpton, 1961.)

Dible, J. Henry. *Dible and Davie's Pathology.* (J. and A. Churchill, 1950.)

Pinniger, J. L. *Pathology.* (Baillière, Tindall and Cox, 1964.)

Thomson, A. D. and Cotton, R. E. *Lecture Notes on Pathology.* (Blackwell Scientific Publications, 1968.)

Turk, D. C. and Porter, I. A. *A Short Textbook of Microbiology.* (English Universities Press, 1965.)

PHARMACOLOGY

Bailey, Rosemary E. *Pharmacology for Nurses.* (Baillière, Tindall and Cassell, 1963.)

Sears, W. G. *Materia Medica for Nurses.* (Edward Arnold Ltd., 1966.)

RADIOLOGY

British Authors. *A Textbook of X-ray Diagnosis* (edit. by Shanks, S. C. and Kerley, P). Vol. I, 1957. Vol. II, 1962. Vol. III, 1958. Vol. IV. 1959. (H. K. Lewis Ltd.)

Caffey, John. *Paediatric X-ray Diagnosis.* (The Year Book Publishers, 1968.)

Chesney, D. N. and M. O. *Care of the Patient in Diagnostic Radiography.* (Blackwell Scientific Publications, 1962.)

Clark, K. C. *Positioning in Radiography.* Eighth Edition. (Ilford Ltd., and Wm. Heinemann Medical Books Ltd., 1964.)

Emmett, J. L. *Clinical Urography.* (Saunders, 1964.)

Ingram, Frank L. *Radiology of the Teeth and Jaws.* (Edward Arnold, 1964.)

Lodge, Thomas. *Recent Advances in Radiology,* 3rd Edition. (J. and A. Churchill Ltd., 1955.)

Lodge, Thomas (edit. by). *Recent Advances in Radiology.* 4th Edition. (J. and A. Churchill, 1964.)

McLaren, J. W. (edit. by). *Modern Trends in Diagnostic Radiology.* (Butterworths, 1960.)

Middlemiss, H. *Tropical Radiology.* (Wm. Heinemann Medical Books Ltd., 1961.)

Pugh, D. G. *Roentgenologic Diagnosis of Diseases of Bone.* (Williams and Wilkins, 1951.)

SURGERY, OPHTHALMOLOGY, OTO-RHINO-LARYNGOLOGY, ORTHOPAEDICS AND UROLOGY

Adams, J. Crawford. *Outline of Orthopaedics.* (E. and S. Livingstone, 1967.)

Badenoch, A. W. *Manual of Urology.* (Wm. Heinemann Medical Books Ltd., 1953.)

Illingworth, Sir Charles. *A Short Textbook of Surgery.* (J. and A. Churchill, 1965.)

Martin-Doyle, J. L. C. *A Synopsis of Ophthalmology.* (John Wright & Sons Ltd., 1967.)

Miller, A., Slade, N., and Leather, H. M. *A Synopsis of Renal Diseases and Urology.* (John Wright & Sons, 1966.)

Reading, Philip. *Common Diseases of the Ear, Nose and Throat.* (J. and A. Churchill Ltd., 1966.)

Robinson, J. O. *Surgery.* (Longmans, Green & Co., 1965.)

Wiles, P. and Sweetman, R. *Essentials of Orthopaedics.* (J. and A. Churchill, 1965.)

TERMINOLOGY

Roberts, Ffrangcon. *Medical Terms. Their Origin and Construction.* Fourth Edition. (Wm. Heinemann Medical Books Ltd., 1966.)

JOURNALS

The British Medical Journal (British Medical Association).
The British Journal of Radiology (British Institute of Radiology).
Clinical Radiology. (E. and S. Livingstone.)

Glossary

SOME PREFIXES AND SUFFIXES, AND OTHER COMPONENTS OF MEDICAL WORDS

TABLE 1

Usage of some General Prefixes, Suffixes and other word components in Medicine

This table shows some of the ways in which a number of prefixes and suffixes and other components of a general nature, are used in medical words. Common usages, given here, may differ in some instances from original literal meanings.

Components of words referring to the organs and tissues of the body are not included in Table 1; but the meanings of a number of these are indicated in Table 2 of this Appendix.

Prefix, suffix or other component	Senses in which commonly used	Examples
a-	absence of.	*aplasia,* absence of growth.
ab-	away from.	*abduct,* move away from the median plane.
ad-	towards.	*adduct,* move towards the median plane.
andr-	male.	*androgens,* male hormones.
ante-	before.	*ante-natal,* before birth.
anti-	opposed to.	*antihistamine,* a drug acting in opposition to histamine.
bi-	two.	*bilateral*—on both sides.
bio-	life.	*biopsy*—visual examination (usually microscopic) of tissue from a living subject.
calc-	calcium.	*calcification*—deposition of calcium salts in the tissues.
circum-	around.	*circumduct,* move in a circle.
con-	together with.	*congenital,* together with (i.e. present at) birth.
dys-	difficult, disordered.	*dysplasia,* disordered growth.
e-	out.	*evert,* turn outwards.

Prefix, suffix or other component	Senses in which commonly used	Examples
-ectomy-	cutting out, removal.	*splenectomy,* removal of the spleen.
end-	inside, inner.	*endothelium,* the inner lining of various body structures.
epi-	upon.	*epidermis,* on the skin, hence the outer layer of skin.
extra-	outside.	*extra-uterine,* outside the uterus.
gen-	referring to production, birth or reproduction.	*genitalia,* reproductive organs.
-genic	producing.	*pathogenic,* disease producing.
-graphy	recording.	*radiography,* recording by use of ionizing radiations.
gyn-	female.	*gynaecology*—study of diseases of women.
haem-	blood.	*haemorrhage*—bleeding.
hemi-	half.	*hemiplegia,* paralysis of half of the body.
hydro-	fluid.	*hydrothorax*—fluid in the thorax.
hyper-	above, in excess of normal.	*hypertrophy*—growth in excess of normal.
hypo-	beneath, less than normal.	*hypodermic,* beneath the skin. *hypoplasia,* growth of a degree less than normal.
in-	in.	*inverted,* turned inwards (also, upside down).
intra-	within.	*intracranial,* within the cranium.
iso-	same.	*isotopes,* differing forms of the same element, possessing the same chemical properties and the same atomic number (but differing atomic weights).
-itis	inflammation.	*osteitis*—inflammation of bone.
macro-	large.	*macroradiography,* direct enlargement radiography.
mal-	bad.	*malunited,* badly united.
mega-	big.	*megacolon,* enlarged colon.
men-	month.	*menopause,* cessation of the monthly periods.
micro-	small.	*microcephalic,* having a small head.
multi-	many.	*multicentric,* in many centres.

Prefix, suffix or other component	Senses in which commonly used	Examples
-natal	birth.	*neonatal,* newly born.
neo-	new.	*neoplasm,* new growth.
-oid	like.	*osteoid,* like bone.
-ology	science.	*radiology*—the science of radiation, esp. referring to medical use of ionizing radiations.
-oma	tumour.	*osteoma,* tumour of bone.
-orrhoea	flow, discharge.	*otorrhoea,* a discharge from the ear.
-osis	a condition of, or to indicate a degenerative disorder.	*diverticulosis*—a condition or having diverticula. *spondylosis*—a degenerative spinal disorder.
-ostomy	making an opening into.	*cholecystostomy*—making an opening into the gall-bladder and inserting a tube for drainage.
-otomy	cutting into or through.	*osteotomy*—cutting through a bone.
per-	through.	*pertrochanteric,* through the femoral trochanters.
peri-	around.	*periapical,* around the apex of a tooth root.
pneumo-	} air (or other gas).	*pneumoperitoneum*—air in the peritoneal cavity.
pneu-mato-		*pneumaturia*—gas in the urine
poly-	many.	*polyarthritis,* inflammation of many joints.
post-	after.	*post-natal,* after birth.
pre-	before.	*pre-cancer,* a condition which is a forerunner of cancer.
pro-	before, in front.	*prothrombin,* a precursor of thrombin, a substance concerned in the clotting of the blood.
pseudo-	false.	*pseudo-angina,* a condition simulating angina.
psych-	mind.	*psychogenic*—produced in the mind.
py-	pus.	*pyuria,* pus in the urine.
quadri-	four.	*quadriplegia*—paralysis of all four limbs.

Prefix, suffix or other component	Senses in which commonly used	Examples
radio-	radiation.	*radioactive,* emitting ionizing radiations.
retro-	behind.	*retrosternal.*
sub-	below.	*subnormal,* below normal.
supra-	above.	*supracondylar,* above the condyles.
tox-	poison.	*toxin,* a poisonous substance.
tri-	three.	*tri-iodide,* a compound with three iodine atoms in its *molecule.*
ultra-	beyond.	*ultrasonics,* sound vibrations beyond the audible range.
uni-	one.	*unilateral,* on one side.
-uria	urine.	*albuminuria,* albumen in the urine.

TABLE 2

Some Components of Words Referring to Body Structures

Component	Pertaining to
aden-	gland(s).
angi-	vessel(s) (esp. blood vessel).
arthr-	joint(s).
aur-	ear(s).
cardi-	heart, or cardiac orifice of the stomach.
caud-	tail, hence the lower part of the human body.
cephal-	head.
cholangi-	bile-ducts.
chole-	biliary system.
cholecyst-	gall-bladder.
choledoch-	common bile duct.
chondr-	cartilage.
col-	colon.
cyst-	bladder (esp. urinary bladder).
dactyl-	finger(s).
derm-	skin.
encephal-	brain.
enter-	intestine.
epiphysi-	epiphysis(es).
fibro-	fibrous connective tissue.
gastr-	stomach.
gloss-	tongue.
hepat-	liver.
hyster-	uterus.
lien-	spleen.
lymphangi-	lymph vessels.
lymph-	lymphatic system.
mamm-, mast-	breast.
myel-	bone marrow or spinal cord.
myo-	muscle(s).
nephr-	kidney(s).
ocul-	eye.
ophthalm-	eye.
orchi-, orchid-	testis(es).
or-	mouth.
oste-	bone(s).
ot-	ear(s).
phleb-	vein(s).

Component	Pertaining to
pneumon-	lung.
port-	portal vein.
proct-	rectum.
pyel-	kidney pelvis(es).
pyle-	portal vein
ren-	kidney(s).
rhin-	nose.
salping-	uterine tube(s).
sial-	salivary gland(s).
spondyl-	vetebra(ae).
vesic-	urinary bladder.

11

TABLE 3

List of some Important Abbreviations which are
used in Medical Notes

A.P.H.	ante partum haemorrhage.	*G.U.*	gastric ulcer, genito-urinary.
A.P.M.	anterior poliomyelitis.	*Hb.*	haemoglobin.
A.S.D.	atrial septal defect.	*H.V.*	hallux valgus.
B.I.	bony injury.	*I.C.P.*	intracranial pressure.
B.M.R.	basal metabolic rate.	*I.D.K.*	internal derangement of the knee joint.
B.P.	blood pressure, British Pharmacopoea.	*I.O.F.B.*	intra-ocular foreign body.
B.S.R.	basal sedimentation rate.	*I.S.Q.*	"in status quo", i.e. unchanged.
C.D.H.	congenital dislocation of the hip joint.	*I.P.P.R.*	intermittent positive pressure respiration.
C.S.O.M.	chronic suppurative otitis media.	*I.P.P.V.*	intermittent positive pressure ventilation.
C.T.	cerebral tumour or coronary thrombosis.	*I.U.C.D.*	intra-uterine contraceptive device.
D. & C.	uterine dilatation and currettage.	*I.U.D.*	intra-uterine death (or intra-uterine contraceptive device).
D.D.A.	Dangerous Drugs Act.		
D.L.E.	disseminated lupus erythematosus.	*I.V.*	intravenous.
		K.U.B.	kidneys, ureter and bladder.
D.S.	disseminated sclerosis.		
D.U.	duodenal ulcer.	*L.B.*	loose body.
D. & V.	diarrhoea and vomiting.	*M.P.V.*	metatarsus primus varus.
D.X.R.T.	deep X-ray therapy.	*M.S.*	mitral stenosis.
E.C.G.	electro-cardiography.	*N.A.D.*	no abnormality demonstrated.
E.D.D.	expected date of delivery (childbirth).		
		N.G.	new growth.
E.E.G.	electro-encephalography.	*N.Y.D.*	not yet diagnosed.
		O.A.	osteoarthritis.
E.N.T.	ear, nose and throat.	*O.T.*	occupational therapy.
E.S.R.	erythrocyte sedimentation rate.	*P.I.D.*	prolapsed intevertebral disc.
E.U.A.	examination under anaesthesia.	*P.M.*	post mortem.
F.B.	foreign body.	*P.P.H.*	post-partum haemorrhage.

G.P.I.	general paralysis of the insane.	*P.R.*	by (through) the rectum.
P.U.	peptic ulcer.	*T.B.*	tuberculosis or tubercle bacilli.
P.U.O.	pyrexia of unknown origin.	*T.P.R.*	temperature, pulse and respiration.
P.V.	by (through) the vagina.	*T's and A's.*	tonsils and adenoids.
R.B.C.	red blood cells.	*U.G.*	urogenital.
R.E.	rectal examination.	*V.D.*	venereal disease.
Rh.	rhesus factor.	*V.E.*	vaginal examination.
R.T.	radiotherapy.	*V.S.D.*	ventricular septal defect.
Ski.	skiagraph, i.e. a radiograph.	*V.V's.*	varicose veins.
S.M.R.	submucous resection of nasal septum.	*W.B.C.*	white blood cells.
		W.R.	Wassermann reaction.
S.O.B.	shortness of breath.	*X.R.*	X-ray.
S.O.L.	space-occupying lesion.		
T.A.B.	vaccine against typhoid and paratyphoid A. B. & C. fevers.		

Index

Index

Index

Index

Index

This book is to be returned on or before the last date stamped below.